A Dictionary of Dermatologic Terms

FOURTH EDITION

A Dictionary of Dermatologic Terms

FOURTH EDITION

Edited by

ROBERT L. CARTER, B.S., M.D.

Consultant Dermatologist
Fairfax Hospital
Falls Church, Virginia

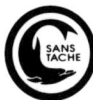

WILLIAMS & WILKINS
BALTIMORE · HONG KONG · LONDON · MUNICH
PHILADELPHIA · SYDNEY · TOKYO

SANS TACHE

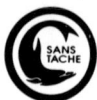

Editor: Fran Witthauer
Cover Design: Dan Pfisterer
Production: Adele Boyd-Lanham

Williams & Wilkins
428 East Preston Street
Baltimore, Maryland 21202, USA

Copyright © 1992   by Miles Inc.

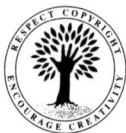

Accurate indications, adverse reactions, and dosage schedules for drugs are provided
in this book, but it is possible that they may change. The reader is urged to review the
package information data of the manufacturers of the medications mentioned.

Printed in the United States of America

First printing 1968

ISBN: 0-683-01469-2

92 93 94 95
1 2 3 4 5 6 7 8 9 10

DEDICATION

It is a singular honor to dedicate the Fourth Edition of this dictionary (formerly *A Dictionary of Dermatological Words, Terms, and Phrases*) to Dr. Morris Leider, the original author. His brilliant mind is reflected throughout its pages. The contribution he made to the clarity of dermatological thought is so evident in this lexicon.

Dr. Leider, with Dr. Morris Rosenblum, the other initial co-author, made the dictionary a classic. We all remain in their debt. These gentlemen are deceased and did not contribute to the revision of this Fourth Edition.

Robert I. Carter, M.D.

PREFACE

It has been an enormous pleasure to try to bring this lexicon up to date as it is so inherently rich in content. The authors, Morris Leider, M.D., and Morris Rosenblum, PhD., combined their abundantly creative talents over a period of twenty-five years into this work which resulted in three excellent editions. I trust the reader will find this Fourth Edition an enjoyable and instructive contribution to the rich dermatological literature.

I owe thanks and appreciation to so many individuals for their generous and enthusiastic assistance.

My total thanks goes to William French of Westwood-Squibb Pharmaceuticals, Inc. for his belief in this dictionary and the resulting outstanding commitment to underwrite the dictionary. Without his firm's truly generous financial support, it would not have been possible. Westwood-Squibb is a world leader in its support of dermatology. I appreciate the help of Kingsley Davis, Professional Medical Representative, Westwood-Squibb.

My special thanks to Karen Kapeluck for much assistance with the new manuscript, to Mary Ella Carter for her tireless efforts to bring this edition to publication, and to Cherie Stamper for all her assistance and patience over the last few years.

William Sawchuck, M.D., very kindly reviewed a brief portion of the manuscript.

I am very grateful to Janet Connell of International Computaprint Corporation for so many helpful suggestions and guidance with the book.

Many, many thanks also to so many others through my twenty years in dermatology who have so kindly given me their encouragement and enlightened guidance . . . especially John McSorely, M.D., and Joseph Penner, M.D. Thanks to Charles

Aaronson, M.D., Lee Blakley, M.D., and James Rotchford, M.D.

I would like to acknowledge sincere appreciation to William Hensyl of Williams & Wilkens for his encouragement in the development of this dictionary.

Effort has been made to credit sources properly for the use of previously published material. Some credits are missing and for that I apologize. If brought to my attention, the omission will be corrected.

ACKNOWLEDGMENTS

It would not have been possible to publish this dictionary without the complete and generous cooperation of Westwood-Squibb Pharmaceuticals, Buffalo, New York.

I gratefully acknowledge Miles, Inc. for permitting use of the original material.

R.L.C.

GUIDE TO PRONUNCIATION, SUPPLEMENTARY LEXICAL NOTES, AND ANGLICIZATION OF LATIN WORDS

Guide to Pronunciation

ă—hăt	ŏ—hŏt	ch—church [chûrch]
ā—hāte	ō—hōme	'l—model [mŏd'l]
â—hâre	ô—hôrn	'm—chasm [kăz'm]
ä—härt	ōō—hōōd	'n—license [lī's'ns]
	ōō—hōōt	ng—sing, singer
ĕ—hĕn	oi—hoist	[sĭng; sĭng'ẽr]
ē—hē	ou—house	ngg—finger, linger
ẽ—hẽr		[fĭng'gẽr; lĭng'gẽr]
	ŭ—hŭt	
ĭ- hĭt	ū—hūge	y—yet [yĕt]
ī—hīde	û—hûrl	zh—measure [mĕzh'ẽr]

The symbol ə, known as the schwa (from the name of a Hebrew symbol of pronunciation) indicates a weakened, faint and indistinct vowel sound, as follows:

a—mitral [mī'trəl]	o—method [mĕth'əd]
e—system [sĭs'təm]	lesion [lē'zhən]
i—cavity [kă'və-tē]	u—nevus [nē'vəs]

The pronunciation of modern foreign words is merely approximated by the use of the above symbols, for example:

ng for French nasal n and m—rond ([rông], d'emblée [dängblā']. (The g is silent as in *sing*.)

ōō for French u—vésicule [vāsēkōōl'].

Since the syllables of French words are supposed to be uttered with practically equal force but with a slight stress on the last (or the one before that if the last is ə), we have left the word undivided into syllables in the guide to its pronunciation within the square brackets and have placed an accent mark after the required syllable (virtually always the final one).

Some German sounds are represented as follows:

kh for ch (whether pronounced with a hiss or with what represents a heavy aspirate)—Ich [ēkh]

o͞o for short u and short ü—burg [bo͞org], Lützen [lo͞ots′ĕn]

o͞o for long u and long ü—buch [bo͞okh], Schüller [sho͞ol′ĕr].

v for w—wucher [vo͞o′khĕr].

Supplementary Lexical Notes

In the case of Greek, Latin and most Latinized words, the present tendency is to anglicize them, but there seems to be no uniform practice. For the most part we have used the so-called English method as set down in *Webster's New International Dictionary,* Second Edition. We have used this system to achieve some measure of consistency. Aware of current trends, we have, however, included some variations, notably that of considering *i* of terminal *-ia* long. The first appearance of the full word in the pronunciation guide within square brackets indicates the pronunciation of that word according to the English method; variations appear on either side. A single example will illustrate the procedure that we have followed. The pronunciation of the Latin word *canis,* dog, or of a (the) dog, is represented in its entry as follows: [kä′-, kă′-, kā′nĭs, -nəs]. The full word, kā′nĭs, denotes the pronunciation according to the English method, the variations on either side of the full word show either an approximation of the Roman system (the way in which we think the Romans pronounced Latin) or an anglicization (as in the use of schwa for i in the final syllable). Preference is not indicated; any of the methods should be considered good for such words. Division into syllables generally follows English analogies.

Turning back to English itself (but not as a foreign language), we have given the pronunciation of some words as they are pronounced by the British, e.g., *capillary*, pronounced kăp′ə-lĕr′ē in the American manner and kə-pĭl′ə-rĭ in the British manner.

For the sake of simplicity and ease of understanding, we have used a small number of diacritical marks and only one kind of accent mark (′) to indicate both primary and secondary stress. For all words (except Greek, Latin and Latinized as noted above), preference is indicated by the first full appearance of the word as divided into syllables and marked within square brackets.

There are no fixed rules for division into syllables to indicate pronunciation. The "syllable-dividers" themselves belong to different schools; the same word can be found divided up differently in three different authorities. We, too, are not in accord with any one system of division into syllables to indicate pronunciation. The length of the vowel, the nature of the consonants surrounding it, the position of the accent, the length of the word, physiological considerations, practice, usage, the way in which speakers pronounce these words—all these factors have been taken into account. We may differ in many instances from other dictionaries, but the system and method we use have their rationale and we have been consistent, as far as possible.

We have put down basic pronunciations for prefixes, suffixes and combining forms that are listed individually, but it must be understood that these change according to the nature of the rest of the word. For example, *acro-* is pronounced ăk′rō in *acromegaly*, ă-krŏ′ in *Acropolis* and ăk′rə in *acronym*. Likewise, according to Webster's Third, at least ten different pronunciations exist for *-sia* and *-sian*. Hence, selectivity is certainly in order.

If the pronunciation of a word appearing inside a long term or a cross-reference is not given in situ, it will be found in the independent entry of that word. Also, in such cases, variants of the pronunciation will be found in the separate entry of the particular word, if not given in the entry of the longer title.

We have taken due cognizance of changing trends in pronunciation. There is a growing tendency to slur vowels, long as well as short, and to use schwa almost at will without indicating a marked vowel as an alternate. We have retained many of these "displaced" vowels, either disregarding the schwa or setting it down merely as an unpreferred alternate. For example, although *adiposis* is marked in some dictionaries as ăd′ə-pō′səs, we have given ăd′ĭ-pō′sĭs the preferred position.

Another trend, which we consider all to the good because it is more realistic, concerns the pronunciation of terminal *e* in some words, terminal *y* in all words and *i* before a vowel in certain combinations. For example, the *e* of *acne* and *acme* is marked as a short i (ĭ) in some dictionaries but as a long e (ē), and properly so, in the latest ones. Likewise, the final *y* of words like *liberty* and *philology* is marked as a short i in the older dictionaries but as both ē and ĭ in the newer ones, with ē preferred. Finally, the *i* in *-ia*, once marked only as ĭ, is now marked as long e (ē) and occasionally also as y, e.g., *mania* [mā′nē-ə, mā′nyə], *arthropathia* [är′thrō-păth′ē-ə]; similar lengthening may take place before other vowels, e.g., *facies* [fā′shē-ēz, fā′shēz]. We have retained or discarded the short i (ĭ) in similar words according to the frequency of its current use.

As used in this work, the words *classical* and *classicized* mean in the style of Greek or Latin, usually the latter, to which the word *Latinized* also applies. The expression *New Latin* indicates a word coinage made after the medieval period. Such words may be classicized words formed from English words or may be adaptations of words used by the Greeks and Romans. Unless otherwise noted, the form of classicized and New Latin words is in the nominative singular according to the rules of Latin declensions. For example, when we say that *bullosa* is the feminine singular of a New Latin adjective, it is understood that it is in the

xv Supplementary Lexical Notes

nominative case. Other cases of Latin declensions found in medical terms are the genitive, which basically indicates possession or an adjectival relationship, e.g., singular, *capilli*, literally of a hair, plural, *capillorum*, literally of the hairs, of the hair, *capitis*, of the head, *unguium*, of the nails; the accusative, when used as an object of certain prepositions, e.g., *in cutem*, into the skin; and the ablative, also when used after certain prepositions, e.g., *ab igne*, literally from fire, hence, caused by fire.

Additional terms used in this work to indicate the language from which a word is derived are:

Late Latin, which refers to Latin of the period from about the third to the end of the sixth century A.D.

Vulgar Latin, the language of the *vulgus*, crowd, people; Latin as spoken by the uneducated masses.

Old English, or *Anglo-Saxon*, which refers to the period from about 450 to 1100.

Middle English, which refers to about 1100 to 1500.

Old French, which refers to the period from the ninth to the sixteenth century.

Germanic, or *Teutonic,* which, as used here, refers to German and kindred languages before about 1500, i.e., older German.

Gothic, an East Germanic language, as known through a biblical translation of the fourth century A.D.

Old High German, a Germanic, or Teutonic language, known from documents before the twelfth century.

Old Norse, a North Germanic language of the period through the middle of the fourteenth century.

Afrikaans, also known as *Cape Dutch* and *Taal*, a South African language that developed from Dutch after the sixteenth century, an official language of the Union of South Africa.

Celtic, a medieval language spoken in Brittany, Cornwall, Ireland and Wales, the ancestor of modern Breton, Cornish, Gaelic and Welsh.

Hindi, a language of many parts of India, an official language of many states of India, especially in the north.

Sanskrit, an ancient language of India, the classical literary language of India, with many roots akin to those in Latin and Greek.

Indo-European, the ancestor of all the languages listed above and of many more, including most of those spoken in Europe, India, Persia and Afghanistan; an unrecorded language of prehistoric times which has been reconstructed by scientific philological deductions from correspondences among known derived languages. Indo-European roots are indicated by an asterisk (e.g., **kar*) to show that they are hypothetical.

Anglicization of Latin Words

Numerous Latin words, terms, phrases, and even longer expressions are still frequently spoken and written, especially in learned, legal, and scientific—particularly medical—discourse. Time was, when much more Latin was used in the so-called learned professions, and in those bygone days Latin was pronounced in what was taken to be a correct ancient Roman manner. From internal evidence in extant Latin literature, by application of certain phonetic laws, and from researches in other linguistic phenomena, modern scholars have determined how Latin must have been pronounced at different periods to approximations as good as possible for a language that is no longer "living." Thus, many years past, when Latin was taught extensively and intensively in the higher schools of Great Britain and the United States, the pronunciation of Latin words by formally educated persons, even if they were not professional Latinists, was by what is called the Roman method, i.e., what is thought to have been standard during the two centuries around the lifetime of Christ (100 B.C. to A.D. 100). As the teaching of Latin waned (it is nearly extinct in present-day school curricula), the Roman method began to be replaced for practical, logical, and aesthetic reasons by an English method in which Latin words are pronounced according to certain rules that make the sounds of their letters correspond in a consistent way to the pronunciations of the same letters in current standard English. And, in keeping with the Roman habit, every letter of anglicized Latin words is pronounced, except for a few borrowed from Greek, in which occasional letters are silent.

It has come to pass, however, that by now most speakers of English, having occasion to utter Latin words, know neither the Roman nor the English method distinctively and, in the main, mix up the two methods of pronunciation. It may matter little in what way, Roman or anglicized, a single Latin word is said; challenged, a speaker may deviously or honestly claim that he or she is speaking in one way or the other. When, however, it comes to terms and phrases of several words, it is not so easy to cover inconsistency or cloak ignorance. Lawyers and other professionals, as much as physicians, are remiss in this regard. One would think that at least those tags of Latin that already are or are nearly adopted into English—because they are so commonly said—would be pronounced correctly in the English manner. It is not so. More people who should know better say dä′tə or dā′tə, and think the word is singular in grammatical number, then say dā′tə and know it is the plural of dā′təm. For another example, the Roman way of pronouncing *per se* is pēr′sā; the anglicized, pûr′sē. Most speakers tend to say pûr′sā, which is half in the English manner and half in the Roman. Nothing good can come of that. Still another, more egregious, example is *curriculum vitae*. If an ancient Roman had had to use this term, he or she would have said kōō-rĭ′kōō-lōōm wē′tī. Again, most speakers nowadays say kə or kū-rĭ′kū-lūm vē′tī, which is anglicized up to and through the *v*. Consistency in anglicization demands kə or kū-rĭ′kū-lūm vī′tē.

The matter of pronunciation according to a consistent standard is of some scholarly importance in dermatology because so many of the titles of cutaneous conditions are in classical or New Latin. Therefore, we enter here a few rules that govern anglicization of Latin words, especially of those Latin or Latinized words that are to be found in this dictionary and of some others that are generally mispronounced.

The vowels *a, e, i, o,* and *u* always have a long sound when they end an accented syllable. Examples are *labium* [lā′bĭ-əm], *pedis* [pē′dĭs], *angina* [ăn-jī′nə], *scrotum* [skrō′təm], and *pubes* [pū′bēz]. Otherwise they are usually short, variously different or may be long.

A final *i* is almost always long, e.g., *pili* [pī′lī] and *nasi* [nā′zī].

At the end of a word, *es* is pronounced like *ese* in *these,* e.g., *comedones* [kōm-ə-dō′nēz] and *diagnoses* [dī′ăg-nō′sēz].

The diphthong and digraph æ is pronounced like long *e.* Most speakers stumble over it. We have just given an example in *curriculum vitae.* A good way to clarify in mind the English method in this respect is to recall the plurals of *alumnus* and *alumna,* namely, *alumni* and *alumnae.* It happens that the pronunciation of the terminal letters *i* and æ is exactly opposite in the Roman and English methods, and this is what makes for more confusion. In either method, there must be a difference in pronunciation of the terminal vowels in order to specify gender. The way to determine the difference in English is to recall the rule given above about terminal *i* pronounced long and then to perceive that terminal æ must be pronounced differently, namely, like long *e.* Thus, at a class reunion of a coeducational school, men can know to shake hands with the *alumni* [ă-lūm′nī] and kiss the alumnae [ă-lūm′nē], assuming all graduates are conformist. Women may do either, neither, or both, graciously.

With few exceptions, the pronunciation of consonants is the same in both the Roman and English methods.

The letter *c* is pronounced like *s* in *saint* before *e, i, y,* and the diphthong æ. Examples are *cerulæ* [sē-rōōl′ē], *cimi-*

cosis [sĭm′ĭ-kō′sĭs], *cyanosis* [sī′ə-nō′sĭs], and *verrucae* [vĕ-rōō′sē]. When *c* stands before *i* and another vowel and follows or ends an accented syllable, it has the sound of *sh* or *s* as above. An example is found in the two ways of pronouncing *alopecia* [ăl′ō-pē′shē-ə, sē-ə]. Before the vowels *a*, *o*, and *u*, *c* is pronounced like *k*, e.g., *capitis* [kăp′ĭ-tĭs], *corium* [kō′rĭ-əm], and *cutis* [kū′tĭs]. Double *cc* is pronounced like *k* before *a*, *o*, and *u*, e.g., *buccal* [būk′′l], *buccolabial* [būk′ō-lā′bĭ-əl], and *coccus* [kō′kəs]; but double *cc* is pronounced *ks* before *e* and *i*, e.g., *access* [ăk′sĕs] and *cocci* [kōk′sī].

The pronunciation of *ch* is *k*, e.g., *cheilitis* [kī-lī′tĭs] and *cheiropompholyx* [kī′rō-pŏm′fō-lĭks].

The consonant *g* is pronounced soft, i.e., like *j*, before *e*, *i*, *y*, and the diphthong æ; otherwise it is pronounced like *g* in *get*. Examples of soft *g* are in *congenita* [kōn-jĕn′ə-tə] and *gyrata* [jī-rā′tə], and an example of both soft and hard *g* is in *gigantica* [jī-găn′tĭ-kə].

The usual sound of *s* is sibilant as in *sin*. There are, however, several important exceptions in which its sibilance is as of *z*. Examples are in *albicans* [ăl′-bĭ-kănz], *herpes* [hûr′pez], and *rosacea* [rō-zā′shē-ə]. There is no agreement on the pronunciation of *s* in the noun ending -*sia* as in *achromasia*, in which it is variously pronounced *s*, *sh*, *z*, and *zh*. Double *ss* has the usual sound of single *s*, e.g., *glossitis* [glō-sī′tĭs].

The letter *p* is silent when it is initial before *n* in words derived from Greek relating to breath [*pneuma*], for example in *pneumonia* [nū-mō′nĭ-ə], but it is not silent before *n* when it is internal in related words, for example, in *apnea* [ăp′nē-ə] and *dyspnea* [dĭsp′nē-ə]. The combination *ph* is pronounced *f*, unless followed by *th*, wherewith it is silent, e.g., *phimosis* [fī-mō′sĭs] and *phlegmon* [flĕg′mōn], and *phthiriasis* [thĭ-rī′ə-sĭs] and *phthisis* [thī′sĭs]. All of these words are borrowings or derivatives from Greek.

The sound of *t* is exceptionally *sh* when it follows an accented syllable and precedes *i* and another vowel. Examples are *gentian* [gĕn'shən], *patient* [pā'shənt], *induratio* [ĭn'dū-rā'shĭ-ō], and *preputium* [prē-pū'shĭ-əm].

There are many matters about the pronunciation of Latin words that we have not treated exhaustively because we have limited ourselves mainly to medical—particularly to dermatological—words. It has not been possible to consider every letter of the alphabet in all pronunciations, historical variations, and influences arising from accentuation and syllabification. Nor are we able to note that there are different methods of pronouncing Latin words in some European countries and in the practice of the Roman Catholic Church. With respect to the latter points, we would warn that if one hears a learned continental speaker pronounce a Latin word in a manner that sounds outlandish, it is more than polite to assume that the speaker is following conventions adapted and peculiar to his or her native tongue rather than that he or she is mangling language. For example, whereas *Cicero* is pronounced kĭ'kĕ-rō in Roman and sĭs'ə-rō in English, it is sēsārō' in French, chē'chā-rō in Italian, thē'thā-rō or sē'sā-rō in Spanish, and tsē'tsē-rō in German.

Morris Rosenblum, Ph.D.
Deceased

Lecturer
Classical Languages and Comparative Literature
Queens College
Brooklyn College
City College of the City University of New York

Associate
Department of Greek and Latin
Columbia University.

CONTENTS

A

A as a capital letter is sometimes used as an identifier, e.g., vitamin A.

a [ă], **a-** [ă, ə], **ab** [ăb], **ab-** [ăb, əb], **abs, abs-** [ăbs] are different forms of a Latin preposition and prefix with a basic meaning of from or away from, and, in some terms, an extended meaning of on account of or in consequence of. As a preposition with this latter sense, some of these forms are found in titles like *erythema a calore,* and *erythema ab igne,* and as a prefix with the basic meaning, in words like *avert, abrasion* and *abscess. A* and *a-* are used only before consonants, the others before consonants and vowels.

a- [ă, ə, ā], **an-** [ăn] are forms of a negative Greek prefix called alpha privative, similar in force to Latin *in-* and English *un-.* Both *a-* and *an-* are attached to words and word elements of Greek and Latin ancestry; *a-* is used before consonants, e.g., *amelanotic,* whereas, for the sake of euphony, *an-* is used before vowels and sometimes *h,* e.g., *anergy, anhidrosis.* Both forms denote lack, absence or negation of whatever is indicated in the rest of the word, e.g., *achromia,* colorlessness, *anergy,* nonreactivity, *anhydrous,* waterless. Often, partial rather than complete lack, absence or negation is the fact, e.g., *anemia* means less blood than normal rather than absolute bloodlessness.

Å is the symbol for Ångström unit, a length equal to one ten-millionth of a millimeter (or one hundred-millionth of a centimeter or about one two-hundred-and-fifty-millionth of an inch). The modern tendency is to use nanometers instead of Ångström units to designate electromagnetic wave lengths. A nanometer is one billionth (10^{-9}) of a meter or 10 Ångström units. Used mainly in physics to measure and designate wave lengths of electromagnetic energy, it is of dermatologic importance because the skin, as an exteriorized organ, is affected by electromagnetic energy of various wave lengths. Since *Å* and *ö* are separate and distinct letters in the Swedish alphabet, they should, strictly speaking, always appear with the superscripts. On the other hand, if one were to follow the usual convention about eponymously designated units of physics like *ampere, gauss, ohm, volt,* etc., one should write *angstrom* with no further adornments.

ab, ab-. See *a*.

abiotrophy [ăb'ĭ-ŏt'rō-fē] literally means a condition (*-y*) in which there has been failure (*a-*) of adequate nourishment (*-troph-*) of life (*-bio-*). The word has been applied to incomplete development of structures in dysplastic processes of embryonal or genetic nature, e.g., in Marfan's syndrome, in which elastic tissue or ground substance is defective.

abrasion [ăb-rā'zhən, ă-, ə-brā'zhən] is literally a rubbing (*ras-*, from *radere*, rub) away, off (*ab-*). The word may be applied to any amount of superficial removal of epithelium, usually by mechanical friction, that results in oozing and crusting.

Abrikossov's tumor [ă-brē-kôs'ŭf] Granular-cell myoblastoma.

abs, abs-. See *a*.

abscedens [ăb-sē'dĕnz] is a Latin present participle that means departing (*abscedere*, to go away). The word is used exclusively in the title *folliculitis et perifolliculitis abscedens et suffodiens* and conveys the sense of dissolution, discharge and slough of tissue. (*Suffodiens*, which see, means digging under, channeling or burrowing.)

abscess [ăb'sĕs] is related to *abscedens* etymologically and derives directly from the Latin noun *abscessus*, a departure or separation. A circumscribed collection of pus. A cavity formed by liquefaction necrosis within solid tissue. (*Stedman's*)

abscess, cold. *Cold abscess* carries the connotation of no "heat" or no acute inflammation in localized and necrotizing processes, such as are seen in tuberculosis of organs like the skin, bones and lymph nodes, or structures like joints. Discharge of particulate matter rather than free flow of pus is characteristic. Actinomycosis, syphilis and other granulomatous diseases may show similar phenomena.

abscess, micro-, (Munro's [mŭn-rōz'], **Pautrier's** [pōtrēāz']). These designations, partly descriptive of histologic process and partly eponymic, would be even better as *micro-abscess of psoriasis* and *micro-abscess of mycosis fungoides* respectively to describe the minute collections of leukocytic elements found in the epidermis in those diseases.

abscess, sterile [stĕr'l, -əl, -ĭl]. *Sterile abscess* connotes demarcated inflammatory process containing pus caused by inanimate agents, or, if caused by micro-organisms, containing pus that is finally free of living micro-organisms.

absolute anergy. See *anergy, absolute*.

abtropfung [ăb-trŏp′fōōng] is a German noun that means a dropping (-*tropfung*) off or down (*ab-*). It is used to describe the proliferative extension, or streaming, of cells of junctional nevi from the dermo-epidermal junction into the corium.

acanth(o)- [ăk′ăn-thō, ə-kăn′thō] is a combining form derived from the Greek word for a thorn or prickle. In dermatology the element finds use in forming words describing conditions of the prickle-cell layer of the epidermis.

acantholysis [ăk′ăn-thŏl′ĭ-sĭs, -ə-səs] means dissolution or separation (-*lysis*) of intercellular bridges in the prickle-cell layer of the epidermis (*acantho-*). The process is seen strikingly in pemphigus vulgaris, wherein intercellular bridges seem to have melted away. Compare *acanthorrhexis*.

acantholytic [ə-kăn′thə, ăk′ăn-thō-lĭt′ĭk] is an adjective meaning pertaining or relating to acantholysis.

acantholytic acanthoma a benign tumor of epidermal keratinocytes that exhibits various histologic patterns. This is a newly recognized solitary benign cutaneous tumor. Median age of patients is sixty years. Differential diagnosis; keratosis and basal cell carcinoma. Histology shows hyperkeratosis, papillomatosis, acanthosis and acantholysis throughout the malpighian layer with variable perivascular lymphohistiocytic infiltrate in the superficial corium. (Brownstein)

acanthoma [ăk′ăn-thō′mə] is used to designate gross or microscopic hypertrophy (-*oma*) of the prickle-cell layer of the epidermis (*acanth-*) in a localized, rather than diffuse (compare *acanthosis*) fashion. The word may be used in a generic way for any neoplastic process (benign or malignant) in which the prickle-cell layer is increased in local mass. Thus verrucae, molluscum contagiosum, kerato acanthoma and basal- and squamous-cell epithelioma are all acanthomata. As a practical measure, *acanthoma* can be employed as a grossly descriptive word of a clinically visible process of the above sorts while histologic resolution of the precise type of process is in progress. As soon as resolution is made, the more meaningful differentiating title is more communicative. The plural of this word is *acanthomata* after the ancient Greek fashion or *acanthomas* in the modern English manner.

acanthorrhexis [ə-kăn′thə-, ăk′ăn-thō-rĕk′sĭs] means rupture (-*rrhexis*) of the intercellular bridges of the prickle-cell layer of the epidermis (*acantho-*). This phenomenon is seen in "tension" vesicles of bullae, i.e., processes in which intercellular edema seems to rise until intercellular bridges seem to be torn apart. Conditions like primary irritant dermatitis and allergic contact dermatitis show acanthorrhexis. Compare *acantholysis*.

acanthosis [ăk′ăn-thō′sĭs] is used commonly to designate a condition (-*osis*) of diffuse rather than localized hypertrophy (compare *acanthoma*) of the prickle-cell layer of the epidermis (*acantho-*). Psoriasis shows a good example of the process under the microscope. The word can also be used to describe a condition of gross "thorniness," as in the following title.

acanthosis nigricans [nī′grĭ-, nĭg′rĭ-kănz] is the title of a characteristic dermatosis that is marked by tan to blackish (*nigricans,* present participle of a Latin verb, meaning turning black) verrucous excrescences, particularly in the axillae, then variably in the other great folds of intertriginous regions, and in most extensive development, in the fine ridges and furrows of the skin. There is a juvenile or benign form that is in the nature of a nevus, a pseudo-form that is related to the effects of endocrinopathy or obesity in the great folds of the body and a malignant form that bespeaks overt, covert or eventual internal carcinomatosis.

acanthotic [ăk′ăn-thŏt′ĭk] is an adjective meaning pertaining or relating to acanthosis.

acar- [ăk′ər] a combining form, derives from Greek via Latin *acarus,* a mite, and signifies things relating to mites and ticks. See *acarus*.

acariasis [ăk′ə-rī′ə-sĭs] is a general term for a condition (-*iasis*) caused by any mite or tick. This term is in more common use than *acarinosis, acariosis* or *acarodermatitis*.

acariosis [ə-kăr′ĭ-ō′sĭs, -ē-ō′sĭs] is still another term for a condition (-*osis*) caused by any mite or tick. It is less used than *acariasis*.

acatalasia a rare inherited deficiency of catalase in erythrocytes (acatalasemia) and other tissues. In some subjects acatalasia is associated with severe gangrenous lesions of the oral cavity and destruction of alveolar bone (Takahara's disease). (Wyngaarden)

All the teeth may be lost with destruction of the jaw in the worst type. Heals post puberty. (Takahara)

-acea [ā′shē-ə, -sē-ə, -shə], **-aceae** [ā′sē-ē], **-aceous** [ā′shəs], **-aceus** [ā′shē-əs, -sē-əs] are suffixes, three of Latin form and one (-*aceous*) English, meaning like, in the nature of, or composed of. For example, we find -*acea* (Latin feminine singular) in *rosacea* (rosy) and *amiantacea* (like asbestos) and as a neuter plural in nouns like *Crustacea* (related to *crusta*, a shell, thence a class of Arthropods); -*aceae* (plural of -*acea*) in *Moniliaceae* (like a string of beads, in mycology a family of certain fungi); -*aceous* in *foliaceous* (in the nature of leaves, as in *foliaceous pemphigus*); *-aceus* (Latin masculine singular) in *foliaceus* (*pemphigus foliaceus*).

Achard-Thiers syndrome [äshär′; tyâr] Diabetes, hypertension, and hirsutism in women.

acne [ăk′nē] is a word whose origin is obscure. There is a Greek word (*achne*) nearly like it with meanings like chaff, lint, particle, and efflorescence, but it is not certain that it is the source word. The Greek word *akme* and Latin *acme* (high point) are perhaps a little closer—very little—to the clinical facts about some lesions of the disease, but it is difficult to account plausibly for the switch from *m* to *n* in this instance. Perhaps it was corrupted by a transcribing error. Whatever its origin, *acne* is a well-established, short and useful word to designate the common dermatosis and, with modifying adjectives, further to distinguish variant, related or simulating conditions. The dermatosis and its variants so designated are notable for a primary or special lesion that is named the *comedo* or *blackhead*, and secondary or evolutionary lesions upon the comedo that are principally inflammatory papules, pustules, odd abscesses and encystments. Variations of this process are so numerous in amount, site, intensity and cause that *acne* has acquired perhaps the longest list of modifying adjectives to designate those variations, rivaled only by *eczema* and *dermatitis*. Some conditions with *acne* in their titles are merely acneform rather than truly acneic. Following are several titles containing the word *acne*, many of which we think are still interesting, needed or useful at the present time.

acne bacillus [bə-sĭl′əs] is the nontechnical term for the gram-positive, anaerobic rod that is commonly found in the comedones and pustules of acne. It was originally named *Bacillus acnes* (*acnes* is the genitive singular of *acne*), then *Corynebacterium acnes* and now *Propionibacterium acnes*. It was once held, probably not firmly, to be the cause of acne. Today it is known to be one of the normal saprophytic floras of the skin.

acne cheloidalis [kē′loi-dā′lĭs, -dä′lĭs, -dăl′ĭs] and **acné chéloïdique** [ăknä′ kālōēdēk′]. The first is a classicized title, the second, a French title. See *acne, keloid*.

acne, comedo [kŏm′ē-dō, -ə-dō]. *Comedo acne* is descriptive of ordinary acne that consists principally of blackheads with very little inflammatory reaction in and about them.

acne conglobata [kŏn′glō-bā′tə, kŏn-glō′bə-tə], or **conglobate** [kŏn-, kən-glō′bāt, kŏng′glō-bāt] **acne,** describes a form of acne that is sufficiently common, serious and distinctive to deserve special designation. *Conglobate* means gathered into balls (Latin *globus*, ball). The important features are pea- to nut-sized abscesses or cysts, with intercommunicating sinuses, which contain a thick, stringy, mucoid content, and which leave, upon resolution, deeply pitted or irregularly elevated scars traversed by keloidal "bridges."

acne cystica [sĭs'tĭ-kə], or **cystic** [sĭs'tĭk] **acne,** is descriptive of acne process in which inflammatory encystments are the most prominent feature. *Acne conglobata* is related and suggests more of the same process.

acné excoriée des jeunes filles [äknā' ĕkskəryā' dā zhŭn fēy'] is an expressive phrase in French which describes a type of acne in which acneform lesions are compulsively touched, pressed, squeezed and picked, in short, excoriated. Its literal translation is "excoriated acne of young girls." The acne need not be severe, but the compulsion to pick is uncontrollable. In well-developed cases, superficial crusts or scabs and fine scars or atrophy are more prominent than blackheads, papules, pustules and cysts. The condition is more common in young girls, who need not be so young in years, merely immature; boys too are victims of the physical and psychologic complex.

acne fulminans An uncommon, acute, ulcerative type of acne accompanied by fever and musculoskeletal manifestations. It occurs almost exclusively in adolescent boys. Only about fifty patients have been reported. (Troupe et al)

acne, keloid [kē'loid]. *Keloid acne* is the anglicized title, and *acne keloidalis* [kē'loi-dā'lĭs, -dä'lĭs, -dăl'ĭs] is the classicized title of the condition that is equally well, or better, known as *dermatitis papillaris capillitii*. *Folliculitis keloidalis* is still another equivalent title and is perhaps more accurately expressive of the nature of the process since it appears to be a pyoderma in and around the pilosebaceous structures that eventuates in keloidal scarring. The commonest site of the affliction is the nape of the neck, and the next most common is the junction of the lower lip and chin. Blacks are highly susceptible.

acne miliaris [mĭl'ĭ-ā'rĭs, -ä'rĭs, -ē-ăr'ĭs], or **miliary** [mĭl'ĭ-ĕr'ē, -ĭ, mĭl'ē-ĕr'ē, -ĭ, mĭl'yə-rē, -rĭ] **acne,** designates acneform process that consists largely of pinpoint- to pinhead-sized milia (whiteheads). See *miliaris* and *miliary*.

acne nectrotica [nē-krŏt'ĭ-kə] is Unna's original term for what is now better known as *acne varioliformis*. The adjective (*necrotica*, New Latin from Greek, meaning causing death) is descriptive of the destructive nature of the papular process, but the substantive (*acne*) is misleading since the condition is not predicated upon comedones, but is probably a pyoderma.

acne necrotica(ns) miliaris [nē-krŏt′ĭ-kə, -kănz mĭl′ĭ-ā′rĭs] is a title that designates a pruritic or pustular eruption of the scalp. Again the adjectives are descriptive of the destructive nature (*necrotica* and *necroticans*, New Latin present participle, meaning causing death) and small size (*miliaris*) of the lesions but the substantive (*acne*) is misleading because this process is most likely a pyoderma.

acne neonatorum [nē-ō-nə-tō′rəm, -nä-tôr′ŭm] is a simple and useful term to designate the occurrence of acneform lesions in the newborn (*neonatorum*, New Latin, meaning of the newborn) or infants. Usually a localized process of grouped comedones or a sparse sprinkling of comedones is the appearance. Some cases may be in the nature of a nevus (nevus comedonicus); others may be drug eruptions from iodides or bromides taken by the mother prenatally, or postnatally during the nursing period; and still others may be truly precocious acne vulgaris of the usual complex endocrinologic and/or other causes.

acne, occupational [ŏk′ū-pā′shən-əl]. *Occupational acne* is a moderately useful term to communicate the idea of acneform process acquired in certain industrial situations like those involving frequent contact with oils, tars and chlorinated products.

acne papulosa [păp′ū-lō′sə], or **papular** [păp′ū-lər] **acne,** is a descriptive title of acne process which consists principally of comedones that appear as moderately inflamed papules.

acne pustulosa [pŭs′tū-lō′sə], or **pustular** [pŭs′tū-lər] **acne,** is a descriptive title of acne process in which local and moderate suppuration of comedones is a predominant feature. Severer grades of this process verge on *acne conglobata.*

acne rosacea [rō-zā′shē-ə, -sē-ə, -shə] is a descriptive title of rosaceous process when inflammatory papules and pustules reminiscent of acne are a prominent feature. The process, of course, is not ordinary acne. *Rosacea* in this title is an adjective meaning rosy. It becomes a noun when used alone to designate the condition, and this may be better in order to get away from the idea of acne. Complications include rhinophyma, blepharitis, conjunctivitis, episcleritis, iritis, and keratitis.

"acne surgery" [sûr′jẽr-ē, sər′jə-rē, -rĭ] refers to the practice of comedo extraction, and incision and drainage of pustules, abscesses and cysts of the severer grades of the acne process.

acne, tropical [trŏp′ĭ-kəl, -ə-kəl]. *Tropical acne* is a useful term because it designates an unusually severe form of acne that occurs in hot, humid climates. The severity lies not only in intensity of inflammatory process in the form of pustules and conglobate abscesses but in extent of process. The chest in entirety, parts of the abdomen, shoulders, upper parts of the arms and entire back, buttocks and even upper parts of the legs may be involved.

acne varioliformis [vā′rĭ-, văr′ĭ-ō-lĭ-fôr′mĭs] is a title which is apt in its adjective (*varioliformis*, resembling smallpox), but misleading in its substantive (*acne*). The uncommon condition, also called acne frontalis, consists of crusted or scabbed papulo-pustular lesions which tend to occur in the scalp and brow (especially along the anterior and temporo-parietal hairline) and heal with scarring that is reminiscent of smallpox. The condition may be a tuberculid (compare *acnitis*) or an odd pyoderma but is surely not of the nature of acne. There is a long and useless synonymy for the condition.

acne vulgaris [vŭl-gā′rĭs, -gä′rĭs, -găr′ĭs] is the common (*vulgaris*, of the crowd) or ordinary variety of acne. It is still useful to use this complete title for average cases with the understanding that nothing derogatory is implied in the classical adjective.

acneform [ăk′nə-fôrm] and **acneiform** [ăk-nē′ĭ-fôrm] are adjectives meaning resembling, appearing like or having the form of acne or of the lesions of acne. *Acneform* itself is a useful word, but the *i* in *acneiform* seems to be an unnecessary insert that may lead to confusion, since *ei* may be mistaken for a diphthong. Hence, on grounds of simplicity in spelling, pronunciation and printing or writing, *acneform* ought to be the preferred form. The same applies to the following entry.

acneforme and **acneiforme** are the neuter singular of a New Latin adjective which appears in the title *ulerythema acne(i)forme*. See *acneform*, above.

acnegen [ăk′nə-jən] denotes a substance that promotes or gives rise to (-*gen*) acne.

acnegenic [ăk′nə-jĕn′ĭk] is the adjective from *acnegen* and means promoting or giving rise to acne.

acneic [ăk-nē′ĭk] is a moderately useful adjective from *acne*. However, *acne* itself, though a noun, is short enough to serve as its own adjective as is a common habit of short nouns.

acneiform eruptions are characterized by papules and pustules resembling acne lesions, not necessarily confined to the usual sites of acne vulgaris. The eruptions are distinguished by their sudden onset, usually in a patient well past adolescence. This condition is not infrequently associated with the use of systemic corticosteroids. (Andrews)

acnes [ăk′nēz], meaning of acne, is the genitive singular (Greek declension carried over into New Latin) of *acne.*

acquired hypertrichosis lanuginosa (malignant down) the sudden onset of excessive growth of fine, long, unpigmented fetal hair (lanugo) over the face, trunk and limbs, has been associated with breast, uterine, pancreatic, pulmonary and gastrointestinal carcinomas as well as lymphomas. (Frank Parker)

acquisita [ăk′wĭ-sī′tə, -sē′tə, ə-kwĭz′ĭ-tə] and **acquisitum** [ăk′wĭ-sī′təm, -sē-təm, -tōōm, ə-kwĭz′ĭ-təm] are respectively the feminine singular and the neuter singular of a Latin perfect passive participle used as an adjective and meaning acquired. They appear in the titles *epidermolysis acquisita* and *leukoderma acquisitum centrifugum.*

acro- [ăk′rō] is a combining form taken from Greek that refers to extremities, tips or high points, or to things stretched out, extended, lengthened or pointed. In ancient Greece, *acropolis* designated a high point in a city (*-polis*), a hill or flat, high district usually used as a fortress or a site for a temple. Specifically, *the Acropolis* refers to the famous rocky eminence in Athens on which the Parthenon and other renowned buildings of the past still stand. (Akron, Ohio, being a city on a hill, derives its name in the same pointed way.) A large number of more or less useful words describing conditions and phenomena of, on or about the extremities of the body particularly, but also of the vertex of the scalp, tip of the nose and rims of the ears can be made with this element as will be seen from the following entries.

acrochordon [ăk′rō-kôr′dən] literally means something (*-on,* Greek noun ending) in the form of an extended (*acro-*) string or cord (*-chord-*). In modern times it is a somewhat pretentious designation for a cutaneous tag or fibroma pendulum.

acrodermatitis [ăk′rō-dûr′mə-tī′tĭs, -tē′tĭs] is a comprehensive word for an inflammatory condition of the skin (*-dermatitis*) of the extremities (*acro-*).

acrodermatitis chronica atrophicans [krŏn′ĭ-kə ə-trŏf′ĭ-kănz, -trō′fĭ-kănz] is the title of a characteristic condition that starts as inflammatory plaques on or around the knees, elbows and/or elsewhere. Atrophy that has been likened in appearance to wrinkled cigarette paper is an eventuation. In some cases the condition is a prodrome of a lymphoma.

These are the late skin lesions of Lyme disease. Often recognized in Europe but not in the United States, they are infiltrated violaceous plaques or nodules most often on exterior surfaces which become atrophic. (S.E. Malawista)

acrodermatitis continua [kŏn-tĭn′ū-ə, -ōō-ə] is a title in classical form for an inflammatory dermatosis affecting the toes, sometimes the feet, fingers, hands and neighboring areas, that appears like an intractable pyoderma or like a combination of purulence and psoriasis. An autosomal recessive trait caused by defective intestinal absorption of zinc. Treatment with zinc sulfate by mouth corrects the disease.

acrodermatitis enteropathica [ĕn′tĕr-, ĕn′tĕr-ə-păth′ĭ-kə] is another inflammatory dermatosis that appears like a cross between psoriasis (heavy scaling), epidermolysis bullosa (blisters and crusts on hands, feet, knees and elbows) and superficial pyoderma or fungous (monilial) infection (oozing, crusting, erythema and margination of lesions). A characteristic alopecia is part of the cutaneous picture and gastro-enteropathy is a systemic accompaniment. Due to deficiency of zinc absorption.

acrodermatitis papulosa infantum [pă′pōō-lō′sə ĭnfăn′-tŭm]. Gianotti-Crosti disease.

acrodynia [ăk′rō-dĭn′ē-ə, -ĭ-ə, dī′nē-ə, -nĭ-ə] literally means a painful (-odyn-) condition (-ia) of the extremities, tips or high points (acr-) of the body. The word is applied to a disease which has also been titled *dermatopolyneuritis, erythredema* and *pink disease* and some of whose signs and symptoms may be derived from the literal meanings of all the titles. In typical cases the fingers and toes, hands and feet, sometimes nose and cheeks, are pink, red or dusky purple, swollen, painful and tender. The skin is also cold and clammy. There is constitutional disturbance in the form of anorexia, insomnia, gastrointestinal upset and great general discomfort. The condition is seen in infants between the ages of one and two years. Mercury poisoning has been proved or strongly implicated as cause in many cases.

acrokeratoelastoidosis a secondary dermal disorder of elastic tissue (one of the dermal elastoses). A rare, autosomal, dominantly inherited condition in which firm, shiny papules are seen at the periphery of the palms and soles with some extension to the dorsa of the fingers and the sides of the feet. The essential histologic feature in the papules consists of diminution and fragmentation of the elastic fibers, especially in the deeper portions of the dermis. (Costa; Jung et al; (Lever))

acrokeratosis [ăk′rō-kĕr-ə-tō′sĭs] means a state (-*osis*) of (excessive) cornification (-*kerat-*) on the extremities (*acro-*). It appears in the following titles:

acrokeratosis neoplastica Bazex syndrome a cutaneous marker of malignancy presenting with hyperkeratoses of the extremities, i.e., thickening of the skin of the palms and soles which later spreads to the body. This has been reported as associated with both primary and metastatic carcinomas.

acrokeratosis verruciformis [vē-roo′sĭ-fôr′mĭs] refers to a characteristic genodermatosis in which wart-like (*verruciformis*) excrescences of horn (-*kerat-*) develop on the hands and feet (extremities, *acro-*).

acronym [ăk′rə-nĭm]. An acronym is a word formed from the initial letter or letters of each of the members of a succession of words or of the important parts of compound terms. The word is derived from *acro-* and Greek -*onym*, name. Acronyms are a form of abbreviation sparingly used years ago. In recent years, however, acronyms by the thousands have been created and the habit of creating them is developing unreasonably. The phenomenon is not, however, entirely unhealthy. There is legitimate need for acronyms and legitimate practice of formation of acronyms in disciplines like chemistry and in industries like the pharmaceutical where the requirement for short terms of chemicals and drugs is great. Even when it is reasonable, one may hope that the acronym explosion will not result in a babel of permutations and combinations that will require computers and other electronic devices to devise and decipher. To give examples of the nature of the problems, consider acronyms that make common words or a succession of letters that are not standard words but that can be articulated easily, e.g., *AIDS* (**a**uto-immune **d**eficiency **s**yndrome). What, then, should be done with *ACTH* (**a**dreno**c**ortico**t**ropic **h**ormone)? We pose the problems without attempting solutions.

acropustulosis of infancy recurrent crops of pustules or vesicopustules seen mainly on the distal extremities. May begin at birth, during the first year or unusual to start later (Ingber & Sandburch). Clears spontaneously in a few years (Jarratt & Ramsdell).

acrosclerosis [ăk′rō-sklē-rō′sĭs, -sklĕr-ō′sĭs, -sklə-rō′sĭs] literally means a state (-*osis*) of hardening (-*sclero-*) of the extremities (*acro-*). The word is applied to a sclerodermatous condition of the hands and fingers, feet and toes and sometimes the face, that is not quite like ordinary diffuse scleroderma, but relates to more appreciable vascular dysfunction (as from Raynaud's disease).

acrosyringium [ăk′rō-sĭ-rĭn′jĭ-əm] designates the last part (*acro-*, end, top) of the duct (*syringium*, a tube) of a sweat gland. The word is applied to the intraepidermal portion of the duct of a sweat gland.

actin-, actino- [ăk′tĭn, ăk′tĭ-nō] pertain to rays or beams of light (from Greek *aktis*, ray). These word elements are used to make words that apply to visible and ultraviolet light of natural (solar) or artificial sources.

actinic [ăk-tĭn′ĭk] is an adjective meaning relating or pertaining to rays or beams of light.

actinic keratosis [kĕr′ə-tō′sĭs] describes damage to the skin in the form of hyperkeratosis and scaling attributable to injury caused by prolonged exposure to sunshine in susceptible persons, i.e., the fair-skinned, blue-eyed. Solar and senile keratosis are alternate titles.

actinic prurigo (Hutchinson's summer prurigo) onset often before puberty; common among American Indians. It shows primarily prurigo-like papules but there may also be eczematous patches. Most severe in summer but occurs throughout the year. Involves exposed and covered parts of the skin. Chronic in nature. (Lever)

actinic reticuloid is an idiopathic, severe, chronic photodermatosis, which occurs most often in men, middle-aged or older. It is characterized by infiltrated, erythematous, shiny plaques on an eczematous background on exposed areas, often with involvement of covered sites and occasional progression to generalized erythroderma. Patients have a history of erythroderma. They react to UVA, UVB, and visible light. Contact dermatitis plays a major role. The dermal infiltrate has been shown to be primarily suppressor T cells.

actinism [ăk′tĭn-ĭz'm] is a condition (*-ism*) relating to or resulting from the action of electromagnetic energy of the order of visible and ultraviolet light (*actin-*).

actino-. See *actin-*.

actinodermatitis [ăk′tĭ-nō-dûr′mə-tī′tĭs, -tē′tĭs] is a reasonable, general designation for any inflammatory condition of the skin (*-dermatitis*) caused by visible or ultraviolet (*actino-*) light.

actinodermatosis [ăk′tĭ-nō-dûr′mə-tō′sĭs] means any pathologic condition of the skin (*-dermatosis*) attributable to the action of visible or ultraviolet light (*actino-*).

Actinomyces bovis [ăk′tĭ-nō-mī′sēz bō′vĭs] (of the cow), **Actinomyces hominis** [hŏm′ĭ-, hō′mĭ-nĭs] (of humans) and **Actinomyces**

israelii [ĭz-rā′lē-ī] (eponymic of a person's name) are specific micro-organisms of the genus.

actinomycosis is a chronic suppurative and granulomatous bacterial infection characterized by contiguous spread, abscess formation, and sinuses that discharge grains ("sulfur granules"). There are four clinical forms: cervicofacial ("lumpy jaw"), thoracic, abdominal, and disseminated. (Drutz)

actinomycotic [ăk′tĭ-nō-mī-kŏt′ĭk] is an adjective meaning pertaining or relating to actinomycosis.

actinotherapy [ăk′tĭ-nō-thĕr′ə-pē, -pĭ] means treatment (*-therapy*) by visible or ultraviolet light (*actino-*) from a natural source (sun) or an artificial source of roughly equivalent spectrum.

acuminata, acuminatae, acuminatus, acuminatum [ə-kū′ mĭ-nā′tə, -nä′tə; -nā′tē; -nā′təs, -tŭs, -tōōs; -nā′təm, -tŭm] are forms of a Latin adjective that means pointed. The different endings denote different gender and number, e.g., *verruca acuminata* (feminine singular), *verrucae acuminatae* (feminine plural), *licen ruber acuminatus* (masculine singular), *condyloma acuminatum* (neuter singular), *condylomata acuminata* (neuter plural).

acuminate [ə-kū′mĭ-nāt, -mə-nət] is an adjective meaning rendered sharp or pointed (from the Latin adjective *acuminatus*, pointed or sharpened).

acuminate warts [wôrts] are verrucous formations that localize on and around the genitalia and anus. Individual wart units, when not too macerated, are more or less pointed, filiform or digitate. Usually the real thing is not so sharp as *acuminate* would suggest.

acupuncture [ăk′ū-pŭnk-chŭr] literally means pricking (*-puncture*) with a sharp point or needle (*acu-*). The word could be applied to ordinary injections of everyday medical practice. However, it is reserved for the ancient Chinese practice of sticking and twirling needles into elaborately worked-out spots or "points" on the body that are said to be along "channels" called "meridians" in order to achieve temporary anesthesia for surgical operations and enduring relief in painful conditions like the arthrititides and neuropathies. So many have attested to its efficacy that it is under intensive research and clinical application almost everywhere now. Even if that efficacy is more than illusory or delusory, we still lack a rational explanation of the mechanism of action.

acuta [ə-kū′tə] and **acutum** [ə-kū′təm, -tŭm, -tōōm] are respectively the feminine singular and neuter singular of a Latin adjective (see *acute*) meaning acute, sharpened. They appear in titles written in classical form, e.g., *parapsoriasis acuta* and *ulcus vulvae acutum*.

acute [ə-kūt′] derives from Latin *acutus*, perfect passive participle of *acuere*, to sharpen. It thus carries several connotations relating to sharpness, namely, sudden, brief, and severe. In some connotations it is also antonymous to *chronic*. Many dermatoses carry the word as part of their titles, e.g., *acute disseminated lupus erythematosus, acute pemphigus, acute urticaria*, etc.

acute cutaneous lupus erythematosis (ACLE) is characterized by erythema and/or edema of the skin or the presence of vasculitic lesions. These lesions tend to occur almost exclusively in patients with systemic lupus erythematosis (SLE). Malar erythema, or "butterfly" rash, is a typical example of this type of reaction. Resolution of these lesions, like those of systemic cutaneous lupus erythematosis, is without scar formation but pigmentary abnormalities can occur. This eruption has been associated with a more significant systemic disease, but there is not a characteristic pattern of involvement. (J.P. Callen)

acutum. See *acuta*.

ad-, -ad [ăd] are respectively a prefix and a suffix derived from the Latin preposition *ad*, meaning to or toward. In English words *ad-* retains the force that it has as a prefix in Latin words, to wit, direction, change to, intensification. It changes to *ac-, af-, ag-* and *al-* before word elements beginning with *c, f, g* and *l*, e.g., *accede, affix, aggregate* and *allocate*. The use of *-ad* as a suffix is not found in classical Latin; it was adopted as a method of forming certain adverbs in anatomy and zoology, e.g., *cephalad* (toward the head or anterior), *caudad* (toward the tail or posterior), *dorsad* (dorsally, toward the back). There is still another suffix *-ad*, which is of Greek origin. It comes from the genitive *-ados* of the feminine noun ending *-as*. From this derivation words are formed that designate aggregates (e.g., *myriad*, ten thousand) or members of a class (e.g., *trichomonad*).

adamantinoma [ăd′ə-măn′tĭ-nō′mə] refers to a tumor (*-oma*) of the jaw that arises from remains of the enamel organ of a tooth. The word derives from a Greek word element (*adamantin-*) meaning unconquerable, and therefore by extension, the hardest substance. The word *diamond* is so derived.

Addison's disease [ăd′ĭ-sən] Hypoadrenalism. Caused by a hypofunction of the adrenal cortex, is characterized by weakness, hypotension, and hyperpigmentation of the skin and oral mucosa. The hyperpigmentation is most pronounced in the areas of the skin exposed to the sun, at sites of pressure, and on the genitalia. Pigmentation of the oral mucosa usually is patchy. (Lever)

The hyperpigmentation is the result of an increased activity of melanocytes, without an increase in their number. (Szabo) This is caused by increased concentrations of beta MSH (melanocyte-stimulating hormone) in the serum.

adenitis [ăd'n-ī'tĭs, -ē'tĭs, ăd'ə-nī'tĭs] means inflammation (*-itis*) of a gland (*aden-*). It must be understood that a lymph gland (node) is usually meant.

adenoid [ăd'n'oid, ăd'ə-noid] means pertaining to, in the nature of, resembling, of or like (*-oid*) a lymph gland or node (*aden-*).

adenoides [ăd'n-oi'dēz, ăd'ə-noi'dēz] is an adjective in classical Greek form equal to *adenoid*. It occurs in the title *epithelioma adenoides cysticum*.

adenoma [ăd'n-ō'mə, ăd'ə-nō'mə] means hypertrophy or tumefaction (*-oma*) of a gland (*aden-*). The term is used in this sense in both gross and microscopic areas of viewing. Without qualification there is no connotation of malignancy.

adenoma, sebaceous [sə-, sē-bā'shəs]. *Sebaceous adenoma* refers to hypertrophy or benign hyperplasia of a sebaceous gland.

adenoma sebaceum [sē-bā'shē-əm, -sē-əm, -shəm] describes the dermatologic component of a dysplastic complex which includes, in its completest expression (epiloia), gliomatous proliferation in the central nervous system (tuberous sclerosis) that may be attended by mental deficiency and epileptic convulsions, and neoplasias of the kidneys, intestines and sometimes other viscera. The cutaneous picture consists of pinhead to match-head sized papules of yellowish, waxy or reddish color, more or less symmetrically distributed on the cheeks, nose, chin and brow. Histologically, the lesions consist of tissue that is fibroblastic and/or hemangiomatous. The sebaceous glands per se are not involved, which makes the adjective *sebaceum* inappropriate. Hypopigmented macules are the most common skin lesions—often best visualized with the use of a Wood's light. Pringle's name is attached to *adenoma sebaceum* in well-developed form when in addition there are subungual and periungual warty fibromas. Balzar's name is also heard in connection with *adenoma sebaceum* but what is meant by this eponym is *epithelioma adenoides cysticum*. As one may expect, in congenital, dysplastic, hereditary, nevoid and neoplastic processes, multiplicity of effects and variability of involvement give rise to nosologic difficulty and confusion.

adermal [ə-dûr′məl] and **adermic** (ə-dûr′mĭk] are adjectives meaning relating to (-al, -ic) lack of (a-) skin (-derm-).

adermia [ə-dûr′mē-ə, -mĭ-ə] literally means a condition (-ia) in which skin (-derm-) is lacking (a-). It is descriptive, then, of appearance as varied as traumatic avulsion of the skin to skin defects of the newborn.

adermia congenita [kən-, kŏn-jĕn′ĭ-tə] is a title in classic form for skin defects of the newborn.

adermic [ə-dûr′mĭk]. See adermal.

adip(o)- [ăd′ə-, ăd′ĭ-pō] is a Latin word element that means relating to fat.

adiponecrosis [ăd′ə-, ăd′ĭ-pō-nē-krō′sĭs, -nĕ-krō′səs] means a condition (-osis) in which fat tissue (adipo-) dies (-necr-).

adiposis dolorosa [ăd′ə-, ăd′ĭ-pō′sĭs, dŏl′ə-, dō′lō-rō′sə] is the title of a condition (-osis) in which the fat (adip-) tissue of the panniculus adiposus, in its excess and redundancy, is painful (dolorosa).

adiposus [ăd′ə-, ăd′ĭ-pō′səs] is a Latin adjective meaning full of fat. It appears in the title panniculus adiposus.

adnexa [ăd-nĕk′sə] is a Latin neuter plural form that means structures that are bound, attached to or in proximity to a main part of reference. With regard to skin, the structures that make up hair, nails, eccrine, sebaceous and apocrine glands are the adnexa. It may have merit to reserve adnexa for the internal hair apparatus, the nail matrix and all the cutaneous glands. The extruded hair shafts and the nail plates might better be termed appendages. The singular, adnexum, refers to any one of the structures but is rarely used.

adnexal [ăd-nĕk′səl] is an adjective meaning pertaining or relating to adnexa.

adnexum [ăd-nĕk′səm]. See adnexa.

adult T-cell leukemia (ATL) has clinical and histologic similarities to cutaneous T-cell lymphoma (CTCL), particularly the Sézary syndrome variant, and appears to be caused by the human T-cell leukemia-lymphoma virus (HTLV). It is ordinarily a fulminant acute illness occurring among young adults, associated with multiorgan involvement and hypercalcemia. (Kaplan)

adult T-cell lymphoma skin lesions are erythroderma, papules and nodules in approximately 2/3 of patients; occurs mainly in blacks in the USA. HTLVI retrovirus antibodies present. Hepatosplenomegaly, osteolytic bone lesions, hypercalcemia are features. (Frank Parker)

adult T-cell lymphoma-leukemia this is one of the cutaneous T-cell lymphomas, associated with human T-cell lymphotropic virus type I (HTLV-I) infection. (Lever)

(a)estival (ēs'-, ĕs'tĭ-vəl, -tə-vəl, ēs'tī-, ĕs-tī'vəl] means pertaining to the summertime (Latin *aestas,* summer). In American convention, the initial digraph is changed to *e* by dropping the *a,* and the word is written *estival.* Compare *aesthetic* and *esthetic,* and see *haem-.*

(a)estivale [ēs'-, ĕs'tĭ-vä'lē, -vä'lē, -văl'ē] **(a)estivalis** [ēs'-, ĕs'tĭ-vä'lĭs, -vä'lĭs, -văl'ĭs] are respectively the neuter singular and the masculine and feminine singular (same form for both) of the Latin adjective from which *(a)estival* is derived. In American medical writing they appear as *estivale* and *estivalis.* The words are used in titles of classical form, e.g., *hydroa (a)estivale* (neuter), *pruritus (a) estivalis* (masculine) and *acne (a)estivalis* (feminine). The plurals are respectively *(a)estivalia* and *(a)estivales.*

agammaglobulinemia [ă-găm'ə-glō-bū-lĭ-nē'mĭ-ə] designates a condition (*-ia*) in which there is a paucity (*a-*) of gamma globulins in the blood (*-em-*). There are genetic (primary) and acquired (secondary) kinds of agammaglobulinemia. (Lever)

agammaglobulinemia ("Swiss" type) stems from hypoplasia of the thymus and of all lymphoid tissue, resulting in both defective, cell-mediated immunity and hypogammaglobulinemia. (Higgs and Wells) There is candidiasis which is generally mild and is often limited to the oral cavity. Death usually occurs before the age of two from severe infections such as viral pneumonia. (Lever)

agenesia [ā'jē-, ā'jə-, ā'jĕn-ē'zhē-ə, -zē-ə, -zhə], or **agenesis, pilorum** [ā-jĕn'ə-səs, ā'jĕn-ē'sĭs pī-lō'rəm, -lôr'ŭm] is a title for failure (*a-*) of hair (*pilorum*) development (*-genesia, -genesis*).

aggressive digital papillary adenoma and adenocarcinoma a rare neoplasm of the sweat gland that can occur as an aggressive digital papillary adenoma (ADPA) or adenocarcinoma (ADPA ca). It presents as a painless mass on the fingers, toes and adjacent palms and soles. Microscopic features resemble breast carcinoma. An ADPA ca has the potential for distant metastases leading to fatality. Recognition is important for they are aggressive tumors and can possibly metastasize. Continuous patient follow-up is necessary. (Kao, Helwig & Graham). Some pathologists may wish to lump these into more generic diagnoses such as eccrine acrospiroma. (Flotte)

agminata [ăg′mĭ-nā′tə, -nä′tə] and **agminated** [ăg′mə-, ăg′mĭ-nāt′ĕd, -ĭd] are respectively a Latin and an English adjective meaning gathered together in a group (from *agmen, agminis,* a collected group in action, army on the march).

agr- [ăgr, āgr] is a word element found in the Greek adjective *agrios,* wild, that denotes severity, wildness or other such quality of disagreeable sensation (pain, itch) and carries additional connotation of seizure (sudden onset and equally sudden cessation) of such sensation. The feminine singular of the complete adjective appears in a title like *prurigo agria* (a condition of severe itching) and the combining form is found in words like *pellagra* (wildly uncomfortable skin), *podagra* (an attack of pain in the foot as from gout) and *mentagrophytes,* which relates etymologically to severe (*-agro-*) sycosiform fungous (*-phytes*) infection of the hair of the chin (*ment-*).

AIDS (the acquired immunodeficiency syndrome) is a life-threatening, opportunistic infection and/or Kaposi's sarcoma, developing in a previously healthy individual, with cellular immunodeficiency due to the HIV (human immunodeficiency virus) infection of the immune system. This is a rapidly progressive disease with high mortality from opportunistic infection or neoplasm. (J.E. Groopman)

ainhum [ān′həm, ĭ-nyūm′] is derived via Portuguese from *ayun,* or *eyun,* a word in Yoruban (language spoken along the eastern Guinea coast, Africa) meaning to saw. A synonymous title that is more descriptive to those who are more familiar with classic than African tongues is *dactylolysis spontanea.* The condition, ethnically limited largely to blacks and regionally limited largely to Africa, is a startling process of slow, progressive, band-like constriction, usually of the proximal phalanges of the small toes, which eventually ends in painless withering or amputation of the digits. Pain may be an accompaniment at times when the process is complicated by secondary infection or mechanical distortion.

alastrim [ə-lăs′trĭm] is a name derived from the Portuguese word *alastrar* (to spread) and given to an exanthematic disease that resembles a mild case of smallpox. Its course and severity are like those of chickenpox. The exact viral relationship of the cause of alastrim and smallpox is not settled. There are many provincial designations like *amaas* (an Afrikaans word), *kaffir pox, milk pox,* etc., that would be best forgotten. Modern terminology favors *variola minor* over all other titles.

alb- [ălb] is a Latin word element denoting the color white.

alba [ăl'bə] is the feminine singular of a Latin adjective meaning white. It appears in the titles *linea alba, miliaria alba, phlegmasia alba* and *pityriasis alba.*

albicans [ăl'bĭ-kănz] is a Latin present participle that means making, turning or becoming white. It appears in the titles *Monilia albicans*, in the more modern *Candida albicans*, where it is something of a redundancy, since *candida* also relates to whiteness, and in *stria albicans.*

albinism [ăl'bĭ-nĭz'm, -bə-nĭz-əm] is white- (*albin-*) -ness (*-ism*) of the skin. The word is usually applied to congenital absence of ability to form melanin, although there is nothing in the word that limits it that way.

An inherited, autosomal recessive disorder of melanin synthesis which affects skin, hair and eyes. It typically presents with congenital milk-white skin, white hair, photophobia, and nystagmus. The term albino is derived from the Latin albus meaning "white." The term albinism should be restricted to those congenital, universal hypomelanoses limited to eye and skin (oculocutaneous albinism) or to the eye alone (ocular albinism). (Fitzpatrick)

albinism, localized [lō'kə-līzd], or **circumscribed** [sûr'kəm-scrībd], describes limited areas of congenital depigmentation.

albino [ăl-bī'nō, -bē'nō] derives from Latin through Portuguese and is the designation for a person afflicted with complete albinism.

Albright's disease or **polyostotic fibrous dysplasia** three or four large, irregularly shaped hyperpigmented macules (often reported to look like the Coast of Maine) are usually found unilaterally distributed on the buttocks or cervical area. (Parker) Also endocrine dysfunction and precocious puberty in females and sometimes in males. (Fitzpatrick) Osteitis fibrosa cystica disseminata; brown-spot syndrome.

Alezzandrini syndrome facial vitiligo, poliosis, deafness and unilateral macular degeneration.

alkaptonuria is a rare disorder in the degradative pathway of phenylalanine and tyrosine metabolism. The genetic defect in the activity of the enzyme homogentisic acid oxidase leads to the accumulation and excessive urinary excretion of homogentisic acid. There is an associated deposition of dark pigment in connective tissues (ochronosis) and a particular form of degenerative arthritis. (Wyngaarden) The pigmentation may be noticed in the cartilage of the nose, the sclera and ears.

algia [ăl′jə, -jē-ə, -jĭ-ə] is a Greek word element denoting a state of pain, e.g., dermatalgia (a painful condition of the skin) and causalgia (a condition of burning sensation; *caus*- is from a Greek root meaning to burn, as in *caustic*).

Alibert's disease [älēbĕr′]. Several: keloid, leishmaniasis tropica, sycosis barbae, mycosis fungoides.

allergic [ə-lûr′jĭk] is the adjective from *allergy*. It can be used alone in a formation like *an allergic manifestation* or followed by a preposition in a construction like *allergic to penicillin*. There are two uses of the word that are deplorable, namely, 1) as a noun to designate a person with an allergic state, and 2) as a general adjective with the meaning of disagreeably reactive. The use of *allergic* as a noun distinguishes no one since everybody who has lived more than one to three weeks (the incubation period to the development of an allergic state) has allergic transformations to some things. Everybody is, therefore, an "allergic." What is usually meant by *allergic* when it is used to designate a person is *atopic*, i.e., one who has, or has a potential for, allergic states that are of the atopic variety. See *atopy* and related words.

allergic contact dermatitis caused by chemical agents that elicit type IV delayed hypersensitivity reaction on skin. The contact precedes rash by two or more days; in both instances site and configuration of eczema reaction conform to site of contact with exogenous substances (plants, medicaments, cosmetics, metals); patch tests. (Frank Parker)
 Usually due to delayed hypersensitivity reaction, type IV, with latent periods of a few days to greatly prolonged periods. May also be due to a primary irritant substance resulting in inflammation either after the first or repeated contacts.

allergic eczema [ĕk′sə-mə, ĕg-zē′mə] is a poor title because both words mean different things to different users. Those who equate allergy with atopy, and eczema with any erythematous and oozing or crusting eruption, seem to apply the title to atopic dermatitis. If one qualifies eczema with a requirement that the process be fundamentally in the epidermis, then the title is not apt for atopic dermatitis. The most reasonable use of it would be for a dermatitis predicated upon allergic sensitization to simple chemical contactants. Such an eruption is allergic and eczematous both clinically and histologically. The dermatitis caused, for example, by sensitization and exposure to poison ivy fulfills the requirements of this title. It is not, however, so used. See entry following.

allergic eczematous contact (-type) dermatitis. See *allergic eczematous dermatitis*.

allergic eczematous dermatitis [ĕg-zĕm′ə-təs dûr′mə- tī′tĭs, -tē′tĭs] is, in our opinion, the best title for what is frequently designated as *allergic eczematous contact (-type) dermatitis* or simply *contact dermatitis*. It states the allergic mechanism and the eczematous clinical appearance. It omits *contact (-type)*, which lengthens the title in an ungainly way and introduces difficulty in understanding when the approach of the allergen is not from without but from within.

allergic granulomatosis (Churg-Strauss syndrome) About two-thirds of the patients have cutaneous lesions. A systemic disease in which a necrotizing vasculitis is seen in association with necrotizing granulomas. Respiratory symptoms, usually asthma, precede the onset of allergic granulomatosis. Pronounced eosinophilia both in the circulating blood and in the lesions, the presence of pulmonary infiltrations, involvement of small arteries and veins, and the presence of palisading granulomas with central necrosis extravascularly in the connective tissue are found. Two types of cutaneous lesions occur, hemorrhagic lesions varying from petechia to extensive ecchymoses, sometimes accompanied by necrotic ulcers, and cutaneous-subcutaneous nodules. (Lever)

allergic stomatitis [stō′mə-tī′tĭs, -tē′tĭs] is a simple title for what is comparable in the mouth to allergic eczematous dermatitis.

"allergic" vasculitis. See *palpable purpura.*

allergy immediate-type hypersensitivity consists of two types: one is anaphylactic reactions or reaginic hypersensitivity and another type is Arthus-type reaction. Both types of immediate hypersensitivity are caused by antibodies; however, the mechanisms of the reactions are entirely different. Anaphylactic reactions are caused by the reaction of antigen with cell-bound antibodies, while Arthus-type reactions are caused by preformed antigen-antibody complexes. Hay fever or allergic rhinitis is recognized as the human counterpart of anaphylactic reactions in animals. (Ishizaka & Ishizaka)

allergy or **hypersensitivity** the detrimental consequences to the host of the immune response. This is a clinical judgement and does not imply that the basic pathways leading to immunity, beneficial to the host, or hypersensitivity are different. (Austen)

"alligator boy" [ăl′ə-gā′tĕr boi] and **alligator skin** describe, in an exaggerated way, the victim and the condition of a severe grade of ichthyosis. Compare *sauriasis.*

Allodermanyssus [ăl′ō-dûr′mə-nĭs′əs] is a New Latin formation from Greek word elements meaning a changed, different or abnormal (*allo-*) pricker (*-nyssus*) of the skin (*-derma-*). The word names a genus of mites, bloodsucking and parasitic, on rodents. One species, *A. sanguineus* (bloody) transmits to humans the agent (*Rickettsia akari*) of rickettsialpox.

alopecia [ăl′ə-, ăl′ō-pē′shē-ə, -shĭ-ə, -shə], when unqualified, is used to designate loss of hair in any amount up to complete baldness. It derives via Latin from the Greek word for fox (*alopex*), an animal that commonly suffers a mange which causes hair loss. The etymological subtleties of the word are not useful to pursue further. *Alopecia* is well-established in dermatologic talk and writing; modified with appropriate adjectives, it is widely used as follows:

alopecia areata [ā′rē-ā′tə, ăr′ē-ăt′ə, är′ē-ä′tə] means baldness (*alopecia*) in circumscribed spots (*areata* a classical adjective from the noun *area*, a limited space). The title is used for a characteristic condition in which there is fairly sudden hair fall in one or more spots on the scalp, beard, eyebrows and other hairy places. The falling hairs are characteristic too in their "exclamation point" formation at the end that leaves the scalp. The baldness is complete but the skin of the affected site appears normal. Regrowth is the rule in a matter of months to one year; occasionally progression to total, generalized and universal hair fall occurs. Considered to be an autoimmune disease.

alopecia cicatrisata [sĭk′ə-trĭ-sā′tə, -sä′tə] denotes a baldness (*alopecia*) attended by scarring (*cicatrisata*) of the skin of the site, especially a form that occurs in a diamond-shaped patch around the vertex.

alopecia circumscripta [sûr′kəm-skrĭp′tə] simply says loss of hair in a circumscribed way. It can encompass alopecia areata, alopecia mucinosa and any other loss of hair that is sharply limited in extent.

alopecia generalisata [jĕn′ĕr-ăl-ĭ-sā′tə, -sä′tə] is the title for loss of all the hair of the body. In complete cases there is nary a one to split. The process seems to be an extreme extension of alopecia areata. The prognosis for recovery is poor; cause and cure are not known. *Alopecia universalis* is synonymous.

alopecia liminaris frontalis [lĭm′ĭ-nā′rĭs, -nä′rĭs frŏn-tā′lĭs, -tä′lĭs, -tăl′ĭs] is the title for loss of hair shafts, not loss of hair proper, at the margin (*liminaris*, from Latin *limen*, threshold) in the frontal region. The condition is an artifact caused by too tight binding of the hair from front backward. It is common in black children who have tufts of hair tightly braided. Of course, other arrangements of tight hair dress may cause patterns of loss other than frontal. The principle, however, is the same. Injury to hair bulbs and permanent alopecia are consequences of long practice of such pull on hair shafts.

alopecia, male pattern [māl′ păt′ərn]. *Male pattern baldness* is a recent coinage to describe frontal recession of scalp hair or loss of hair that starts on the vertex and continues until no more than a temporo occipital fringe of hair is left.

alopecia, "moth-eaten" [môth′ēt′n]. "Moth-eaten" baldness is a characteristic patchy loss of hair in the temporo-parietal and occipital regions of the scalp that occurs in secondary syphilis.

alopecia mucinosa [mū′sĭ-nō′sə] is a title for a condition characterized clinically by patches of erythema and alopecia commonly on the face and histologically by the appearance of mucin in and about the hair apparatus, which is the more abnormal for swollen follicular walls. When not *sui generis*, the condition is seen in association with lymphomas or as a forerunner thereof. *Follicular mucinosis* is an alternate title.

alopecia neoplastica areas of scarring alopecia in the scalp due to underlying metastatic carcinoma as from a breast cancer. The induration and atrophy simulates alopecia areata. (Frank Parker)

alopecia totalis [tō-tā′lĭs, -tä′lĭs, -tăl′ĭs] sounds as if it ought to mean loss of hair all over—which well it might. It must be learned, however, that total loss of hair of the scalp alone is meant, whereas *alopecia generalisata* and *alopecia universalis* are applied to loss of all hair everywhere. Alopecia totalis is an extension of alopecia areata on the scalp.

alopecia universalis [ū′nĭ-vĕr-sā′lĭs, -sä′lĭs, -săl′ĭs] is synonymous with *alopecia generalisata* and more forcibly denotes loss of hair everywhere.

alpha [ăl′fə], or α, the Greek symbol for it, is frequently used as an identifier, e.g., alpha or α rays, globulin, etc.

amebiasis cutis [ăm′ē-bī′ə-sĭs kū′tĭs] is the title for infection of the skin with *Ameba histolytica*. The lesions consist of indolent and long-enduring ulcers from which the organism can be recovered for microscopic identification.

amebic ulcer [ə-mē′bĭk ŭl′sər, -sēr] is a simple designation of the principal lesion of amebiasis cutis.

amelanotic [ə-mĕl′ə-nŏt′ĭk] is an adjective that means lacking (*a-*) in melanin.

amelanotic melanoma [mĕl′ə-nō′mə] describes malignant melanoma in which there has occurred failure of melanogenesis. There is an obvious verbal inconsistency in this title.

amiantacea [ăm′ē-, ăm′ĭ-, -ăn-tā′shē-ə, -sē-ə, -shə] is a New Latin coinage (from Greek via classical Latin noun *amiantus*, asbestos) of a feminine singular adjective meaning in the nature of (*-acea*) asbestos (*amiant-*). It is found in the title *tinea amiantacea*.

amiantaceous [ăm′ē-ăn-tā′shəs] is the English equivalent of *amiantacea* with the same meaning of in the nature of asbestos. It would be used descriptively in a phrase like *an amiantaceous crust*.

amiodarone pigmentation. Amiodarone is an iodinated, adrenergic blocker used in the treatment of tachyarrhythmias. In long-term high-dose use causes a slate blue discoloration of sun-exposed skin, especially in the face, in about ten percent of the cases. (Trimble et al; Lever)

amyloid [ăm′ĭ-loid] means starch- (*amyl-*, from Greek and Latin word for starch) -like (*-oid*). The word is used both as an adjective and a noun. It was coined to suggest the starch-like behavior of some materials of the ground substance or of tissue when treated with sulfuric acid and iodine. Amyloid has three distinct components: protein-derived amyloid fibers, a glycoprotein P component, and ground substance. (Andrews, 8th Edition, Arnold/Odom/James)

amyloid degeneration [dĭ-, də-, dē-jĕn′ə-rā′shən] refers to physical and tinctorial change that occurs in amyloidosis and many other conditions, particularly the chronic inflammatory. The tinctorial change is best demonstrated by special strains that act selectively on amyloid.

amyloid diseases comprise a group of conditions of diverse causes characterized by the accumulation of ultrastructurally fibrillar material in various tissues such that vital organ function is compromised. The associated disease states may be inflammatory, hereditary, or neoplastic and the deposition can be local or systemic. The clinical outcome may be benign or as malignant as the most aggressive of neoplasms. (Joel N. Buxbaum, 18th Ed. *Cecil Textbook of Medicine*, Wyngaarden & Smith, eds. W.B. Saunders Co.)

amyloidosis [ăm′ĭ-loi-dō′sĭs] is a condition (*-osis*) in which amyloid is detectably present in tissues. There are systemic and organ-localized forms of amyloidosis.

amyloidosis cutis [kū′tĭs] is the title for the clinical condition (*-osis*) in which amyloid is deposited in the skin (*cutis*). This title is more generic than *lichen amyloidosus*, which specifies the papular character of the dermatosis.

amyloidosus [ăm'ĭ-loi-dō'səs] is the masculine singular form of a New Latin adjective literally meaning full of (-*osus*) amyloid. It appears in a title in classical form like *lichen amyloidosus*.

an- is a form of alpha privative used before words of Greek origin beginning with a vowel. See *a-*.

ana- [ăn'ə] is a prefix (from Greek) of diverse meanings, namely, up, upward, again, over again, back, against, more than, etc. Medical words employing this prefix sound ridiculous if the right meaning or shade of meaning is not appreciated. An important meaning in words of dermatologic interest is back or against in the sense of opposite, reduced, or reversed, and in any of these senses the prefix begins to have some of the force of alpha privative. See *anaphylaxis* and *anatoxin*. For the meaning of up, upward or over again, see *anagen*.

an(a)emicus [ə-nē'mĭ-kəs] is the masculine singular form of a New Latin adjective meaning blood- (-*aem-* or -*em-*) -less (*an-*). Anemicus is the usual American spelling. The adjective appears in the title *n(a)evus an(a)emicus*.

anagen [ăn'ə-jĕn] could mean literally growing or developing (-*gen*) up, upward or over again (*ana-*). It is applied to that stage of hair development marked by continuous growth.

anagen effluvium or **toxic alopecia** occurs if hair growth is disrupted during anagen. The newly synthesized hair shaft is weakened and the hair breaks readily. Thinning may be extreme, occurring within a few weeks of an insult, involving all 80 percent of follicles in anagen on the scalp. Chemotherapeutic agents, especially Adriamycin and related agents exert their effect on rapidly growing cells in the hair bulb and commonly cause anagen hair damage in cancer patients receiving chemotherapy. Radiotherapy to the scalp area does the same thing. Retinoids and hypervitaminosis A cause hair loss owing to their interference with keratinization. (Frank Parker)

anaphylactic [ăn'ə-fĭ-lăk'tĭk] is an adjective meaning pertaining or relating to (-*ic*) loss (*ana-*) of protection (-*phylact-*, from Greek via Latin).

anaphylactic crisis or **shock** designates the clinical event of anaphylaxis in laboratory animals. Depending on the species, combinations of dyspnea, edema, urticaria, itching and scratching, gastrointestinal dysfunction (vomiting, diarrhea) and cardiovascular dysfunction (hyper- and hypotonia) may be seen.

anaphylactogen [ăn′ə-fĭ-lăk′tō-jən, -tə-jən, -jĕn] is an allergen that is capable of inducing an anaphylactic state and then eliciting anaphylactic crisis or shock.

anaphylactoid [ăn′ə-fĭ-lăk′toid] is an adjective meaning like or resembling (-oid) anaphylaxis.

anaphylaxis [ăn′ə-fĭ-lăk′sĭs] presents a bit of an etymological problem. The prefix ana- has meanings of up, back and over again; -phylaxis relates to protection. The wedding of the two elements with these meanings makes little sense unless one makes an extension of the back meaning of ana- to the plausibility of reduced, reversed or opposite of. Anaphylaxis then means the opposite of protection, i.e., vulnerability or susceptibility to harm, and this best fits the facts.

The most dramatic allergic drug reaction or IgE-mediated hypersensitivity. Penicillin is the most common drug to produce anaphylaxis but many other drugs or diagnostic agents (such as Bromsulphalein) can produce this life-threatening reaction. A history of penicillin allergy increases the risk of this reaction occurring, but most of the patients dying of penicillin-induced anaphylaxis have no history of penicillin allergy. (Nies)

Xylocaine may cause anaphylaxis. Dermatologists need to watch out for the latter. Be sure to get a thorough history of any untoward reactions and avoid the use of Xylocaine if positive.

anaphylaxis (systemic) the most dramatic example of an immediate hypersensitivity reaction. These are uncommon, usually unexpected and occasionally fatal. They occur in previously sensitized individuals after re-exposure to foreign antigens or low molecular weight substances that act as haptens. These reactions are mediated by IgE antibody, begin a few minutes after antigen exposure, and result from the release of basophil and mast-cell mediators. (Lichtenstein) It may range clinically from evanescent urticaria to severe cardiovascular collapse, apnea, convulsions and death.

anaplasia [ăn′ə-plā′zhē-ə, -zē-ə, -zhə] is easily memorable by understanding ana- to mean reversion. The word then comes to mean reversion of growth (-plasia), i.e., reversion to the embryonal or undifferentiated state.

anatomic tubercle [ăn′ə-tŏm′ĭk tōō′-, tū′bĕr-k'l, -bər-kəl], or **wart** [wôrt], is a term applied to re-infection with the tubercle bacillus under circumstances of performing anatomic dissections or autopsies. The lesion is actually a tuberculous chancre comparable to what happens in the second phase of Koch's fundamental experiment. It is essentially tuberculosis cutis verrucosa. Usually located on a finger or hand, it consists of a tumid process that is heavily crusted or hyperkeratotic. *Prosector's wart* and *butcher's tubercle* are synonymous terms. See *tuberculosis cutis verrucosa.*

anatoxin [ăn′ə-tŏk′sĭn] is partially detoxified toxin. The word was coined to designate toxins that have been altered by some manner of processing so that "poison" quality has been reduced but antigenicity retained. Note how in this instance *ana-* must mean reduced.

androgenetic alopecia or **male pattern alopecia** literally hair loss due to androgens. Androgen-induced hair loss in men is the most common cause of alopecia in males and also occurs in women. The condition is largely genetically determined. The other essential component is the effect of androgen on the hair follicle. In patients with this form of alopecia there is increased conversion of testosterone to dihydrotestosterone at the follicular level, possibly mediated by the enzyme, 5 alpha reductase. The resulting high local levels of dihydrotestosterone are then believed to be responsible for the involution of the hair follicles, although the precise mechanism is still the subject of investigation. (Frank Parker)

anemicus [ə-nē′mĭ-kəs]. See *an(a)emicus.*

anesthetic leprosy. See *leprosy.*

anetoderma (macular atrophy) is characterized by atrophic patches located mainly on the upper trunk. The skin of the patches is thin, blue-white, and bulges slightly. The lesions may give the palpating finger the same sensation as a hernial orifice. Two types are generally distinguished: the Jadassohn type, in which the atrophic lesions initially appear red and, on histologic examination, show an inflammatory infiltrate, and the Schweninger-Buzzi type, which clinically is noninflammatory from the beginning. (Lever)

angiitis [ăn′jē-ī′tĭs, -ē′tĭs] means inflammation (*-itis*) of blood vessels (*angi-*).

angiitis necrotizing. See *necrotizing angiitis.*

angina [ăn-jī′nə, ăn′jĭ-nə] means strangulation (from the Latin noun *angina*, quinsy; the verb is *angere*, to choke, to cause or suffer pain). The word has been used for quinsy and for any feeling of distress, particularly of a suffocative nature, in the throat or chest (e.g., angina pectoris).

angina, herpetic [hər-, hûr-pĕt′ĭk]. *Herpetic angina* refers to soreness of the throat caused by infection with the virus of herpes simplex.

angina, Ludwig's (lōōd'vĭgz, -wĭgz]. *Ludwig's angina* is an eponymic designation for the type of stomatitis and pharyngitis that sometimes develops in agranulocytic states.

angina, Vincent's [vĭn'sĕnts]. *Vincent's angina* is an eponymic designation for a type of stomatitis and pharyngitis that is thought to be caused synergistically by a specifc spirillum and fusiform bacillus.

angio- [ăn'jē-o, ăn'gĭ-o] is a combining form from Greek and relates to a vessel, more often of blood, but also of lymph. Many useful words, more than are given below, can be made with this element.

angioblastic lymphadenopathy. Immunologically mediated, this often fatal disorder is characterized by proliferation of plasmacytoid immunoblasts and plasma cells. Fever, malaise, weight loss, hepatosplenomegaly and generalized lymphadenopathy are accompanied in many cases by a generalized, maculopapular, purpuric and occasional exfoliative erythroderma. (Frank Parker)

angioedema evanescent areas of cutaneous edema involving the face, genitalia or hands and feet. Laryngeal edema can occur and may be a serious event requiring emergency medical intervention. Anaphylaxis is a severe and life-threatening form of this disorder. Drug reaction is a frequent cause of this Type I hypersensitivity. A less common condition is hereditary angioedema, an autosomal dominant disorder in which there is uncontrolled complement activation, due to a deficiency of C1 esterase inhibitor. (Patterson & Blaylock)

angioedema-urticaria-eosinophilia syndrome a new syndrome which is related to the action of the eosinophil major basic protein. (Fitzpatrick et al)

angioid [ăn'jē-oid] is an adjective meaning like or resembling (*-oid*) blood vessels (*angi-*).

angioid streaks [strēks] describes a certain appearance on the retinae of some individuals afflicted with pseudoxanthoma elasticum. The precise nature of the streaks, which look like blood vessels (*angioid*), is not decided. Some think they are caused by changes comparable to those occurring in the skin, namely, degeneration of elastic fibers.

angiokeratoma [ăn'jē-ō'kĕr'ə-tō'mə] is a tumor (*-oma*) consisting of vascular elements (*angio-*) covered by hyperkeratotic (*-kerat-*) epidermis.

angiokeratoma corporis diffusum (Fabry's disease) [kôr'pō-rĭs, -pô-rĭs dĭ-fū'səm]. (Glycosphingolipidosis) A metabolic X-linked disease often with striking cutaneous lesions, telangiectases/keratotic angiomas, scattered widely over the body. This is an inborn error of glycosphingolipid metabolism due to a deficiency of the enzyme, alpha-galactosidase-A. Glycosphingolipid accumulates in the lysomes especially of the cardiovascular-renal system. Pain, lancinating episodes in the extremities with fever, angina and myocardial infarction, congestive heart failure and cardiomegaly may ensue. Renal involvement with hypertension is frequent.

Ocular lesions may be present in the cornea (clouding), conjuntiva, retina and other portions of the eye. Attempts have been made at treatment by substitution of the missing enzyme. (*Cecil Textbook of Medicine* 18th Edition, W.B. Saunders Co., Wyngaarden & Smith, Editors)

angiokeratoma (Fordyce) [fôr′dīs] is a species of vascular papules that commonly stud the scrotum and less often the vulva. Hyperkeratosis is not marked on these lesions or in these sites.

angiokeratoma (Mibelli) [mē-bĕl′lē] is a form seen on fingers, hands, toes and feet. The lesions have been aptly described as telangiectatic warts.

angiolupoid [ăn′jē-ō-lōō′poid] is a word coined to designate a rare type of granuloma located on the nose, usually on a side, which in purplish color and telangiectasia suggests hypervascularity (*angio-*). A granulomatous process in the nature of sarcoidosis or the bacillary-barren tuberculids.

angioma [ăn′jē-ō′mə, -jĭ-ō′mə] is a neoplasia or neoplasm (*-oma*) of blood vessels. While the word strictly applies to lymph-vessel neoplasia as well, usually *lymphangioma* is used distinctively, whereas *hemangioma* is understood when *angioma* alone is said or written.

angioma, capillary [kăp′ĭ-lĕr′ē, kə-pĭl′ə-rĭ]. *Capillary angioma* refers to exceedingly superficial types like spider nevi and nevus flammeus.

angioma cavernosum [kăv′ĕr-nō′səm] is neoplasia of blood vessels in which the elements are large, deep and thick-walled.

angioma, senile [sē′nĭl, -n′l]. *Senile angioma* refers to small, superficial telangiectasias that appear in the aged.

angioma serpiginosum [sĕr-pĭj′ĭ-nō′səm] is title for a rare neoplasia of blood vessels that is marked by punctate formations ("cayenne pepper" spots) and progression of the process in a fashion that gives the impression that the developing condition creeps (*serpiginosum*).

angioma simplex [sĭm′plĕks] is a title for nevus flammeus nuchae.

angioma, strawberry [strô′bĕr′ē, -ĭ]. *Strawberry angioma is applied to the common, raised, strawberry-sized and colored, superficial hemangioma seen in the newborn and infants.*

angioma, superficial [sōō′pĕr-fĭsh′əl]. *Superficial angioma distinguishes neoplasias of blood vessels in which the elements are smallish, not deep and thin-walled.*

angiomatosis [ăn′jē-ō′mə-tō′sĭs] is a generic word for a condition (*-osis*) marked by blood vessel (*angio-*) proliferation (*-mat-*) of any degree.

angioneurotic edema [ĭ-, ē-, ə-dē′mə] is the term applied to a form of whealing in which the hive or hives are large, deep and relatively long-enduring. A common site for such an event is on the face about the eyes or lips, but the process may occur anywhere.

angiosarcoma [ăn′jĭ-ō-sär-kō′mə] designates a characteristic malignant neoplasia (*-sarcoma*) of blood vessels (*angio-*).

Ångström unit [ăng′strəm ū′nĭt]. See *Å*.

an(h)idrosis [ăn′(h)ĭ-drō′sĭs] from its Greek word elements, means a state (*-osis*) of absence (*an-*) of sweat or sweating (*-hidr-, -idr-*). Retention or omission of the parenthesized *h* need bring beads of sweat to no brow. It is optional. *Anhydrosis is not a synonym because it means lack (*an-*) of water (*-hydr-*), not of sweat (*-hidr-* or *-idr-*). That the combining element meaning water has a *y* in it can be fixed in mind from the words hydrant and hydraulic.* See (*h*)*idro-* and *hidrosis*.

an(h)idrosis, thermal [thûr′məl], or **thermogenic** [thûr′mō-jĕn′ĭk]. *Thermal,* or *thermogenic, an (h)idrosis designates failure of the sweat function consequent upon the prolonged effects of high temperature and high humidity. The condition is the result of severe and long enduring prickly heat. The clinical complex is termed the sweat-retention syndrome. Tropical an (h)idrotic asthenia is an alternative title.*

an(h)idrotic [ăn′(h)ĭ-drŏt′ĭk] as an adjective means pertaining or related to an(h)idrosis, and as a noun it designates an agent that reduces or stops sweating.

anhidrotic ectodermal dysplasia a congenital disorder with hair loss, short stature, abnormal teeth; an X-linked recessive disorder. Patients have a characteristic facies (frontal bossing) and intolerance to heat. A sex-linked recessive condition occurring only in males. From birth the serious nature is suspected from the altered cranial physiognomy, with abnormalities about the eyes and near absence of teeth in both dentitions. The skin is dry, thin and shows prominence of the subcutaneous vessels. There is a near absence of eccrine sweat glands but not the apocrine sweat glands. Later hair over the head may be scanty and, at puberty, axillary and genital hair does not appear. Patients are often mentally retarded and spastic. (R.D. Adams)

ankylosis spondylitis rheumatoid arthritis of the spine, known as Marie-Strümpell disease.

annular [ăn′ū-lĕr, ăn′yə-lər] is an adjective from Latin *annulus,* a ring, and means circular, round or like a ring. See *annulare.*

annular erythema [ĕr′ĭ-thē′mə] describes a form of persistent edema and erythema in which the process circles normal skin.

annular syphilid [sĭf′ĭ-lĭd] is a useful descriptive term for a characteristic lesion of syphilis. Since syphilis has many lesions of different morphology, distinctive terms serve well. This one occurred commonly, when syphilis was common on the face, especially in Blacks. The raised, round border of the process is what justifies *annular.*

annulare [ăn′ū-lā′re, -lä′rē, -lăr′ē], **annularis** [-rĭs, -lä′rĭs, -lăr′ĭs] and **annulati** [-lā′tī, -lä′tē] are respectively the neuter and feminine singular of the Latin adjective *an* (*n*)*ularis,* meaning annular, shaped like a signet ring, and the nominative masculine plural of the Latin adjective *an* (*n*)*ulatus,* furnished or decorated with a ring, hence ringed. They are used in titles that are written in classical form with correct correspondence of gender, e.g., *granuloma annulare* (neuter), *purpura annularis telangiectodes* (feminine), *pili annulati* (masculine plural).

anonychia [ăn′ə-nĭk′ē-ə, -ĭ-ə] is the condition (*-ia*) of absence (*an-*) of nails (*-onych-*). The term is usually applied to the congenital phenomenon, but it can be used in clear context for acquired, temporary or permanent loss of nails.

anserina [ăn′sə-, ăn′sĕr-, ăn′sĕ-rī′nə] is the feminine singular form of a Latin adjective meaning related to a goose, goose-like. It is used in the title *cutis anserina* (gooseflesh, literally goose skin), which, to those who know plucked geese, aptly describes the papulation of the skin that occurs upon sudden chilling or other stimulation that leads to contraction of the arrectores pilorum.

anthrax [ăn′thrăks] is the disease caused by *Bacillus anthracis.* The word is a transliteration of a Greek word meaning coal. The condition was described and named by Hippocrates, apparently after the appearance of the primary lesion in the stage when a black eschar develops on the carbuncle. The "coal" idea is carried over into

Latin (*carbunculus*, a little coal, whence *carbuncle*) and into French (*charbon* = *anthrax*). Koch discovered the causative organism in 1876 and with it was able for the first time to fulfill those criteria of proof of infectious cause that have since been known as *Koch's postulates*.

ant(i)- [ănt, ăn′tē, -tī, -tĭ, -tə] is a prefix taken from Greek and meaning against. In ancient Greek, *ant-* was used almost invariably in combination with a word or word element beginning with a vowel. However, in the formation of new English words *anti-* is often affixed to a word or word element beginning with a vowel, e.g., *antieczematous, anti-inflammatory* and *anti-urticarial*. *Anti-* is euphonious whether the *i* is pronounced long or short before combining forms that begin with a consonant, but it is awkward and uneconomical before elements beginning with a vowel. Therefore, the question of printing a hyphen between two vowels, each of which has to be pronounced, can be avoided by writing and saying *anteczematous, antinflammatory* and *anturticarial*. The practice is well established in older words such as *Antarctic, antacid, antagonize, antonym*, etc. See entry, *hyphen, use of.* (Only one pronunciation of *anti-* is given in the words below beginning with it; the others are possible.)

antibody [ăn′tĭ-bŏd′ē] is a substance that reacts in some biologic manner with another substance designated as antigen.

antifungal [ăn′tĭ-fŭng′gəl] means acting or operating against fungi. It is applied to agents or procedures used for this purpose.

antigen [ăn′tĭ-, ăn′tə-jĕn, -jən, -jĭn] has to be derived etymologically to mean something producing (*-gen*) against (*anti-*) something. It is an allergen that stimulates production of specifically directed antibody as it induces an allergic transformation.

antigen, Frei [frī]. Frei antigen was originally made by crudely processing pus from buboes of lymphogranuloma inguinale and was used as a test for the disease. Nowadays the virus of the disease is grown on chick embryo and then the infected tissue is processed in a simple manner. When positive, the material causes a tuberculin-type reaction.

antigen, Kveim [kvām] is made by crudely processing sarcoid tissue and is used as a test for sarcoidosis. When positive, the material causes a papule to develop in four to six weeks. See *Kveim antigen.*

antigenic [ăn′tĭ-jĕn′ĭk] is an adjective meaning pertaining or relating to antigen.

3

antigenicity [ăn′tĭ-jĕn-ĭs′ə-tē] denotes the ability of a substance to be an antigen.

antihidrotic [ăn′tē-hĭ-drŏt′ĭk] as an adjective denotes sweat-inhibiting property. It is also used as a noun to designate a substance that inhibits sweating. See *an (h)idrotic* for a synonymous word.

antihistamine [ăn′tĭ-hĭs′tə-mēn] designates an agent which antagonizes the pharmacologic action of histamine. *Antihistaminic* used as a noun is an alternate form.

antihistaminic [ăn′tē-hĭs-tə-mĭn′ĭk] as an adjective means acting or operating against histamine. Since the action is not directed specifically and chemically against histamine, the truer meaning would be acting or operating against what histamine causes, particularly whealing. The word is also used as a noun to designate a substance which is antihistaminic. See *antihistamine*.

ant(i)inflammatory [ănt′-, ăn′tĭ-ĭn-flăm′ə-tôr′ē, -ĭ, -tĕr-ē, -ĭ] means acting against (*ant-*, *anti-*) inflammation. The shorter form is to be preferred.

antiluetic [ăn′tē-lōō-ĕt′ĭk, -lū-ĕt′ĭk] is used synonymously with *antisyphilitic*. Literally, as an adjective it relates to action and as a noun it denotes an agent against (*anti-*) plague (-*lue-*, from Latin *lues*, plague).

antiparasitic [ăn′tē-păr-ə-sĭt′ĭk] is an adjective that means acting or operating against parasites. Although class of parasites is not specified in the word, metazoal parasites are implied. The word is also used as a noun to specify an agent used for the purpose.

antiperspirant [ăn′tē-pĕr-spīr′ənt] is an adjective that means acting or operating against sweating. It is also used as a noun to designate an agent used for the purpose.

antipruritic [ăn′tĭ-prōōr-ĭt′ĭk] is an adjective that means acting or operating against itching. It is also used as a noun to designate an agent used for the purpose.

antipsoriatic [ăn′tĭ-sôr′ē-ăt′ĭk, -sō′rē-ăt′ĭk] is an adjective that means acting or operating against psoriasis. It is also used to designate an agent used for the purpose.

antiscabetic [ăn′tē-skă-bĕt′ĭk, -skə-bĕt′ĭk] is alternate for *antiscabietic*. See strictures under *scabetic*.

antiscabietic [ăn′tē-skā-bē-ĕt′ĭk] is an adjective that means acting or operating against scabies or against scabietic mites. It is also used as a noun to designate an agent used for the purpose.

antiseborrheic [ăn′tĭ-sĕb′ō-rē′ĭk] is an adjective that means acting or operating against seborrhea or seborrheic dermatitis. It is also used as a noun to designate an agent used for the purpose.

antiseptic [ăn′tĭ-sĕp′tĭk] is an adjective that means acting or operating against sepsis, i.e., against pyogenic or toxin-producing organisms. It is also used as a noun to designate an agent used for the purpose.

antitoxin [ăn′tē-tŏk′sĭn] is an antibody that neutralizes an antigen that is a toxin (in specific correspondence). Antibody formed in response to antigenic poisonous substances of biologic origin, such as bacterial exotoxins. (*Stedman's*)

antivenom [ăn′tĭ-vĕn′əm] is an antibody that neutralizes venom (in specific correspondence). Venom is poison produced by a snake, a spider or other metazoa.

Apert's syndrome [äpĕr′]. Acrocephalosyndactyly. Autosomal dominant disorder shows synostosis of the hands, feet, carpi, tarsi, cervical vertebrae, and skull. There are distorted facial features and the second, third and fourth fingers are fused into a bony mass with a single nail. Oculocutaneous albinism and severe acne vulgaris may be features. (Andrews, *Diseases of the Skin*, 8th Ed., Arnold/Odom/James, Saunders Co.)

aphtha [ăf′thə] is derived from Greek via Latin. The word was and is now used to designate a characteristic lesion of the mouth which starts as a painful, red macule and evolves into an intensely painful ulcer that eventually heals spontaneously in one, two or three weeks only to recur unpredictably. Neither cause, prophylaxis nor cure is known.

aphthosis [ăf-thō′sĭs] is a title to designate the condition (*-osis*) in which aphthae or lesions like aphthae appear on the conjunctivae, in the mouth (and possibly further along the gastro-intestinal tract) and in and about the genitals. *Behçet's syndrome* is eponymic.

aphthous [ăf′thəs] is an adjective meaning relating to or characterized by aphthae.

aphthous stomatitis [stō′mə-tī′tĭs, -tē′tĭs] is an inflammatory condition (*-itis*) of the mouth (*stoma-*) marked by several or numerous aphthae.

aplasia [ă-, ə-plā′zhē-ə, -zē-ə, zhə] means a condition (*-ia*) of failure or lack (*a-*) of full development or growth (*-plas-*, from a Greek word pertaining to molding, shaping).

aplasia cutis congenita [kŭ'tĭs kŏn-jĕn'ĭ-tə] is an obvious title for a condition of underdevelopment of the skin apparent at birth. One might imagine from the title that underdevelopment of the entire skin is meant, but this is not the fact. The title is applied to what is more prosaically known as skin defects of the newborn and designates areas (usually on the scalp) of clean ulcers with granulation that ultimately heal by scarring in the usual fashion. Perhaps an amended title like *aplasia cutis congenita circumscripta*, or *areata*, would be better.

apocrine [ăp'ō-krīn, -krēn, -krĭn] is an adjective that means separating (*-crine*) from or away from (*apo-*). It was coined apparently to denote a kind of separation of structure such as occurs in apocrine glands and the mammary glands. The tips of the glandular cells seem to degenerate into a fatty substance which is then discharged with the rest of the secretory product of the gland.

apocrine cystadenoma apocrine retention cyst, a single benign nevoid tumor occurring usually on the face. This is a dome-shaped, smooth-surfaced, translucent nodule, frequently pigmented. These are a benign, adenomatous cystic proliferation of the apocrine glands. When feasible simple excision is the treatment. (Andrews)

apostematosa [ăp'ō-stĕm'ə-tō'sə] is the feminine singular of a New Latin adjective formed from Greek elements and meaning full of (*-osa*) abscess formation (*apostemat-*). It appears in the title *cheilitis glandularis apostematosa*.

appendages [ə-pĕn'dĭj-əz] are things that hang (*-pend-*) attached (*ap-* = *ad-*). In dermatology, the word ought to be applied to the nail plates and particularly to the extruded hair shafts. Loosely, the word is also applied to internal structures, like the matrix of the nail, the pilosebaceous apparatus and the apocrine and sweat glands. For the latter, *adnexa* is the better word.

apple-jelly nodule [ăp'l-jĕl'ē nŏd'ūl, nŏj'ool] is the papule found in plaques of lupus vulgaris which, especially under diascopy, has a brownish shade of color that is reminiscent of apple jelly. Although not originally intended, the term could also apply to the soft consistency of such lesions.

aquagenic urticaria [ă'kwă-jĕn'ĭk ûr'tĭ-kâr'ē-ə] is a good example of bad coinage. It says water- (*aqua-*) producing (*-genic*) urticaria, whereas urticaria produced by water was intended. *Aquagenous urticaria* would have been verbally exact. The same kind of mistake was made with *iatrogenic* (see *-gen*). Nevertheless, does aquagenic urticaria mean a whealing produced by 1) H_2O as a chemical entity that is a primary urticariogenic substance comparable to others like histamine; or 2) a substance that, through interaction with water, becomes a primary urticariogenic substance or urticariogenic after sensitization; or 3) the warmth of water in a bath or the stroke of water in a shower? The first possibility is incredible; the second would make it cholinergic urticaria; the third would make it dermographism. The concept of the title is fuzzy. An urticariogenic substance resulting from interaction of water and sebum has been hypothesized. If this should be true, it still would not make water *per se* urticariogenic in a primary way or secondarily upon sensitization. If water in itself could be or become urticariogenic, a person afflicted would not last long, since we are all mostly water.

arachnidism [ə-răk′nĭd-ĭz′m, -nĭ-dĭz′m] designates the reaction or state (*-ism*) consequent upon the bite of a venomous member of the *Arachnida*, particularly a spider.
Brown recluse spider bites.

arachnodactylia [ə-răk′nō-dăk-tĭl′ē-ə, -ĭ-ə] is a condition (*-ia*) in which the fingers and toes (*-dactyl-*) are long and resemble the legs of a spider (*arachno-*, with *-o-* as a connecting insert). Compare *aranodactylia*.
In Greek mythology, Arachne was a very skillful weaver who dared challenge the goddess Athena (Minerva) to a weaving contest. Of course, the poor mortal lost and as a punishment for her hubris she was changed into a spider by the goddess. In her metamorphosed state Arachne immediately began to spin webs and is still spinning them, so that to this day her name designates a spider in Greek. To the unromantic the myth is an example of (a)etiology (this word, meaning the study of the causes of phenomena, has its uses in disciplines other than medicine; in the study of legendary and early history it refers to the invention of a story to explain a tradition, custom, practice or the appearance of a form of life). The myth of Arachne attempts to answer the question, "Who came first, the lady or the spider?" (with a bow to F. R. Stockton, author of "The Lady or the Tiger?").

araneidism [ăr′ə-nē′ĭd-ĭz′m] designates the reaction or state (*-ism*) consequent upon the bite of a venomous spider (*araneid-*, from Latin word for a spider). *Arachnidism* is synonymous and more common.

araneus [ə-rā′nē-əs, -rä′nē-əs] is a Latin adjective which denotes what resembles a spider or web (from *aranea*, spider). It appears in the title *nevus araneus*.

aranodactylia [ə-rā′nō-dăk-tĭl′ē-ə, -ĭ-ə] is a condition (*-ia*) in which the fingers (*-dactyl-*) and toes are long and resemble the legs of a spider (*arano-*). *Arachnodactylia* (*arano-* is from Latin; *arachno-*, from Greek) is a more common synonym.

arboviruses are viruses which are maintained in nature principally through biological transmission between susceptible vertebrate hosts by hematophagous arthropods. They multiply and produce viremia in the vertebrates, multiply in the tissue of arthropods, and are passed on to new vertebrates by the bites of arthropods after a period of extrinsic incubation. (WHO)

ARC (AIDS-related complex) Human immunodeficiency virus infection which may range from the asymptomatic carrier state to a generalized lymphadenopathy which may be symptomatic. (J.E. Groopman)

arciform [är′sĭ-fôrm] is an adjective that means shaped (*-form*) in curves (*arci-*) and is used descriptively in the morphology of clinical or histopathologic lesions of the skin. It is usually mispronounced är′kĭ-fôrm, probably because är′sĭ-fôrm, which is correct, sounds so distinctly gluteal.

arcuate [är′kū-āt] is synonymous with *arciform*.

areata [ā′rē-ā′tə, ăr′ē-ăt′ə, är′ē-ä′tə] is the feminine singular of a New Latin adjective meaning limited to a circumscribed area. (The Latin word *area* means a courtyard, and thus by extension, a confined flat space). The adjective appears in titles like *alopecia areata* and *keratolysis exfoliativa areata manuum*.

areate [âr′ē-āt] is the English equivalent of *areata*.

Argyll Robertson pupil [är-gĭl′ rŏb′ĕrt-s'n]. In neurosyphilis, particularly tabes dorsalis, and in some other diseases of the central nervous system, pupils that are small, respond to light slowly or not at all, but converge and contract normally upon accommodation.

argyria [är-jĭr′ē-ə] means a condition (*-ia*) caused by silver (*argyr-*). Silver salts attaining the interior of the body are deposited in the skin about the coils of the sweat glands and in the mucous membranes. The clinical effect is shades of slate gray to blackish color imparted to the skin and mucous membranes, depending upon the amount of silver deposited.

arrector pili [ə-rĕk′tôr, -tər pī′lī, pē′lē] is a Latin term meaning erector (*arrector*) of a hair (*pili*). The plural is *arrectores pilorum* [ăr′ĕk-tō′rēz pĭ-lō′rəm, -lôr′əm]. The structures are organized smooth muscle elements that cradle the sebaceous gland, running from some point of origin at the hair follicle sheath below them upward to some point of insertion at the dermo-epidermal junction.

arteriosclerosis obliterans a vascular disease of the limbs caused by organic arterial obstruction which consists of segmental arteriosclerotic narrowing or obstruction of the lumen in the arteries supplying the limbs. The commonest cause of arterial obstructive disease of the extremities. The symptoms are intermittent claudication, pain at rest, and trophic changes in the involved limb. (H. A. Kontos)

artifact [är′tə-, är′tĭ-făkt] is an alternate of *artefact*, the former being more commonly used. The latter word is derived from Latin *arte*, by art, plus *fact-*, made. The *i* of *artifact* may be due to analogy with words like *artifice, artisan, artificial,* etc. The word is used in dermatology to denote a lesion or disease that is produced deliberately, and usually by agents like fingernails, traumatizing metal instruments or caustic chemicals. There is a sense of "human-made" or "not natural" in *artifact*. "Not natural" must then be conceived of as "not in the usual course of uncontrollable events." Compare the use of *artifact* by anthropologists for the pots and pans, clubs and knives and other fabricated articles of a culture. The word also finds use in histopathology to describe those changes in structure or tinctorial reaction which result from faulty laboratory technique.

artificial [är′tə-fĭsh′əl] is the English adjective that means of or pertaining to an artifact.

aspergillosis [ăs-pûr′jĭ-lō′sĭs] is the word for a condition (*-osis*) of infection with a fungus of the genus *Aspergillus*.

A mycosis, it encompasses a variety of disease processes that share an etiologic relationship with aspergillus species. Three cutaneous forms occur, aspergillus flavus in the immunosuppressed patient causing primary disease, secondary cutaneous aspergillosis from the disseminated disease, and primary disease in the normal host.

Aspergillus [ăs′pĕr-jĭl′əs] is a genus of *Ascomycetes*, some members of which are in the family of *Moniliaceae*. The source of the name is interesting. It apparently derives from a fancied resemblance to the aspergillum (from Latin *aspergere*, to scatter or sprinkle), a somewhat brushlike instrument used in rituals of the Roman Catholic Church to sprinkle holy water.

asteatosis [ə-stē′ə-tō′sĭs] is a word formed from Greek word elements for a condition (*-osis*) in which fat (*-steat-*) is lacking (*a-*). It is used in connection with conditions of the skin in which dryness is associated with faults of sebum or other production of skin lipids. Ichthyosis is such a condition.

astringent [ăs-trĭn′jĕnt] is derived from Latin elements that mean to draw closed or bind fast (*ad - stringere*). As an adjective, the word means binding, contracting, constrictive, or styptic and, as a noun, a substance that has those properties.

ataxia telangiectasia (Louis-Bar syndrome) chromosome breakage syndrome; autosomal recessive condition with increased frequency of malignancy which may be the consequence of alterations in DNA repair process. (Hamerton) A complex syndrome with neurologic, immunologic, endocrinologic, hepatic and cutaneous abnormalities. The most prominent clinical features are progressive cerebellar ataxia, oculocutaneous telangiectasias, chronic sinopulmonary disease and variable humoral and cellular immunodeficiency. Ataxia typically becomes evident soon after the child begins to walk. Telangiectasias usually develop by three to six years of age. Recurrent, usually bacterial, sinopulmonary infections occur in roughly 80 percent of these patients. (Buckley) Death often results from lymphoma-leukemia in the second or third decade of life. (Rosen)

atheroma [ăth′ĕr-ō′mə] literally means a formation or tumor (-*oma*) consisting of a mealy material (*ather-*). It is sometimes used synonymously with *sebaceous*, or *epidermal*, *cyst*, but some would make a distinction and reserve the term *atheroma* for a tumor or cyst whose content is matter that is mainly keratin, rather than matter that is largely lipid. Some of the lumps on the scalp that have long been called wens, when they are not ordinary sebaceous cysts but contain a hard substance, could be designated *atheromata* (plural, as a Greek form, of *atheroma*).

"athlete's foot" [ăth′lĕts foŏt] is a lay term for superficial fungous infections of the feet that has all the disadvantages of folkways. The sporting implication of the term is misleading of cause and pathogenesis. The infection occurs as readily in the unathletic. The phrase gives rise to ridiculous formulations like "athlete's foot of the hands." The mildest stricture we would make is that the term be avoided, and not encouraged by physicians.

atopic [ă-, ə-, ā-tŏp′ĭk] as an adjective relates to atopy, and as a noun to a person who has an atopic expression or is of the atopic habitus.

atopic dermatitis [dûr′mə-tī′tĭs, -tē′tĭs] is the title of a highly characteristic dermatosis that sometimes occurs in atopic individuals and is marked by erythema, oozing and crusting (in the infantile and early childhood phases), and crusting, excoriation and lichenification (especially in adolescent and adult phases). There are notable sites of election, namely the face and flexures (antecubital and popliteal fossae). Pruritus is usually intense; and chronicity and recurrences are notorious.

atopy [ăt′ə-pē, -pĭ] literally means no- (*a-*) -place- (*-top-*) -ness (*-y*). It is amusing to realize that *Utopia*, Sir Thomas More's name for the ideally perfect state, literally means the same thing as *atopy*, a baleful state. That oddity, however, does not vitiate the usefulness of this easily spoken word because it has been given clarifying attributes which make it a designation for that constitutional habitus to acquire, and to transmit the trait or susceptibility to, certain allergic states that express themselves clinically as seasonal rhinitis (hay fever), asthma, some other vague syndromes like migraine and Ménière's disease and a characteristic dermatosis (atopic dermatitis).

atrophicans [ə-trŏf′ĭ-kănz, -trō′fĭ-kănz] is a New Latin present participle (singular and in all genders) which means becoming or turning atrophic. It appears in the following titles of classical form, *acrodermatitis chronica atrophicans* (feminine) and *lichen sclerosus et atrophicans* (masculine).

atrophie blanche [ätrōfē′ blängsh] is a title in French for a process that occurs on the lower portions of the legs of the elderly and consists of small areas of inflammation and necrotization that result in equally small, white (*blanche*) macules of atrophy. Often, nonhealing, painful ulcers form in these white plaques. (Andrews)

atrophoderm(i)a [ăt′rə-fō-dûr′mə, -mē-ə, mĭ-ə] denotes a condition (*-ia*) in which proper development (*-tropho-*) of the skin (*-derma*, *-dermia*) is lacking (*a-*). In either form the term has been used in titles which are unusually long and complex in their classical and other formulations, are descriptive of conditions that are rare and uncertain in distinctiveness and have many alternate forms. *Atrophodermia ulerythematosa* (full of scarring redness) is an example.

atrophy [ăt′rō-, ăt′rə-fē, -fĭ] is straightforward English for a condition (*-y*) in which full development (*-troph-*, literally, nourishment) is failing (*a-*). A variety of titles may be made with the word, as for example:

atrophy, macular [măk′ū-lẽr]. *Macular atrophy* designates spotty (*macular*, from Latin *macula*, spot) atrophy.

atrophy of fat is obvious in meaning.

atrophy, primary. See *primary atrophy.*

atrophy, "wucher," [vōō′khẽr]. *"Wucher"* atrophy is one of those bilingual (German and English) terms that catch on and hang on a long time for want of better. It refers to infiltration of subcutaneous fat with inflammatory cells resulting in pressure atrophy of fat elements. The phenomenon has also been termed *fat-replacement atrophy*, which is not much of an improvement. *Wucher* means interest, usury, profit; its verb, *wuchern*, means to grow rampant and luxuriantly. Hence, its connotation is that of "waxing," as in the expression "the waxing and the waning of the moon." In our context, *wucher* signifies rampant growth or proliferation. The process is seen in some panniculitides.

aurantiasis [ô′răn-tī′ə-sĭs] is a word for a condition (*-iasis*) in which the skin has a golden (*aurant-*) color. The real thing is not so precious as the name would suggest. It is usually applied to the color of the skin that occurs in carotinemia. The word could well enough be used to designate an eruption caused by gold salts, but it is not done. *Chrysoderma* is a synonymous word with the same implications.

aureotherapy [ô′rē-ō-thĕr′ə-pē, -pī] means treatment (*-therapy*) with gold (*aureo-*) compounds.

Auspitz's sign [ou′shpĭts′z sīn] refers to the appearance of pinpoint bleeding observed when the scale of a lesion of psoriasis is forcibly or completely removed. The phenomenon is accounted for by rupture of capillaries which lie high in the papillary dermis beneath a thinned suprapapillary plate.

aut(o)- [ôt′(ō)] is a combining form from Greek *autos*, self, and has a multiplicity of meanings: same, self, self-acting, self-induced, self-regulating, self-causing, etc.

autoantibodies antibodies produced by an animal (or human) that bind to antigens present in its own cells or extracellular proteins. Any immunoglobulin isotype can have autoantibody activity but the development of autoimmune lesions hinges on autoantibodies of particular isotypes. Binding specificities have been found for antigenic determinants in cell nuclei, cytoplasm, cell membranes, plasma proteins, hormones, enzymes, and in receptors for physiological ligands. Autoantigens may be proteins, nucleic acids, phospholipids, lipoproteins, sugars or steroids. The numerous kinds of autoantibodies fall into two main classes, depending on whether they bind to organ-specific or ubiquitous autoantigens. (Schwartz & Datta)

auto-eczematization [ô′tō-ĕg-zĕm′ə-tĭ-zā′shən, -tī-zā′shən] is a word fashioned to designate a concept of the pathomechanism of an eruption that is eczematous in form and that springs up as a result of sensitization to body-own allergens. The spread of process from certain dermatitides of the legs and from other chronic dermatitides to other sites has been explained in this fashion. The explanation is not satisfactory to everybody.

autoerythrocyte sensitization syndrome (Gardner Diamond syndrome) is characterized by the sudden and unexplained appearance of cutaneous purpura, primarily in young to middle-aged women. The purpuric lesions are usually preceded by pain or "burning" and are most commonly found on the extremities. There is either no history of trauma or trauma, if acknowledged is too mild to account for the purpura. The syndrome often first develops shortly after an episode of psychologic or physiologic stress. Nearly all patients with this syndrome have a variety of functional or hysterical complaints. (Fitzpatrick)

autoimmunity the appearance of antibodies in the human directed against self represents an autoimmune response. These autoantibodies may reflect a normal response to tissue antigens which are separated anatomically from the immune system during fetal development and appear later as a consequence of tissue breakdown. Autoantibodies also may arise following abrogation of tolerance in a normal immune system by an exogenous antigen cross-reacting with self or because an abnormal immune system has lost the capacity to distinguish self. Autoantibodies do not necessarily indicate an autoimmune disease. The latter term must be restricted to situations in which the autoimmune response, humoral or cellular, is responsible for tissue injury. (Austen)

autoimmunization the production of antibodies (or of T cells) that react with antigens of one's own tissues, e.g., rheumatoid arthritis. (Schwartz & Datta)

autosomal-recessive severe combined immunodeficiency disorder (SCID). Infants early in life have unremitting infections, otitis, pneumonia, sepsis, diarrhea and skin infections. Growth may appear normal, but extreme wasting quickly develops. Infections with opportunistic organisms results in death.

Low serum immunoglobulin levels are characteristic and no antibody formation occurs following immunization. There is a lack of cellular immune function with lymphopenia and absence of lymphocyte responses to mitogens or allogeneic cells, delayed cutaneous anergy and inability to reject foreign tissues. (Rebecca H. Buckley. *Cecil Textbook of Medicine,* 18th edition. Wyngaarden & Smith, eds. Saunders)

B

B. The capital letter is frequently used as an identifier, e.g., vitamin B.

bacterial septicemia. Gonococcal, streptococcal and Staphylococcus aureus are the most characteristic organisms in this condition, causing deep-seated pustules. Arthritis is frequent in gonococcal septicemia as are acral lesions.

bacterid [băk'tēr-ĭd] is a recent coinage on a poor analogy with well-established -id words like *dermatophytid*, which is itself poorly coined (see specific entry for this word), *tuberculid, syphilid* and *leprid*. The analogy is poor because in the latter instances a lesion of a class (-id) of disease (tuberculosis, syphilis, leprosy) is named, whereas *bacterid* really means a member of the class of bacteria, in short, a bacterium. Nevertheless, the word is found in the title *pustular bacterid*, and those who use the word *bacterid* understand it to mean a lesion of the condition denoted by this title. The implication that has come to be attached to the word is that certain lesions, usually sterile pustules on the hands and feet, are related to distant foci of infection (in teeth, tonsils, appendix, gall bladder, etc.) by unspecified organisms in a manner comparable to, say, dermatophytids and dermatophytosis. There is disupte about the validity of the concept of bacterids and the reality of the condition. The differential diagnostic problem of pustules on hands and feet always involves somewhat less controversial diagnoses, like pustular psoriasis, pompholyx and dermatophytid. It is moot in many minds if there is such an entity as pustular bacterid that is not an instance of one or another of the latter conditions.

Bäfverstedt's syndrome [bāf'vēr-stĕt]. Lymphadenosis benigna cutis; lymphocytoma.

balan-, balano- [băl'ən; bâl'ə-nō], the combining forms from the Greek word for acorn, are used in compound words to denote conditions on or of the glans penis, i.e., the portion of the organ that resembles an acorn. English does not use its own word *acorn* for the anatomic part but employs the disguises of Latin or Greek in medical titles. Latin, French and German, on the other hand, employ their common words for acorn to designate the head of the penis, e.g., *glans* (Latin), *gland* (French), *eichel* (German).

balanitis [băl′ə-nī′tĭs, -nē′tĭs] designates any inflammatory condition (*-itis*) of the glans (*balan-*). There are many balanitides that range in character from apthosis to zona, but the only condition that contains the word in its title follows.

balanitis circumscripta plasma cellularis has the same clinical appearance as erythroplasia of Queyrat or Bowen's disease of the glans penis. Presents as an symptomatic, sharply demarcated bright red, shiny, very slightly infiltrated plaque on the glans penis, or less often, in the coronal sulcus or on the inner surface of the prepuce. (Lever Goette)

balanitis xerotica obliterans [zē-rŏt′ĭ-kə ŏb-lĭt′ĕr-ănz] is a degenerative and sclerosing inflammatory process of the glans that starts near or around the meatus and develops into a dry (*xerotica*) plaque that tends to produce shrinking or stenosis (*obliterans*) of the orifice. The condition is lichen sclerosis et atrophicus.

balano-. See *balan-*.

balanoposthitis [băl′ə-nō-pŏs-thī′tĭs, -thē′tĭs] designates an inflammatory condition (*-itis*) of the prepuce (*-posth-*) of the glans (*balano-*).

    Inflammation and swelling of the prepuce and glans penis often due to candida and or bacterial organisms.

bald [bôld] in Middle English and in cognate words in other languages (Greek, Gothic) has the connotation of white. This sense still appears in *bald eagle* and *piebald*, but the bare word has come to mean devoid of expected adornment, especially hair.

baldness means hairlessness, particularly of the scalp. See *alopecia*.

baldness, male-pattern [māl păt′ĕrn]. *Male-pattern baldness* refers to that type of loss of scalp hair that occurs in men for genetic and endocrinologic reasons. Frontal recession, deep lateral nooks, loss at the vertex and fringe tonsure are common forms.

balloon cells [bə-lōōn sĕls] and **balloon degeneration** [dĭ-, də-, dē-jĕn′ə-rā′shən] are descriptive of a type of intracellular edema of epidermal cells. The word *balloon* suggests a bloated quality. Cells so affected have a homogeneous, eosinophilic cytoplasm, several nuclei and no prickles. The phenomenon is seen in certain viral diseases of the skin, namely, the herpetic and varicelliform.

balm [bäm] is a doublet as a "collapsed form" of *balsam*, which derives via Latin and French from the Greek word *balsamon*, meaning a balsam tree or its fragrant oil or an aromatic herb.

balneotherapy [băl′nē-ō-thĕr′ə-pē, -pī] means treatment (-*therapy*) by baths (*balneo-*). The word encompasses procedures as elaborate as splashing in water at a spa and as simple as immersion or tubbing in more or less medicated waters at home.

balsam [bôl′səm] and **balsamics** [băl-, bôl-săm′ĭks]. See *balm*. In antiquity and up to quite recent times resinous materials from many trees (fir, pine, etc.) generally designated as balsamics were standard pharmacopoeial items prized for their parasiticidal and "healing" properties. They are mixtures of aromatic compounds that are now largely being replaced by refined or synthetic chemicals of known composition and more definable action.

bamboo hair [băm-bōō′ hâr] is descriptive of trichorrhexis nodosa, in which the regular spacing of brush fractures in hair shafts alternating with areas of relatively normal shaft gives a resemblance to bamboo. The condition is seen in Netherton's syndrome and is also termed **trichorrhexis invaginata.**

barbae [bär′bē] is the genitive (possessive) singular case of the Latin word *barba*, beard, and thus means of the beard. Modifying a noun, it designates the structure involved, e.g., *sycosis barbae, tinea barbae.*

barber's itch [bär′bērz ĭch] is an utterly unsatisfactory folk designation for folliculitis of the bearded area that is either pyogenic or fungal. It is so unsatisfactory that one cannot tell from it who is itching, the barber or the barbered. See strictures under *athlete's foot* and *baker's dermatitis.*

barbula hirci [bär′bū-lə hûr′sī] literally means the little beard (*barbula*) of the goat (*hirci*). It has been applied to describe picturesquely heavy tufts of coarse hair that tend to develop on the tragi of the ears of older men.

Barcoo disease or desert sore. Barcoo rot, this is an ulcerative disease found among soldiers and tribespeople in Australia and Burma. Grouped vesicles develop on the extremities which rupture and form chronic ulcers. These may enlarge and be covered with a diphtheritic membrane. Cultures show streptococci, staphylococci, and Corynebacterium diphtheriae. (Andrews, *Diseases of the Skin,* 8th Ed., Arnold/Odom/James, Saunders Co.)

barrier layer [bär′ē-ēr lā′ēr], or **zone** [zōn], designates an indefinite area in the lowest reaches of the stratum corneum that is thought to be what makes the skin so ordinarily impermeable to inanimate materials.

Bart-Pumphrey syndrome [bärt; pŭm'frē]. Deafness, knuckle pads, and leukonychia.

Bart's syndrome autosomal, dominant inheritance, congenital localized defects of the skin, mechanoblisters and nail deformities. Scars are not serious; good outlook.

basal [bā's'l, -z'l, -zəl], **basalar** [bā'zə-, bā'sə-lēr] and **baso-** [bā'sō, -zō] all designate position at a base or refer to a basis. In dermatology the words are used in connection with the basal layer of the epidermis or its cellular contents.

basal-cell carcinoma [kär'sĭ-nō'mə], or **epithelioma** [ĕp'ĭ-thē-lē-ō'mə], refers to malignant neoplasia in which the proliferating cells have structural and tinctorial characteristics of the basal cells of the epidermis and seem to stem from them positionally and developmentally. Modern studies suggest that development from adnexal epithelium is also likely or more likely. They rarely metastasize but have considerable potential for extensive, local destruction. Four clinical types should be recognized: nodular, superficial, pigmented, and scarring or sclerosing basal cell cancers. Diagnosis should be confirmed by biopsy.

   basal-cell nevus syndrome. See *nevus, basal-cell,* and *Gorlin-Goltz syndrome.*

basiloma terebrans [tĕr'ə-, tĕr'ē-brănz] is coinage for a type of basal-cell epithelioma that is invasive in a piercing or boring manner (*terebrans*).

basket-weave vacuolization. See *vacuolization, basket-weave.*

basophilic degeneration [bā'zə-, bā'zō-, bā'sə-, bā'sō-fĭl'ĭk dĭ-, də-, dē-jĕn'ə-rā'shən] refers to change in tinctorial properties of connective tissue (usually of elastic fibers, sometimes of collagen) from the normal pink (eosinophilic, acidophilic) with hemotoxylin-eosin processing to shades of blue (basophilic). The phenomenon is seen in actinism, lupus erythematosus and senile skin.

Bateman's disease [bāt'mən] Molluscum contagiosum and senile purpura.

bathing-trunks nevus [bā'thĭng trŭnks nē'vəs] One almost always hears and sees this homely designation as *bathing-trunk nevus.* One is then led to wonder what a "bathing trunk" is. Garments of paired structures that cover the nether part of the body, e.g., jeans, pants, shorts, slacks, trousers and trunks, have the same spelling in the singular and plural, and are said elliptically for a "pair of . . . ." The same applies to scissors and shears. It would be better to use a term like *giant congenital nevus* for that dreadful hamartoma that consists of junction, compound, and intradermal nevi; that is hairy and frequently neurofibromatous; that may cover the entire pelvic region like bathing trunks or nearly the entire torso (trunk!) like a bathing suit of bygone days; and that may (10 to 15 percent of the time) go on to malignant degeneration (malignant melanoma). Moreover, the condition is often spotty enough, or situated only on the upper portion of the back across the shoulders, or on hands, arms, feet and legs, which has prompted other descriptive titles in terms of garments like scarf, glove, and stocking nevus.

bayonet hair [bā′ə-net, -nət hâr] describes an anomaly of scalp hair shafts in which the free end of a hair seems to emerge tapered from a spindle-shaped swelling below it, giving the whole section resemblance to a bayonet. The phenomenon does not seem to be the result of any disease of the hair apparatus. It is seen in hairs near whorls and at the margins of baldness.

Bazex syndrome or **acrokeratosis paraneoplastica.** A cutaneous marker of malignancy, this is a symmetrical dermatosis that most commonly affects the hands, feet, ears and nose with an erythematous psoriasiform eruption. Later changes involve the cheeks, elbows, and knees with still later changes often involving the central trunk where bullae may be seen. The nails are involved early and severely. There is subungual hyperkeratosis, as well as a flaky white surface to the nail. The nails may be shed. The syndrome is associated with neoplasia of the upper respiratory system, lungs, tongue, and esophagus. (Hazelrigg *Archives*, Dermatol. 113, 1977.)

Bazin's disease [băzăngz′ dĭ- , də-zēz′]. See *erythema induratum.*

BCC is an acronym for *basal-cell carcinoma.*

BCE is an acronym for *basal-cell epithelioma.*

beaded hair [bēd′əd hâr] is quasi-literal English for *monilethrix,* which means a hair (*-thrix*) necklace (*monile-*). Both terms describe a characteristic condition of scalp hair shafts in which alternations of fusiform thickening and normal or less than normal girth along hair shafts produce the effect of a string of beads.

Beau's lines [bōz līnz] are temporary transverse depressions that appear in nail plates and slowly move from matrix to free edge as the nails grow. They follow debilitating illnesses like episodic malnutrition, prolonged febrile illnesses, coronary occlusions, etc., and seem to result from less development of nail keratin during the period of debility. A comparable phenomenon occurs in hair growth and probably in the stratum corneum generally, where the effect is less noticeable. The nail change was first described by Joseph Honoré Simon Beau (1806–1865), a French physician.

beautician [bū-tĭsh′ən] is a word like *cosmetologist* to designate one who gives "beauty" treatments which consist largely of fussing with scalp, hair and nails.

beauty mark [bū′tē märk] is a term used by the laity for common nevi, particularly the pigmented variety and particularly those on the face. Through the ages certain nevi, especially those that are flat, round, dark brown and situated high on a zygoma, have been deemed to enhance appearance. The opinion is so common that from the remotest past to this day women have been simulating "beauty marks" with materials like "court plaster" and topically applied dyes or pigments. Tastes differ, however, and one person's beauty mark is another's blemish.

Becker's nevus [bĕk′ər]. Hyperpigmentation and hypertrichosis as an acquired phenomenon.

bedsore [bed′sôr′] is plain English for *decubitus ulcer* (which see). Sores and ulcers resulting from the friction of bedclothes and the pressure of the skin during prolonged sojourn in bed are common in debilitated states, particularly in extreme old age, chronic malnutrition, strokes and spinal cord injuries.

Behçet's disease is a multi-faceted syndrome characterized by oral and genital ulcerations and ocular abnormalities, including keratitis, optic neuritis, uveitis and hypopyon iritis (pus in the anterior chamber of the eye). The disease has multiple systemic associations that include involvement of the gastrointestinal, cardiovascular, and central nervous systems as well as the joints, blood vessels, and lungs. (Arbesfeld & Kurban). The cause is unknown.

Behçet's syndrome [bĕkh′shĕts sĭn′drōm]. (*Behçet* is a Turkish name. The pronunciation given is close to the way a Turk would utter this name; anglicized versions and approximations are bĕ′chĕts and bā′sĕts.) The name should be pronounced Bĕh′chĕts with heavy aspiration on the first syllable.

bejel [bĕ′jəl] derives from *bajlah*, a colloquial Arabic word for syphilis. It is a treponematosis caused by a micro-organism that is indistinguishable from that of syphilis in darkfield appearance. In its epidemiology, clinical manifestations and course, bejel is much like yaws with respect to chronicity, nonvenereal contagiosity and cutaneous expressions in the form of buttons, granulomas and ulcers.

Nonsyphilitic treponematosis causing skin disease. Disfiguring ulcerations may occur with invasion to bone and other tissue. Bejel is caused by a Treponema that is indistinguishable from the organisms which cause yaws and pinta. Prevalence has been reduced by the use of penicillin. (Thomas Butler)

benign [bē-, bə-nīn′] and **benigna** [bə-, bē-nĭg′nə] are respectively an English adjective and the feminine singular of a Latin adjective meaning kind or gentle. In medicine the words are used as antonyms of *malignant* and *maligna,* and as modifiers to designate a mild form of a disease or a condition that is not serious at all. The Latin form appears in the title *lymphadenosis cutis benigna.*

benign symmetric lipomatosis (Madelung's disease) lipomas which may give a horse-collar appearance due to their distribution in the neck region, also may appear over the trunk and arms.

beriberi [bĕr′ē-bĕr′ē, -ī] is a doubling of the Singhalese word *beri,* which means weak. The reduplication intensifies the sense of weakness, i.e., it conveys the meaning of very or extremely weak. The device of reduplication for emphasis occurs in other languages: English, *so-so,* French, *bonbon,* etc. Sometimes the words are repeated separately and consecutively, as in Shakespeare's *Hamlet:* "O, that this too too solid flesh would melt." In the disease beriberi, the skin shows edema as a clinical expression of deficiency of vitamin B.

berlock [bər′-, bĕr′lŏk] and **berloque** [bĕrlôk′, -lōk′] mean a pendant. They derive from German and French respectively, but their etymology is not definitely known. The modern form of the German word is *berlocke;* the French word has an alternate form *breloque* and another meaning, which is not pertinent here. Original reports of the condition that is now designated as *berlock,* or *berloque, dermatitis* appeared in German and described a "skin condition in berlock-form." In current dermatologic literature one frequently sees misspellings like *berlocque* and *Berloque* (suggesting eponomy).

berlock, or **berloque, dermatitis** [dûr′mə-tī′tĭs, -tē′tĭs] is the unsatisfactory title for that transient inflammatory dermatosis and subsequent temporary pigmentation that sometimes results from light exposure upon skin that has had photosensitizing substances (furocoumarins) deposited upon it. Perfumes are the common source of photosensitizing agents; oil of bergamot is the commonest of such agents. The pendant design occurs when deposition of photosensitizing substance is on the sides of the neck or the suprasternal notch and results in a run onto the bosom. Streaks from behind the ears, variable patterns on the face and arms and bizarre designs anywhere on the body are seen in heavily perfumed persons, particularly women, all depending upon how activating agents and electromagnetic energy come into interaction.

berylliosis exposure to beryllium produces both acute and chronic diseases of the skin and lungs. Some believe beryllium produces irritant or toxic lesions while others contend T-cell mediated delayed hypersensitivity is the pathogenic factor. Acute contact to beryllium may produce papules, vesicles, pustules or eczematous lesions on the face, neck and dorsal aspect of the hands within a few hours or days. Conjunctivitis, rhinopharyngitis, and tracheobronchitis often accompany the cutaneous eruption. Chronic exposure to beryllium results in a granulomatous reaction in the lung, and in cutaneous nodules, presumably from hypersensitivity or foreign body reaction. (J.W. Burnett)

Besnier's disease [běnyā′]. Atopic dermatitis.

beta [bā′tə], the second letter of the Greek alphabet, or β, the Greek symbol for it, is used as an identifier, e.g., beta or β rays.

Biet, collarette of [bēā′]. The peripheral rings of scales that develop around macular lesions of secondary syphilis, in distinction from the scales of the lesions of pityriasis rosea which tend to adhere in their centers as they separate at the peripheries.

biopsy [bī′əp-, bī-ŏp′sē, -sī] derives from Greek word elements that are now taken in combination to mean examination (-*opsy*, viewing) of lately live (*bi-*) material. Moreover, the word is restricted by usage to examination with the microscope of specimens of tissue that have been finely sectioned and variously processed by stains. No one uses *biopsy* in a literal sense of gross inspection of a living organism, for which another word, *bioscopy* [bī-ŏs′kō-pē, -kə-pē, -ī] is used, and rarely at that. One sees and hears *biopsy* used as a verb, noun and adjective. As a verb (*to biopsy*), the taking of a specimen is expressed; as a noun (*take* or *do a biopsy*), the specimen or procedure is specified; as an adjective (*a biopsy specimen*), the kind of specimen or examination is told. *Autopsy* and *necropsy* are comparable words that are used in some similarly special and restrictive senses.

Birt-Hogg-Dubé syndrome dominantly inherited, multiple fibrofolliculomas with trichodiscomas and acrochordons. Myriads of small skin-colored papules develop on the face, trunk and extremities close to a vellus hair. Not associated with underlying medical problems. Treatment is dermabrasion.

birthmark [bûrth′märk′] is a lay term for common pigmented nevi and hemangiomata. The congenital or hereditary factor is well expressed in the word.

Bizzozero's nodes [bĭ-tzō′tzĕ-rō]. Desmosomes.

black-dot ringworm [blăk′dŏt′ rĭng′wûrm′] describes the clinical appearance of tinea capitis caused by *Trichophyton tonsurans* particularly. The breakage of hair shafts close to the scalp produces what looks like a stubble of agminated black dots in the area affected.

black hairy tongue [blăk hâr′ē tŭng], or **lingua nigra** [lĭng′gwə nī′grə], which is Latin for black tongue, is the title for the condition in which hypertrophy of the papillary elements on the dorsum of the tongue and multiplication of ordinarily saprophytic organisms in the site produce a black mat that resembles a Vandyke beard. In many cases the color is not black, but green, yellow, tan, red or polychromatic. The causes of the condition are vague; poor mouth hygiene, nutritional deficiencies and alteration of flora caused by sucking lozenges containing antibiotics have seemed to be causative in many cases.

blackhead [blăk′hĕd′] is the lay term for *comedo*, the primary lesion of acne. The word describes the darkened bit of sebum and keratin that shows at the pilosebaceous ostium. The rest of the formation is, of course, not black, but gray or yellow.

black piedra [Spanish, pyā′drä; English, pē-ā′drə] describes a rare fungous infection of hair shafts caused by *Piedraia hortai*. The clinical appearance is that of black, stone- (*piedra*) -hard concretions of small size surrounding portions of hairs on the scalp, beard and axillae. There is also a white variety of piedra.

black-widow spider [blăk wĭd′ō spī′dĕr, -dər]. See *Latrodectus mactans.*

blain [blān] is an old Anglo-Saxon word for a sore, blister or pustule. It is not used as such in modern writing but persists in *chilblain*, i.e., a sore caused by cold (*chill*).

Blastomyces [blăs′tō-mī′sēz] derives from Greek elements meaning sprouting or budding (*blasto-*) fungus (*-myces*). The word is used to designate genera of yeast-like fungi, e.g., *B. brasiliensis* (of Brazil, Brazilian) and *B. dermatitidis* (genitive of *dermatitis*.)

blastomycetica [blăs′tō-mī-sē′tĭ-kə, -sĕt′ĭ-kə], is the feminine singular of a New Latin adjective meaning relating to the genus *Blastomyces*. It appears in the title *erosio interdigitalis blastomycetica.*

blastomycosis [blăs′tō-mī-kō′sĭs] is clinical infection with one of the pathogenic blastomycetes. There are two varieties caused by different micro-organisms, namely North American blastomycosis caused by *Blastomyces dermatitidis*, and South American blastomycosis caused by *Blastomyces brasiliensis*. The cutaneous lesions of the disease resemble tuberculosis cutis. What is spoken of as European blastomycosis is cryptococcosis.

A systemic mycosis often with skin lesions caused by *Blastomyces dermatitidis*, with primary focus usually in the lungs. When infection disseminates from the lung, a number of cutaneous forms of the disease are seen. The most characteristic is an elevated, verrucous, crusted, varicolored lesion which has a sharply slanting serpiginous border and a tendency towards central healing, with a thin, depigmented, atrophic scar. (Utz and Shadomy)

Caused by *Blastomyces dermatitidis*, farmers and outdoor people inhale the spores and develop pulmonary lesions hematogenously goes to the skin and bones. Skin lesions are enlarging inflammatory papules and plaques with hyperkeratotic crusts, miliary abscesses, draining sinuses, and central healing with scarring. Diagnosis is by culture of the organism. Skin biopsy is often helpful, pseudoepitheliomatous hyperplasia, intraepidermal abscesses and granulomatous dermal infiltrate. Appearance of the organism even with routine stains is characteristic. (Patterson & Blaylock) Treatment is very effective with ketoconazole. (Tomecki et al, *JAAD*, v. 21, no. 6)

bleb [blĕb] means a blister or bubble. It derives from dialectal English along with *blub, blubber, blab*. One tends to use the word to describe a large blister that is rather flaccid.

blemish [blĕm′ĭsh], ultimately derived from a Germanic word meaning to make pale, is used by the laity to describe nevi and some other dysplastic processes that are deemed to be unsightly. Such, however, are the vagaries of human taste and judgment that one person's blemish may be another's beauty mark and vice versa.

blenn(o)- [blĕn′(ō), -(ə)] derives from a Greek word for mucus, but in modern application refers to pus, particularly of gonorrhea.

blennorrhagia [blĕn′ə-rā′jē-ə, -jə] describes a discharge (*-rrhagia*) of pus (*blenno-*) and is applied to gonorrheal discharge.

blennorrhagic [blĕn′ə-rāj′ĭk] and **blennorrhagica (-cum)** [blĕn′ō-rā′jĭ-kə (-kəm)] are adjectives in English and New Latin forms respectively, which relate to discharge (*-rrhag-*) of (gonorrheal) pus (*blenno-*). The Latinized forms of the adjective appear in the title *keratodermia blennorrhagica* (feminine singular), or *keratoderma blennorrhagicum* (neuter singular).

blennorrhea [blĕn′ə-rē′ə] means a flow (*-rrhea*) of pus (*blenno-*). Like *blennorrhagia*, this word is sometimes used as a disguising term for *gonorrhea*.

blepharitis [blĕf′ə-rī′tĭs, -rē′tĭs] designates an inflammatory condition (*-itis*) of the eyelids (*blephar-*). The word is generally applied to that characteristic condition of chronic redness and crumbly crusting at the lid margins that is probably seborrheic dermatitis of the region.

blepharochalasia [blĕf′ə-rō-kăl-ā′zhē-ə, -zē-ə, zhə] and **blepharochalasis** [blĕf′ə-rō-kăl′ə-sĭs] are words that describe sagging, relaxation or slackening (*-chalas-*) of the skin of the eyelids (*blepharo-*). The term is applied to a condition in which the "bags under the eyes" result from structural damage of unknown cause in the skin, rather than to the appearance of the lids in chronic fatigue, or insomnia and other conditions like *neurofibromatosis*.

blister [blĭs′tĕr, -tə(r)] derives from Middle English, Dutch, Old Norse, and Old French words for swelling. In general modern usage any superficial, relatively thin-walled structure containing air or fluid is termed a blister; in dermatology, vesicles and particular bullae are so designated.

Bloch-Sulzberger syndrome [blŏkh; sŭlts′bĕrg-ĕr] Incontinentia pigmenti.

Bloom's syndrome [blōōm]. Telangiectatic erythema (congenital telangiectatic erythema), photosensitivity, and small stature.

Telangiectatic redness of the skin in photoexposed areas and stunted growth; has a low incidence of association with internal malignancy. (Frank Parker)

blotch [blŏch] may derive from Old French *bloche*, a clod of earth, or be an alteration of either of the English words *blot* or *botch*. The formation of the word is also thought to have been influenced by *blister* and *blain*. In any event, *blotch* is applied to any largish, irregular stain or unsightly mass that mars what should otherwise be an evenly colored, smooth surface. In descriptive dermatology, it may be used to describe skin affected by certain erythemas, purpuras and melanotic or other pigmentations or by grouped lesions, especially of rupial blisters and pustules.

blue nevus [blōō nē′vəs] is a collection of intradermal melanocytes large enough to produce a grossly discernible macule or papule of distinctly blue or blue-black color.

blue rubber-bleb nevus syndrome is a rare, hereditary systemic angiomatosis in which blood vessels that are blister-like and that have thin, rubber-like walls and blue color, develop on the skin and endothelial surfaces of internal organs, i.e., the gastrointestinal tract, and may lead to serious gastrointestinal bleeding. (Wheeler)

Bockhart's impetigo [bŏk′härts ĭm′pĕ-tī′gō] is a superficial follicular pyoderma that is notable for persistence.

body louse [bŏd′ē lous] is the common designation for *Pediculus humanus corporis.*

Boeck's sarcoid, scabies [bĕk]. Cutaneous sarcoidosis; Norwegian scabies.

boil as a noun derives from the Germanic languages in which the sense of the parent word is that of a swelling. In modern usage an abscess, especially a pyogenic abscess, is designated by this word. It is also used in parochial titles for the rupial lesions of disease like leishmaniasis, yaws and other exotic granulomas (see *button*).

borderline leprosy [bôr′dĕr-līn′ lĕp′rə-sē] is a form of leprosy in which clinical and histologic differentiation into the major types, lepromatous and tuberculoid, is not distinct. *Indeterminate leprosy* is an alternate term.

Borrelia burgdorferi a tick-borne spirochete, the causative agent of Lyme disease, (borreliosis) which please see.

Borrelia lymphocytoma arises in stage I of the European variant of Lyme borreliosis. Consists of a blue-red nodule with a predilection for soft areas of the skin. The histology resembles that of lymphocytoma of other causes. (Lever)

borreliosis (Lyme disease) caused by the spirochete Borrelia burgdorferi, causes a wide range of disorders from the skin lesions of erythema chronicum migrans to various other difficulties and may result in arthritis and neurologic deficits. As is well known, this class of organisms may produce a bewildering array of signs and symptoms. This spirochete also causes acrodermatitis chronica atrophicans and lymphadenosis benigna cutis.

Vectors are the tiny deer tick, in the eastern U.S., Ixodes dammini; in the West, the black-legged tick, Ixodes pacificus; and in the southeastern U.S., Ixodes ricinus.

Early treatment with the appropriate antibiotic greatly reduces later serious sequelae of this disease.

Borst-Jadassohn epithelioma [bôrst; yä′dä-sōn]. Intraepidermal acanthoma.

botryomycosis [bŏt′rē-ō-mī-kō′sĭs] literally means a fungous condition (-*mycosis*) whose lesions appear in grape-like clusters (*botryo*-). There is a disease of horses that has this title; among human beings it has been applied to a rare form of staphylococcic infection in which pustules and small abscesses gather in clusters.

Bouchard's nodes are osteoarthritic disfigurements of the proximal interphalangeal joints of the hands, i.e., equivalent to Heberden's nodes of osteoarthritis which involve the distal interphalangeal joints.

bovis [bō′vĭs] is the genitive singular of the Latin word *bos*, cow (ox, bull) and means of the cow. See *Actinomyces bovis*.

Bowenoid [bō′ən-oid] is an eponymous adjective used to designate histologic changes in the epidermis that resemble those seen in Bowen's disease.

Bowenoid papulosis Solitary or multiple, small, pigmented or flesh-colored papules occurring on the genitalia or perianal area of young persons. Usually diagnosed as warts or nevi. Histologically they have features suggestive of carcinoma in situ which it is not. (Patterson and Blaylock) Associated with human papilloma virus 16 (HPV-16).

Bowen's disease [bō′ənz, -ĕnz dĭ-, də-zēz′] is an eponymic designation for an intra-epidermal, malignant neoplasia that is fairly characteristic clinically and highly characteristic histologically. Clinically, it appears as an erythematous, crusted plaque and histologically, it is marked by abnormal proliferation (many mitoses) and maldevelopment of epidermal cells in the form of variations in size and shape, multinucleation, vacuolization and dyskeratosis.

Brocq's disease [brŏk]. Several: lichen chronicus simplex (see *Vidal's disease*); parapsoriasis variegata; érythrose pigmentaire péribuccale.

broken veins [brō′k′n, -kən vānz] is a lay term for *telangiectasis*. Like so many other vernacular expressions, it is misleading without having any compensating virtues. One may imagine that a "burst" of capillary vessels as in a nevus araneus was corrupted to *broken*.

brom(h)idrosiphobia [brŏm′hĭ-, brō′mĭ-drō′sĭ-phō′bē-ə] is a word for unwarranted fear (-*phobia*) of a condition (-*osi*- for -*osis*) of foul (*brom*-) sweat or sweating (-*hidr*-, -*idr*-). The condition is, of course, psychiatric rather than dermatologic.

brom(h)idrosis [brŏm′hĭ-, brō′mĭ-drō′sĭs] is the condition (-*osis*) in which sweat or sweating (-*hidr*-, -*idr*-) is foul (*brom*-). The worst odors may be described as acrid, alliaceous (garlicky or oniony), butyric (buttery), caprylic (goaty), caseous (cheesy) or fetid. Even odors that are floral or fruity (like those of aldehydes) seem to be obnoxious.

bromism Bromide intoxication is primarily a chronic disorder manifested by neurological and dermatologic changes. The neurological signs and symptoms include headache, agitation, weakness, slurred speech, confusion, delusional ideations, hallucinations and, if severe, stupor and coma. Dermatologic changes include acneiform lesions pre-dominantly on the face and trunk, as well as the more severe pyoderma gangrenosum-like lesion bromoderma. (Rothenberg et al)

bromoderma [brō′mō-dûr′mə] designates a condition of the skin (-*derma*) caused by drugs containing bromine. The clinical forms are usually acneform, furunculoid, carbunculoid and granulomatous eruptions.

Bruch's membrane [brŏŏkh]. The structure seen as angioid streaks in pseudoxanthoma elasticum.

bubo [boō′-, bū′bō] derives through Latin from *boubon*, the Greek word for the groin. The plural is *buboes* [bu′bōz]. Nowadays the word *bubo* is applied to swollen and inflamed inguinal lymph nodes, particularly those of the venereal diseases (chancroid, lymphogranuloma, venereum and syphilis). Palpable lymphadenopathy in the groin resulting from pyogenic process and from the leukoses are not usually referred to by the word, although there is no inherent reason why *bubo* cannot then be used. An enlarged lymph node in regions other than the inguinal cannot be called a bubo without violating etymologic subtlety.

bubonic [bū-bŏn′ĭk] could be used to designate the anatomic region or other characteristics of the groin (*bubon-*) but it is rarely so used in modern times. The word is used almost exclusively in the vernacular designation of the dread infection caused by *Pasteurella pestis* (bubonic plague), in which inguinal adenopathy is prominent.

bubonulus [boō′-, bū-bŏn′ū-ləs] is a New Latin diminutive of *bubo*. However, the word is applied not to a swollen lymph node of small size but to abscess-like swellings that occur along lymph vessels in diseases like gonorrhea and sporotrichosis.

buffalo hump [bŭf′ă-lō hŭmp] describes, picturesquely, hyperplasia of adipose tissue at the root of the neck posteriorly, and on the upper portion of the back, that develops in Cushing's disease and in adrenocorticosteroid therapy when dosage is high.

bulla [bo͞ol-, bŭl′ə], a blister, derives directly from the Latin word *bulla*, meaning anything that becomes round by swelling, like a bubble. The plural is *bullae* [bo͞ol′-, bŭl′ē]. In modern usage a large blister is implied within a frame of reference that is either gross or microscopic.

bullosa [bo͞ol-, bŭl-ō′sə] and **bullosum** [bo͞ol-, bŭl-ō′səm] are respectively the feminine singular and neuter singular of a New Latin adjective meaning full of (*-osa*, *-osum*) blisters (*bull-*). They appear in titles like *epidermolysis bullosa* and *erythema multiforme bullosum*.

bullosis [bo͞ol-, bŭl-ō′sĭs] means a pathologic condition (*-osis*) characterized by bullae. It is a rather inelegant word that is best used as a nonce word in the company of dermatologists who are less likely to sneer at their own specialistic jargon. It is notable that we also speak of *pustulosis* but not *maculosis* or *vesiculosis*.

bullosum. See *bullosa*.

bullous [bo͞ol′-, bŭl′əs] is the adjective from *bulla* and means full of blisters.

bullous impetigo [ĭm′pĕ-tī′gō] designates a clinical form of superficial pyoderma in which the roofs of pustules remain unbroken and the lesions appear as bullae more or less tense or flaccid with pus.

A vesiculobullous disease which may start with erythema and vesicles eventuating into bullae. Usually due to beta hemolytic streptococci infection.

bullous pemphigoid [bo͞ol′əs pĕm′fĭ-goid] a disease of the elderly, is an autoimmune disorder in which large tense blisters occur on normal or erythematous skin, often in the groin, axillae, and flexural areas. About one-third may have oral lesions. Skin biopsy shows a subepidermal blister. Direct immunofluorescence reveals deposition of IgG immunoglobulin and complement. Circulating antibodies are present in two-thirds of patients. The prognosis is good. (Frank Parker)

The title is defective in that it is tautological. It literally says a blistering (bullous) blister-like condition (pemphigoid).

Burkitt's lymphoma [bûr′kĭt]. A rare monoclonal B cell neoplasm first seen as rapidly growing jaw tumors and abdominal masses in Ugandan children. The Epstein-Barr virus (EBV) is present in almost 90 percent of African Burkitt's lymphoma but less than half of nonendemic cases. Specific chromosomal translocations have also been identified in Burkitt's lymphoma. It is classified as a high-grade small noncleaved cell malignant lymphoma. Diagnosis must be established by biopsy. (Carol S. Portlock)

burn [bûrn] generally brings to mind instantaneous and painful injury caused by heat, but many other forms of injury that may be delayed and even painless for a while and caused by forms of energy other than heat are referred to by this word. Thus, one may speak of burns caused by heat, chemicals, friction, electricity and electromagnetic energy (ultraviolet and X rays). Burns are conventionally designated for clinical convenience as follows:

burn, first-degree, connotes erythema and edema.

burn, second-degree, connotes erythema, edema and vesiculation.

burn, third-degree, connotes erythema, edema and loss of tissue.

burrow [bûr′ō] is the special lesion of some superficial infestations like scabies and creeping eruption. It is an excavation in the stratum corneum of variable size and shape that houses a metazoal parasite. Synonymous words are *channel, cuniculus, gallery, passage* and *tunnel.*

Buschke's disease [boōosh′kēz, dĭ-, də-zēz′]. See *scleredema adultorum.*

Buschke and Lowenstein [boōosh′kē; lō′wĕn-shtīn] giant condyloma accuminata. This is the type that often eventuates into squamous cell carcinoma. Verrucous carcinoma of the glans or foreskin in the male and of the vulvae and perianal region in the female.

Buschke-Ollendorf sign, disease [boōosh′kē; ōl′lĕn-dôrf]. The sign is tenderness of papular lesions of secondary syphilis; the disease is dermatofibromatosis lenticularis disseminata.

Buschke-Ollendorff syndrome connective tissue nevi (hamartomas) found in presence of osteopoikilosis.

butterfly area [bŭt′ér-flī âr′ē-ə] designates the anatomic region across the nose and on the adjacent areas of the cheeks. A lesion spread over the region resembles a butterfly at rest. Lupus erythematosus, particularly the acute, systemic variety, is notable for involving the site.

button [bŭt′n, -ən] comes into English dermatologic jargon from the French *bouton,* bud, button, which in everyday French is also used as we would use the words *boil, pimple* or *sore.* In more highly technical applications the word (in English or French) is modified by a North African, Mid- or Far-Eastern place name to designate chancriform, furuncular or rupial lesions of yaws, cutaneous leishmaniasis, and some other exotic granulomas. Thus, one finds, especially in the reports of medical officers of late colonial powers, "buttons (and boils or sores) of Aleppo, Amboyna, Cairo, Delhi, Gafsa, the Nile, the Orient, Yemen," etc. In modern times, as a result of better diagnostic means and because colonialism has become so odious, such designations are better avoided because they tend to have a faintly pejorative implication, or if used at all, let them be unmistakably picturesque descriptions.

C

C. The capital letter is frequently used as an identifier, e.g., C-reactive protein.

café au lait [kăfā′ ō lĕ′] is French for coffee with milk. The beverage is something that tourists gulp and epicures sniff at. In dermatology the phrase is used to express color, i.e., a shade of brown such as results from mixing coffee and milk.

café au lait spots are those pigmented (brown) patches that are seen as part of the clinical appearance of neurofibromatosis. The color is produced by melanin, and melanocytes are indeed more abundant than usual in the site of the phenomenon.

Calabar swelling(s) [kăl′ə-băr′ swĕl′ĭng(z)] is another example of a regional designation, this time for loaiasis. Calabar is a town and river in southern Nigeria.

Seen in loiasis (Loa loa) subcutaneous filarial infection endemic to African vector horsefly. Localized area of erythema and angioedema occurs mainly on the extremities, lasts a few days and regresses. Probably localized hypersensitivity to the adult worm. (Eric A. Ottesen, *Cecil Textbook of Medicine*)

calcifying epithelioma of Malherbe [kăl′sĭ-fī′ĭng ĕp′ĭ-thē-lē-ō′mə ŏv măl′ĕrb′]. See *pilomatrixoma*.

calcinosis [kăl′sĭ-nō′sĭs] means a pathologic condition (*-osis*) in which calcium (*calcin-*) in abnormal amounts has been deposited where it does not belong.

calcinosis cutis [kū′tĭs] describes the deposition of calcium in abnormal amounts in the skin, such as occurs in scleroderma, some chronic inflammatory processes and in some neo-, meta- and dysplastic conditions.

callositas [kə-lŏs′ĭ-tăs, -ə-tăs], the Latin word for hardness of the skin, designates simple hypertrophy of the stratum corneum in the form of mature keratin. The effect is usually the result of pressure and friction; the palms and soles are common sites but no part of the skin is exempt from the possibility, given the cause. Some persons have a congenital predisposition to the effect and suffer it to a greater extent than average on ordinary, or even less than ordinary, provocation. *Callosity, callus, clavus* and *corn* are nearly synonymous words.

callosity [kă-lŏs′ə-tē, -tĭ] is the English equivalent of *callositas*. This word is a little more restricted than the parent word in suggesting simple hyperkeratinization in a localized area, rather than the phenomenon in general. See *callositas, callus, clavus* and *corn*.

callous [kăl′əs] is an adjective meaning hardened, having the characteristics of, or like a callus.

callus [kăl′əs], designating hypertrophy of the stratum corneum in localized areas, is a word taken over directly from Latin *callus* (alternate form, *callum*) meaning hardened skin (sometimes hardened flesh) of animals. See *callositas, callosity, clavus* and *corn*.

calor [kăl′ôr, -ēr, kā′lôr] is a Latin word for heat. In former times it was freely used for *fever*. The ablative case of *calor* appears in the title *erythema a calore*.

Campbell de Morgan spots [kăm′bĕl dē Môr′gən] ruby spots, senile angiomas, capillary angiomas.

cancer [kăn′sēr, -sər] derives directly from the Latin word for a crab. Latin writers on medicine, like Celsus, used the word to denote "a crawling, eating, suppurating ulcer; malignant tumor." Perhaps the ungainly crawl of the crab with its claw-like appendages suggested applicability of the word to the relatively slow, invasive progression of malignant proliferation. However, Galen has another explanation for the use of a word meaning crab in this application. He and other Greek writers used *karkinos*, a Greek word which also means crab and to which *cancer* is etymologically related, to denote a type of eating sore or ulcer. According to him, the word *karkinos* was used because of a resemblance between the appearance of the swollen veins surrounding the affected area to a crab's claws.

Both *karkinos* and *cancer* go back to an Indo-European root, *kar,* meaning hard (also found in Sanskrit). The *n* in *cancer* in place of the *r* in *karkinos* is accounted for by the deduction that in Indo-European there was an alternate form, *kan.* Such an alternation of letters, especially where *l, n* and *r* are involved, is considered normal in Indo-European. The name used for this linguistic phenomenon is *alternation* or *dissimilation.* Among examples of dissimilation (from *r* to *n*) are the Latin word (also used in English) *carmen,* song, from the Latin root *can-,* sing, from which are derived English *cantor, canticle, chant,* French *chanson, chanter,* etc., and (from *r* to *l*) English *pilgrim,* from Latin *peregrinus* (dissimilation of the first *r*) foreigner, stranger, hence, a wanderer. For an example of alternation of *n* to *l*, see under *lymph-*.

cancer en cuirasse [ŏng kwērās′] (the modifying phrase is French) describes cancerous process that is like or in the form of (*en*) a breastplate of armor (*cuirasse*). Certain extensive malignancies of the breast produce the appearance of this piece of armor. It is of interest that the word *cuirasse* derives from *corium*, the Latin word for leather, and that protective garments were originally made of leather. *Carcinoma en cuirasse* is an alternate term.

canceri- [kăn′sēr-ĭ, -sər-ī] is a combining form from the Latin word *cancer* with the *i* as a joining insert or link vowel. See *cancero-*, *cancri-*, *carcino-* and notes under *zosteriform*.

cancericidal [kăn′sēr-, kăn′sər-ĭ-sīd′əl, -sīd′l] is a new word formation that has been forced by recent developments in cancer therapy. It may be used as an adjective to describe agents (e.g., drugs) or agencies (e.g., x-rays) that destroy (Latin -*cid*-, kill) cancers, or as a noun to denote such an agent or agency. *Cancerocidal* and *cancricidal* are alternate formations.

cancero- [kăn′sēr-, kăn′sər-ō] is a combining form from the Latin word *cancer* with *o* as a joining insert or link vowel. See *canceri*, *cancri-*, and *carcino-*.

cancerocidal [kăn′sēr-, kăn′sər-ō-sīd′əl, -sīd′l]. See *cancericidal* and *cancricidal*.

cancerophobia [kăn′sēr-, kăn′sər-ō-phō′bē-ə], or **cancerphobia**, means unreasonable fear (-*phobia*) of cancer. The *o* is an insert for the sake of euphony or a link vowel. See notes under *zosteriform*.

cancerous [kăn′sēr-, kăn′sər-əs] is an adjective meaning related to, like, or affected by cancer.

cancri- [kăng′krī] is still another combining form from the word *cancer* (even as far back as Late Latin *e* was dropped from *cancero-* resulting in a formation like *cancroma* for *canceroma*) or *cancri-* may come from the New Latin form *cancrum*. See *canceri-*, *cancero-* and *carcino-*; for comments on these forms and on the connecting vowels *i* and *o* see under *zosteriform*.

cancricidal [kăng′krī-sīd′əl, -sīd′l]. See *cancericidal* and *cancerocidal*.

Candida [kăn′dĭ-də] designates a genus (-*ida*) of dermatropic fungi that are characterized by a sort of whiteness (*cand-*) in culture. The word is replacing *Monilia*.

    Candida is the feminine singular of a Latin adjective meaning white; -*ida* is a suffix commonly used in nomenclature and taxonomy to mean a group. On rule, then, the word for the genus of fungi in point could have been *Candidida*. The adapters of *Candida* perhaps saw in the word a ready-made, fortuitous and felicitous fusion of the elements meaning white and class.

Candida albicans [ăl′bĭ-kănz] is a particular species of the genus. The combination makes a tautology by describing a "whiteness" (*candida*) "turning white" (*albicans*).

candidiasis [kăn′dĭ-dī′ə-sĭs] names the condition (*-iasis*) caused by any pathogenic member of the genus *Candida*, most commonly by *Candida albicans*. *Moniliasis* is the older but still quite current alternate.

Due to Candida albicans, also called monilia or moniliasis. Satellite lesions are characteristic, often scaly collarette type, surrounding a beefy red area. Frequent in the groin and intertriginous areas.

candidid [kăn′dĭ-dĭd] designates a lesion within the family (*-id*) of possible lesions of candidiasis. There is a tendency to restrict *-id* words to refer to lesions of an infectious disease that are "secondary" to the primary lesion or complex, especially those that occur sporadically, are sterile of specific micro-organisms and are based on an allergic mechanism. This tendency rests on mistaken etymological and immunologic reasons that are treated under the entry *-id*. *Moniliid* is an alternate word.

canis [kā′-, kă-, kā′nĭs, -nəs], genitive singular of Latin *canis*, dog, means of the dog. It appears in a title like *Microsporon canis*.

canities [kə-nĭsh′ĭ-ēz, -ē-ēz, -nĭsh′ēz] is a direct borrowing of the Latin word meaning hoariness, gray- or grayish-white color, and, by extension, gray hair. As used today, *canities* describes gray, or graying, scalp hair.

canities unguium [ŭng′gwĭ-əm] means whiteness (*canities*) of nails (*unguium*). *Leukonychia* (from Greek) is the commoner designation.

canker sore [kăng′kĕr sôr] is the lay term for an aphtha. *Canker* derives from Latin (*cancer*) via Old French and Middle English, like *chancre* from the same original source via French. In this derivation, implication of malignancy or severe ulceration has not persisted.

capillary angioma [kăp′ə-lĕr′ē, -ĭ, kə-pĭl′ə-rĭ, -rē ăn′jē-ō′mə] denotes a neoplasia of blood vessels (*angioma*) that consists of the smallest units.

capillitii [kăp′ə-lĭsh′ĭ-ī] is the genitive singular of the Late Latin word *capillitium* and means of the hair. It appears in the title *dermatitis papillaris capillitii*. See *crinis* for other words pertaining to hair.

capitis [kăp′ə-, kăp′ĭ-tĭs], genitive singular of Latin *caput*, head, means of the head. It appears in a title like *tinea capitis*.

capsulatum [kăp′sū-lā′təm] is a New Latin neuter singular adjectival formation from *capsula*, a small box, and means encapsulated, i.e., surrounded, encased, as by or in a protective cover. It appears in a designation like *Histoplasma capsulatum*.

carate [kä-rä′tē, kə-rä′tē] is a word in Quechua, an Indian language of Peru, meaning brown ("liver") spots. It is used synonymously with Spanish *pinta* to designate a treponematosis caused by *T. carateum*.

carbuncle [kär′bŭng-k'l] derives from Latin *carbunculus*, which means a small (-*unculus*, diminutive) piece of coal (*carb*-). The word is applied now, as *carbunculus* was in ancient times, to the well-known pyogenic process in which multiple abscesses are in close apposition and have interconnecting sinuses. We imagine that the red-purple-black (necrotic) swelling with high local temperature and pain suggested a glowing piece of coal to some early discerning observer.

carbuncular [kär-bŭng′kū-lẽr, -kyə-lər] is an adjective meaning of, pertaining to or related to a carbuncle.

carbunculoid [kär-bŭng′kū-loid′] is an adjective meaning like or resembling a carbuncle.

carbunculosis [kär-bŭng′kū-lō′sĭs] designates the condition (-*osis*) in which a carbuncle, or more than one carbuncle, is present. Poor Job suffered from carbunculosis, among other miseries.

carcino- [kär′sĭ-nō], deriving from the Greek word for a crab, is a combining form that relates to neoplastic malignancy. See *cancer*, *canceri-*, *cancero-* and *cancri-*.

carcinogen [kär′sĭ-nō-jĕn] designates an agent that promotes or gives rise to (-*gen*) cancer.

carcinogenesis [kär′sĭ-nō-jĕn′ə-sĭs] describes the phenomenon of development (-*genesis*) of cancer.

carcinoid [kär′sĭ-noid] literally means like (-*oid*) cancer (*carcin*-). The word is applied to the syndrome in which collections of cells of the chromaffin series form in sites like the gut and give forth excessive amounts of serotonin. The cutaneous mark of the process is a peculiar fleeting flush of the face and chest.

carcinoid syndrome Enterochromaffin (Kulchitsky) cells predominantly in the gastrointestinal mucosa—may produce amines and peptides including serotonin, Bradykinin, histamine and prostaglandins. Carcinoid tumors are relatively common. Those that release sufficient quantities of mediators into the systemic circulation to produce the clinical carcinoid syndrome—flushing often with diarrhea and sometimes with wheezing or cardiac failure are rare. Most common in the appendix and rectum, but these rarely produce the carcinoid syndrome. Also found in the ileum, stomach, bile duct, duodenum, pancreas, lung or even the ovary. A variety of mediators are released. Increased serotonin and excretion of its major metabolite, 5-hydroxyindoleacetic acid (5-HIAA). (Philip E. Cryer, *Cecil Textbook of Medicine* 18th Edition, W.B. Saunders Co., Wyngaarden & Smith)

carcinoma [kär′sĭ-nō′mə] literally means the result of the action (*-ma*) of "crabbing" (*carcino-*), i.e., behaving like a crab (in motion, not complaint). Ordinary uses of the word are too well known to need exposition. See *cancer* (especially for another explanation of derivation). The word **carcinoma** is reserved for malignant neoplasia of epithelial tissues, i.e., epidermis and endothelium. See **sarcoma** for a distinction.

carcinoma en cuirasse. See *cancer en cuirasse.*

carcinoma in situ [sĭ′-, sē′-, sī′tōō] designates limitation or fixation of malignant process to a given place (*in situ*) of origin.

cardio-cutaneous syndrome is described by the eponym LEOPARD syndrome: lentigines, EKG changes, ocular hypertelorism, pulmonary atresia, arterial stenosis, retardation (mental), and dwarfism. The skin finding of lentigines is a most helpful marker for making the diagnosis.

carotenemia [kär′ō-tə-nē′mē-ə, -mĭ-ə], using *carotene* for *carotin*, is the same as *carotinemia.*

carotenosis (carotenemia) a yellowish discoloration of the skin and sclerae from ingestion of high quantities of carrots and other yellow vegetables. Also now is iatrogenic from beta-carotene therapy of photosensitivity disorders and for treatment of erythropoietic protoporphyria.

carotinemia [kär′ō-tĭ-nē′mē-ə, -mĭ-ə] designates the condition (*-ia*) in which excess of the pigment carotin is present in the blood (*-em-*). The cutaneous mark of the condition is a distinctly yellow color imparted to the skin, particularly visible on the palms and soles. Jaundice of hepato-biliary origin and chrysiasis, chrysoderma and aurantiasis caused by deposition of gold salts would enter into differential diagnosis. A related condition is **lycopenemia** that results from ingestion of tomatoes and certain fruits and berries that contain a reddish pigment (lycopene), which is an isomer of carotene. The cutaneous mark is an orange-bronze color.

carotinosis [kär′ō-tĭ-nō′sĭs] has about the same force as *carotinemia* except that it is more general in its sense of a condition (*-osis*) involving excess of the yellow pigment (*carotin-*) in any tissue of the body and showing the resultant yellow color therein.

carpet-tack scale [kär′pət-, -pĭt-, -pĕt-, -tăk′ skāl] describes the spiked undersurface of the scale that can be removed from some well-developed lesions of discoid lupus erythematosus. Owing to hyperkeratosis in and about follicular orifices affected by the process, forcible removal of scales uncovers patulous follicles which contained the horny spines seen on the undersurface of the scale in corresponding position.

Carrion's disease [kär-ryôn′]. Verruga peruana, or verruca peruviana, bartonellos is an infectious disease caused by the bite of the phlebotomus sand fly which transmits a Gram-negative pleomorphic bacterium, *Bartonella bacilliformis*, endemic to the Andes region of South America. There is an acute febrile anemic stage (Oroya fever), joint pains, albuminuria and progressive severe anemia. This is followed in several weeks by a second stage of the disease, a nodular skin eruption (verruga peruana). Usually the latter is a completely benign process.

caruncle [kăr′ŭng-kəl, kə-rŭng′kəl] designates any small (*-uncle*) fleshy (*car-*) mass.

catagen [kăt′ə-jĕn] means a developing (*-gen*) down (*cata-*), i.e., a degeneration. The word is applied to that phase of the hair cycle in which there is a sharp transition from growth (*anagen*) to cessation of growth and inception of an end stage (*telogen*).

cat-scratch [kăt′skrăch′] a bacterial disease that is transmitted by the scratch of a cat. The disease is characterized by a necrotic lesion at the point of the scratch, fever and a macular exanthem. May have a resemblance to *Sporotrichosis*, due to the swollen lymph nodes.

causalgia [kô-săl′-, kô-zăl′jə, -jē-ə, -jĭ-ə] is New Latin from Greek elements that describe a condition (*-ia*) characterized by burning (*caus-*) pain (-alg-). Sensations of burning pain are complained of in skin, and in muscles particularly. *Dermatalgia* is an alternate, not quite equivalent, word.

cautery [kô′tĕr-ē, -ĭ] derives from Greek through the Latin word *cauterium*, a branding iron. The modern instrument is not much different: a piece of metal shaped to any burning purpose and brought to glowing heat is a cautery. The word has been extended to destructive instruments or procedures employing electricity (*electrocautery*) and chemicals (*chemocautery*).

cavernosum [kăv'ēr-nō'səm] is the neuter singular form of the Latin adjective *cavernosus* meaning full of (*-osus*) hollows or cavities (*cavern-*). It appears in the title *angioma cavernosum*.

cavernous [kăv'ēr-nəs, -ə(r)-nəs] is an adjective meaning relating to a cave or hollow (Latin, *caverna*), hence, deep, vast or having many cavities.

cavernous angioma. See *angioma cavernosum*.

cavernous hemangioma [hē-măn'jē-ō'mə] describes vascular neoplasia in which large and deep blood sinuses make up the hamartoma.

cayenne pepper spots [kī-ĕn', kā-ĕn' pĕp'ēr, -ər spŏts] is a term that describes capillaries that appear as tiny, red macules (capillaries) in the condition named *angioma serpiginosum*. Cayenne is the name of an island in French Guiana, South America, and its capital. The region is noted for its pepper.

Cazenave's disease [käzənäv']. Several: lupus erythematosus; pemphigus foliaceus; alopecia areata.

cellular blue nevus [sĕl'ū-lər bloō nē'vəs] is a histopathologist's term, not a clinician's. The illogical intent is to specify by this title a blue nevus with high cellularity of a special sort, namely, spindle-shaped cells with intense melanogenic capability. The ordinary blue nevus is also cellular and melanotic; the cells thereof are morphologically somewhat different, but still cells. *Cellular blue nevus* is an odd way of making a distinction.

cellulitis [sĕl'ū-lī'tĭs, -lē'tĭs] literally means inflammation (*-itis*) of the little cells (*cellul-*). What is really meant, of course, is diffuse inflammation of parenchyma without necrosis or sharp localization of pus.

cementoma [sē', sə'mĕn-tō'mə] is another of those formations with *-oma* (which see) in the sense of tumor. In this instance the word is applied to a neoplasm of the tissue that produces the cementum of teeth. It has nothing to do with that cement that is a building material.

centrifugum [sĕn-trĭf'ū-gəm, -oō-gəm, -ə-gəm] is the neuter singular of a New Latin adjectival formation and means fleeing (*-fugum*) from the center (*centri-*). It appears in the title *leukoderma acquisitum centrifugum.*

cerulae [sē-, sə-rōōl'ē] and **ceruleus** [sē-, sə-rōōl'ē-əs] are the feminine plural and the masculine singular forms respectively of the Latin adjective *caeruleus* (with *ae* simplified in the English adaptation). The Latin adjective means azure, dark blue or dark green (the ancients were not exact in the use of words for color); the modern English word is *cerulean*, meaning sky blue. The forms entered are found in *maculae cerulae* and *nevus fuscoceruleus.*

cerumen [sə-, sē-rōō'mĕn, -mən], a New Latin formation from Latin *cera*, wax, is applied to the product of the specialized apocrine glands of the ear canal.

ceruminal [sə, sē-rōō'mĭ-n'l] and **ceruminous** [sə-, sē-rōō'mĭ-nəs] are adjectives meaning pertaining to or relating to cerumen.

chafe [chāf], **chafing** [chāf'ĭng] are words that derive from Latin elements, via French, meaning to make warm or hot (*calefacere, chauffer*). In English the words are applied to irritation of the skin caused by friction.

chalazion [kə-lā'zē-ŏn, -ən] designates an infectious pustule of one of the specialized glands (Meibomian) of the eyelid. The plural is *chalazia*. Derivation is via Latin from a Greek word meaning a small pimple. *Chalazion* is diminutive of *chalaza*, which means a hard lump or hailstone in classical Greek. *Chalazion* then came to mean, in general, a small hard lump or tubercle.

chalazoderm(i)a [kăl'ə-zō-dûr'mə; -mē-ə] means lax or relaxed (*chalazo-*) skin (*-derma, -dermia*). The derivation is from Greek but not related to that of *chalazion.*

chancre [shăng'kĕr, -kər] derives from Latin (*cancer*) via French. When unmodified, the word is taken to mean the primary lesion of syphilis. When modified by some other word or phrase, e.g., *tuberculous, of sporotrichosis*, it describes the primary lesion of the respective disease in the skin. Therefore, the word has general use to describe the primary lesion of any disease when that lesion evolves into an indolent ulcer with eroding characteristics. In *chancre*, as in *canker*, the modern malignant implications of *cancer* are lost, but the sense of eroding ulceration remains as it no longer does in *canker.*

chancre, hard. *Hard chancre* is applied to the primary complex of syphilis because, when well developed, the periphery of the lesion, gingerly felt with gloved fingers, has a hard feel.

chancre récidive [rāsēdēv′], or **redux** [rē′dŭks, -dōōks], are titles in French and neo-classical form respectively, meaning recurrent (*récidive*, falling back, relapsing; *redux*, classical Latin, leading back or brought back) chancre. In criminology, a recidivist is a habitual criminal, a repeater in crime.

chancre, soft. *Soft chancre* is applied to a lesion of chancroid. Such an ulcer, unlike the primary complex of syphilis, has a soft feel.

chancriform [shăng′krī-fôrm] describes any lesion that has the form of a persistent ulcer reminiscent of the primary complex of syphilis. The lesions in the skin of the primary complexes of tuberculosis, sporotrichosis, blastomycosis, leprosy and vaccinia are chancriform.

chancriform pyoderma [pī′ō-dûr′mə] is descriptive of a purulent process on the skin that takes the form of a chancre.

chancroid [shăng′kroid] is applied to the venereal disease caused by *Hemophilus ducreyii*. The signs are multiple erosions (soft chancres) and characteristic inguinal adenopathy (buboes) marked by pain, purulence and intense local inflammation.

channel [chăn′əl, -əl] is another word like *burrow, gallery* or *tunnel* to designate an excavation in the stratum corneum that houses an infesting insect or mite.

chapping [chăp′ĭng] is applied to the superficial erythema and scaling of exposed portions of the skin that occur in cold weather and high humidity. It is a temporary xerosis or a sort of first-degree frostbite. The word derives from the Middle English word *chappen*, to crack or open in slits.

Chédiak-Higashi syndrome [chā′dyăk; hē′gä-shē]. Susceptibility to pyogenic infection, photophobia, albinism, hepatosplenomegaly, lymphadenopathy, tendency to leukemia, and malignant lymphomatoses. A fatal disorder also with azurophilic leukocytic inclusions and neurologic abnormalities.

cheilitis [kī-lī′tĭs, -lē′tĭs] designates any inflammatory process (-*itis*) of the oral lips (*cheil-*).

cheilitis exfoliativa [ĕks-fō′lĭ-ə-tī′və] is descriptive of any inflammatory process of the lips (*cheilitis*) that is marked by leaf-like scaling (*exfoliativa*). Cheilitis caused by sensitization and exposure to eczematogenous allergens is marked by exfoliation at some stages and could take the title descriptively, but usually does not. The title is reserved for a persistent cheilitis that is marked by scaling and is of obscure cause. Habitual licking, atopic dermatitis and avitaminosis may be factors in some cases.

cheilitis glandularis apostematosa [glăn′dū-lā′rĭs, -lä′rĭs, -lăr-ĭs ăp′ō-stĕm-ə-tō′sə] describes an inflammatory process of the lips (*cheilitis*) in which minute abscess-like (*apostematosa*) processes develop in the mucous glands. Glue-like discharge and stickiness of the lips that impedes ready opening of the mouth additionally characterize the condition.

cheilitis granulomatosa [grăn′ū-lō′mə-tō′sə] is descriptive of any inflammatory condition of the lips (*cheilitis*) that is marked by granular papulation (*granulomatosa*). Like *cheilitis exfoliativa*, the title is reserved when a clear clause for the appearance is not discernible.

cheilosis [kī-lō′sĭs] designates any abnormal condition (*-osis*) of the oral lips (*cheil-*), inflammatory or not.

ch(e)iropompholyx [kī′rō-pŏm′fō-lĭks] derives from Greek word elements that mean a blistering (*pompholyx*) of the hands (*cheiro-*, *chiro-*). The condition now so named consists of firm, seemingly deep-seated vesicles that characteristically stud the palmar surface of the hands and web surfaces of the fingers. The cause of the condition has to do with the passage of water through the skin, either as sensible or insensible perspiration. *Pustular psoriasis, dermatophytid* and *allergic eczematous dermatitis* frequently figure in differential diagnosis.

cheloid [kē′loid] is sometimes seen in place of *keloid*. There are several Greek words, some beginning with kappa (κ) and one with chi (χ), with meanings like scar, tumor and claw, any one of which could be the source word. Usually, the *kappa* words are transliterated with a *k* and the *chi* words with *ch*. French practice uses *chéloïde*; in English, *keloid* is more often seen. *Chelate* [kē′lāt′] is a related word used in chemistry to describe graphically a compound in which an element is bound within a compound as though by claw-like radicals.

chemocautery,-surgery, -therapy [kĕm′ō-kô′tēr-ē; -sûr′jēr-ē; -thĕr′ə-pē]. *Chemocautery* means burning (*-cautery*) of tissue with chemicals. *Chemosurgery* means about the same thing but suggests combined application of chemicals and the knife as in the Mohs' technique of managing invasive cancers. *Chemotherapy* is the most general word meaning treatment with topically applied chemicals or internally administered drugs. It is used more for drugs administered by mouth or parenterally, especially cytotoxic drugs.

chicken pox [chĭk′ən, -′n pŏks] is the vernacular term for *varicella*. Due to the varicella-zoster virus, one and the same virus, usually causes varicella in children and zoster in adults. The derivation of the term is not certain. There is belief that it came from the mildness of the disease, compared to smallpox perhaps. To this day *chicken* is pejorative, suggesting weakness, timidity or lack of courage. At any rate, the condition is marked by a prodrome of malaise that is followed by fever and an eruption of macules, papules and vesicles. The lesions appear in waves over a period of a few days, then crust and heal in a week or two. The head, face and upper portion of the trunk are sites of predilection. In the course of the cutaneous events, lesions of all types mentioned may be seen at the same time. Most of the process resolves without sequelae but it is common enough for one or more characteristic circular scars to develop, especially on the face.

chigger [chĭg′ĕr, jĭg′ĕr], or **chigga** [chĭg′ə, jĭg′ə], is a word of African origin (Wolof, Yoruba) for *Trombicula irritans*, the harvest mite. It is equated or confused with *chigoe* and *jigger*.

chigoe [chĭg′ō, chĭ′gə, chē′gō, -gə] is a word of Cariban (West Indian, South American) origin for *Tunga penetrans*, the sand flea. It is equated or confused with *chigger* and *jigger*.

chilblain(s) [chĭl′blān(z)] is an Anglo-Saxon word from word elements that mean a sore (*-blain*) or sores (*-blains*) caused by cold (*chil-*).

CHILD syndrome (congenital hemidysplasia with ichthyosiform erythrodermal and limb defects) is a rare striking unilateral ichthyosiform erythroderma ipsilateral underdevelopment of the limbs and brain. Female cases are due to X-linked dominant gene defect which is lethal in the hemizygote male fetus. Also cardiovascular and renal defects. (Cullen)

Chlamydiae. Obligate intracellular parasites but more like bacteria than viruses. *C. trachomatis* is transmitted sexually and it can cause a wide variety of problems from urethritis, cervicitis, to lymphogranuloma venereum, endometritis and salpingitis. Complications include Reiter's syndrome, rectal strictures, infertility, ectopic pregnancy etc. These infections stimulate both a humoral and a cellular immune response. Chlamydia can be treated with a wide variety of antibiotics. (Walter E. Stamm)

chloasma [klō-ăz′mə] derives from Greek word elements that mean the result (*-ma*) of turning green (*chloas-*). The clinical condition to which the word is now attached is patchy hyperpigmentation, especially on the face. However, that hyperpigmentation is not green but tan-brown-black. The cause of the condition is not known. Common location is on the face. May be associated with the use of oral contraceptives.

chloasma gravidarum [grā′və-, grä′vĭ-, grä′vī-, grā′vī-dā′rəm, -dä′rəm] is a title which suggests an endocrinologic mechanism for the condition, especially when its onset occurs during pregnancy.

chloracne [klōr-, klôr-ăk′nē] is applied to the acneform eruption seen in workers who handle chlorinated products (especially in the electrical and related industries).

cholesterosis, extracellular [kō-lĕs′tēr-ō′sĭs ĕks′trə-sĕl′ū-lər]. Extracellular cholesterosis is a rare dyslipoidosis in which cholesterol is deposited in extracellular sites. It is marked by ulcerations of the skin, particularly upon erythematous plaques on the acral areas. Its prognosis is sad.

cholinergic urticaria [kō′lĭn-, kŏl′ĭn-ēr′jĭk ûr′tĭ-kâr-ē-ə] is a characteristic whealing process in which small lesions that do not itch intensely appear under conditions of exertion, excitement or merely environmental heat. Abnormalities of acetylcholine production or metabolism (abnormalities of cholinesterase) are thought to be the biochemical basis of the condition.

chondritis [kŏn-drī′tĭs, -drē′tĭs] designates any inflammatory condition (-itis) of cartilage (chondr-). In those areas where cartilage is immediately subjacent to skin (nose, ears) diseases of this tissue intrude themselves into the purview of dermatology.

chondrodermatitis nodularis chronica helicis [kŏn′drō-dûr′mə-tī′tĭs, -tē′tĭs nŏd′ū-, nō′dū-lā′rĭs, -lä′rĭs, -lăr′ĭs krŏn′ĭ-kə hĕl′ĭ-, hē′lĭ-sĭs] designates a characteristic condition in which the cartilage (chondro-) and overlying skin (-dermat-) are affected by persistent (chronica) inflammation (-itis) and a nodule (nodularis) at the upper rim of the helix (helicis, of the spiral) of the ear. It has been suggested recently that the condition is in the nature of a glomus tumor.

chondrodysplasia punctata (Conradi disease). Skeletal defects stippling of the epiphysis in a paint-splattered pattern is the essential diagnostic feature. Disappears by age three. Three different types appear to exist. Skin finding often consists of ichthyosis, saddle nose; characteristic facies koala bear. Lens opacities.

chondroma [kŏn-drō′mə] designates a neoplasia (-oma) of cartilage (chondr-).

choristoma [kôr′ĭs-tō′mə, kō′rĭs-tō′mə] is a word from Greek elements meaning the result of (-ma) a separation (choristo-). The word is applied to a neoplasia resulting from a displaced anlage. Supernumerary structures like digits and nipples are examples of choristomas. The word is rarely heard or seen but perhaps deserves more currency. Note how much better it is to derive the meaning of the word etymologically by interpreting its Greek-derived elements as the result of (*-ma-*) separation (*choristo-*) rather than as a separated (*chorist-*) tumor (*-oma*). With the latter interpretation it more aptly would designate a metastasis from a malignant neoplasm and would be synonymous with metastasis, which also means a displacement.

chromatophore [krō′mə-tō-fôr′, -fōr′, krō-măt′ə-fōr] designates a macrophage found in the cutis that ingests and carries (*-phore*) pigment (*chromato-*).

chrom(h)idrosis [krō′mĭ-drō′sĭs, krōm′hĭ-drō′sĭs] designates the condition (*-osis*) in which sweat (*-hidr-*, *-idr-*) is colored (*chrom-*). The color may be of the entire spectrum, nearly, but black, red and green are commonest.

chromoblastomycosis [krō′mō-blăs′tō-mĭ-kō′sĭs] is an unsatisfactory designation for a fungous infection (*-mycosis*) caused by certain fungi.

chromomycosis (dermatitis verrucosa) [krō′mō-mī-kō′sĭs] is an infectious species of dermatiaceous fungi such as Phialophora spp., Cladosporium spp. and Hormodendrum spp. It is characterized by warty cutaneous nodules which slowly develop into large ulcerated plaques. The disease usually starts on the foot or lower leg and extends to adjacent areas by lymphatic spread. Chromomycosis has a worldwide distribution, but it is significant that 80 percent of patients are barefooted agricultural workers, mainly adult men, living in subtropical or tropical regions. This is a refractory disease. Treatment of choice appears to be a combination of 5-flucytosine and ketoconazole.

chronic [krŏn′ĭk], derived from a Greek adjective, literally means relating to or concerning (*-ic*) time (*chron-*). The implication of the adjective is "lasting a long time," and when it is opposed to *acute*, the word acquires nuances of sense suggesting things not immediately serious.

chronic bullous disease of childhood is the linear IgA bullous dermatitis of childhood. IgA is seen by direct immunofluorescence at the basement membrane zone. A self-limited, benign disease but may run for years, i.e., from age two or three to puberty. Bullae may be widespread and do involve the mouth. Treated best with sulfapyridine or dapsone. Sometimes topical steroids are sufficient.

chronic discoid lupus erythematosus [dĭs′koid lōō′pəs ĕr′ĭ-thĕm′ə-tō′səs, -thē′mə-tō′səs] describes that form of the disease that is without constitutional symptoms and is marked by long-enduring and disc-shaped lesions that are red, scaly and scarring. Compare *acute, systemic* and *disseminated lupus erythematosus.*

chronic granulomatous disease of children [krŏn′ĭk grăn-ū-lō′mə-təs də-zēz′ ŏv chĭl′drĕn] is a condition characterized by frequent and repeated infections of the skin and other organs that stem from genetic insufficiency of certain enzymes, particularly peroxidase, in leukocytes. Phagocytic capability is preserved but enzymatic destruction of pathogens is failing.

chronic mucocutaneous candidiasis is the widespread tremendously florid form of candida infection of the nails, mucous membranes and skin. This infection is completely unresponsive to routine candida therapy. These patients have multiple immune deficiencies of both immune globulins and T cell function.

chronic radiodermatitis. See under *radiodermatitis.*

chronica and **chronicus** [krŏn′ĭkə; -kəs] are respectively the feminine and masculine singular of a Latin adjective (derived from Greek) and mean chronic. They appear in titles of classical form like *acrodermatitis chronica atrophicans* and *lichen chronicus simplex.*

chrysiasis [krĭs-ī′ə-sĭs] designates any condition (*-iasis*) in which the skin turns golden (yellow) in color. *Chrysoderma* and *aurantiasis* are roughly equivalent words. Carotinemia could be so designated; jaundice, however, would not be specified in this way. A drug eruption, as from gold salts or atabrine, would take the title.

chrysoderma [krĭs′ō-dûr′mə] has about the same force as *chrysiasis* and *aurantiasis* in designating a gold-colored (*chryso-*) skin condition (*-derma*).

cicatrisata [sĭk′ə-trĭ-sā′tə, -trī-sä′tə, -trĭs′ə-tə] is a New Latin spelling of the feminine singular of the perfect participle of a Medieval Latin verb meaning to make a scar; the form itself means scarred. It appears in the title *alopecia cicatrisata.*

cicatrix [sĭk′ə-trĭks, sĭ-kā′trĭks] is the Latin word for a scar or wound. It is used synonymously with *scar.* The plural is *cicatrices* [sĭk′ə-trī′sēz].

cigarette-paper wrinkling [sĭg′ə-rĕt′-pā′pĕr rĭng′klĭng] is descriptive of superficial atrophy which gives the surface of the skin the appearance of cigarette paper that has been subjected to roll-your-own operations. Nowadays cigarettes are "so round, so firm, so fully packed," as the ad used to go, that cigarette paper appears smooth right up to cancer of the lung. The term is applied particularly to the appearance of the skin in acrodermatitis chronica atrophicans.

cimicosis [sĭm′ĭ-, sī′mĭ-kō′sĭs] designates the condition (-*osis*) resulting from bug bites. The word derives from Latin *cimex*, a bug, and is applied particularly to bedbug (*Cimex lectularius*) bites.

circinata [sûr′sī-nā′tə, -nä′tə, -năt′ə] and **circinate** [sûr′sī-nāt′] are respectively the feminine singular of a Latin perfect participle and an English adjective that mean rounded or made round. The Latin form appears in *tinea circinata*, ringworm.

circumscribed [sûr′kəm-skrībd′] is said of lesions that are sharply limited to an area by clean borders.

circumscribed myxedema [mĭks′ə-dē′mə] describes a sharply limited, red-yellow-brown, boggy condition of the skin over the tibias that sometimes occurs before or during hyperthyroidism, after treatment thereof especially, if there is a tendency to recurrence of thyrotoxicosis, and occasionally in seemingly normal or hypothyroid individuals.

circumscribed neurodermatitis [nōō′-, nū′rō-dûr′mə-tī′tĭs, -tē′tĭs] is applied by some to what others call *lichen chronicus simplex*.

circumscribed precancerosis of Dubreuilh [prē′kăn′sēr-ō′sĭs, -sər-ō′sĭs ŏv dōōbrōōē′] is an alternate title for *Hutchinson's freckle*.

circumscripta [sûr′kəm-skrĭp′tə] is the feminine singular of the perfect passive participle of the Latin verb *circumscribere*, literally to write around, to draw a line about or enclose in a circle, and used as an adjective it means circumscribed (which see). It appears in the titles *alopecia circumscripta* and *poliosis circumscripta*.

Civatte's poikiloderma [sīvăt]. Reticulated pigmented poikiloderma affecting the face and neck particularly.

clavus [klā′vəs] is Latin for a metal or wooden nail. Medically, it is used for the type of corn that has a nail-like shape with a broad head and a central spike which seems to be driven into the area in which it forms.

clear cell describes a kind of cell found regularly in and about the basal-cell layer of the normal epidermis. It is thought to be of neuro-ectodermal origin. *Cellule claire, dendritic cell, Langhans' cell, melanocyte* and *tactile cell of Merkel-Ranvier* are terms that are loosely used interchangeably for *clear cell* but used more distinctively by anatomists, physiologists and biochemists who detect differences in cells of this class.

clear cell hidradenoma occurs as a slowly growing, usually solitary nodule. Occasionally, however, several lesions are present. The tumors are firm and measure 0.5 to 2 cm or more in diameter. Some tumors discharge serous material, others tend to ulcerate. (Hashimoto & Lever)

clubbed fingers [klŭbd fĭng′gĕrz, -gərz] is a descriptive term for enlargement, increased convexity, rounding and broadening of the distal phalanges of the fingers as seen in chronic pulmonary diseases. See *Hippocratic fingers*.

Clutton's joints [klŭt′n]. Symmetrical synovitis of the knees in congenital syphilis.

coagulation [kō-ăg′ū-lā′shən] derives from a Latin word meaning curdling. In dermatology, the word is used to describe the effect of bipolar electrosurgery in which tissue substance seems to be curdled by the action of heat generated in that manner.

cocardiform [kō-kär′dĭ-fôrm] is an adjective meaning in the shape of a cockade.

Coccidioides [kŏk-sĭd′ē-oi′dēz] designates micro-organisms that are like (*-oides*) coccidia. *Coccidia* encompasses things in the class (*-idia*) of *cocci*.

Coccidioides immitis [ĭ-mī′tĭs, -mē′tis, ĭ-mĭt′ĭs, ĭm′ĭ-tĭs] is the name of a fungus, elements of which appear like cocci. The Latin word *immitis* specifies that the pathogenicity of this micro-organism is severe (*im-*=*in-*, not, plus *-mitis*, mild).

coccidioidin [kŏk-sĭd′ē-oi′dĭn, -d'n] is an antigen made and used much as tuberculin is made and used.

coccidioidomycosis. A deep fungus infection caused by the spores of *Coccidioides immitis*. Inhalation is the ordinary way of infection.

This fungus infection interestingly can go either way, i.e. from pulmonary to skin or from cutaneous coccidioidomycosis to a systemic form. Prevalent in the southwestern United States. The skin test (coccidioidin) will detect the infection.

Skin lesions include verrucous granulomas, ulcers, cellulitis, abscesses, papulopustules and sinus tracts. A generalized macular exanthem ensues in an appreciable number of patients especially children during the initial period of the disease. "Valley fever" is the manifestation of erythema nodosum, arthralgias and arthritis with erythema multiforme. Diagnosis is made by direct KOH exam of sputum, ulcers, blood, urine, cerebrospinal fluid and bone marrow. Rapidly cultures. Skin test will be positive in days to weeks.

Treatment is with amphotericin B and ketoconozole. (Tomecki et al)

cockade [kŏk-ād′] describes the form of a lesion that is like a rosette or a knot of ribbon. The word comes from the French *cocarde*, a rosette worn as a badge of office or a military decoration. In turn, the French word goes back to an adjective meaning vain derived from *coq*, a cock, rooster. The adjective for *cockade* is *cocardiform*. *Corymbiform* (from Latin *corymbus*, a cluster of fruit or flowers) is a nearly synonymous word.

coil gland [koil glănd] is used synonymously with *eccrine* or *sweat gland*.

cold abscess. See *abscess, cold.*

cold cream [kōld krēm] is a pharmaceutical and cosmetic formation that is designed to "vanish." It is essentially a mixture of an animal fat (e.g., spermaceti) and a sodium salt (e.g., borax). The result tends to be a saponification. When mineral oil is used instead of animal fat, the "vanishing" quality is achieved by addition of dispersing agents. In cosmetic practice, the pretense of use is to beautify the skin by providing emollient and humectant actions.

cold sore(s) [kōld sôr(z)] is colloquial for the lesions of herpes simplex. The association of *cold* is, of course, with the common upper respiratory infection, not external or environmental cold, and that association is not obligatory; other factors e.g., fever, sunburn, local trauma, etc. can activate the virus or induce the condition.

cold urticaria [ûr′tĭ-kâr′ē-ə] is meant to describe whealing caused by external or environmental coldness.

collacin [kŏl′ə-sĭn] designates degenerated material from collagen and elastic fibers (elascin). The word is derived from *kolla*, a Greek word for glue, plus *-in*, a material, as in *lepromin*, with the insertion, for the sake of euphony, of the letter *c*, possibly by analogy with words like *actinomycin* (where, however, *c* belongs as part of the word element *myc-*).

collagen [kŏl′ə-jĕn] is derived from Greek *kolla*, glue, plus *-gen*, giving rise to, and designates the normal fibrillar substance of the connective tissue of the corium.

collagen disease the group of conditions, namely, dermatomyositis, lupus erythematosus, periarteritis nodosa, scleroderma, etc., in which collagen is severely disturbed.

collagenosis [kŏl′ə-jĕn-ō′sĭs] any abnormal condition (*-osis*) of collagen. See *collagen disease.*

collarette of Biet [kŏl′ər-ĕt′ ŏv bēā′] describes the ring of scales that develops around macular lesions of secondary syphilis.

collastin [kə-lăs′tĭn, kŏl′ə-stĭn] is still another degenerated material of collagen plus material from elastic fibers (elastin). See *collacin*.

colliquativa [kŏl-ĭk′-, kō-lĭk′wə-tī′və, -tē′və] and **colliquative** [kŏl-ĭk′, kə-lĭk′wə-tĭv] are respectively the feminine singular of a New Latin adjective and an English adjective meaning tending to liquefaction. The classicized form appears in the title *tuberculosis cutis colliquativa*.

collodion baby [kō-, kə-lō′dē-ŏn, -ən bā′bē] is an aptly picturesque term for the condition more technically known as *lamellar exfoliation of the newborn*. Such an infant at birth looks as if painted with collodion and distorted by the tight grip of the material. The nose is flattened by pressure; the eyelids are pulled into ectropion; the oral and genital lips are also held agape. The condition tends to improve spontaneously in a matter of months by a shedding of the abnormal material. Ichthyotic changes then tend to develop during childhood and finally ameliorate around puberty, adolescence and young adulthood.

colloid [kŏl′oid] bespeaks a material that resembles glue (Greek, *kolla*). In dermatohistopathology, a characteristic tinctorial change of collagen stained with hematoxylin and eosin that results in an amorphous or structureless pinkness is so called.

colloid acne [ăk′nē] is a rare papular dermatosis in which lesions, usually on the face, consist of degenerated collagen.

colloid degeneration [dĭ-, də, dē-jĕn′ĕr-ā′shən] is the simple term for development of colloid.

colloid milium [mĭl′ē-əm] is synonymous with *colloid acne*.

color of lesions and skin. Precise color is hard to convey by ordinary words. Electromagnetic energy begins to stimulate the retina and excite recognition in the range of 2000–8000 Å. Color perception is then described as violet-indigo-blue-green-yellow-orange-red. Absolute white is a combination of the entire spectrum of electromagnetic energy, and absolute black results from absence of any part of the spectrum. It is obvious that the gradations of color, while not infinite, are still too large to be designated by the words that evoke the same remembrance in all normal persons. Individual differences in visual acuity and the anomaly of "color blindness" make communication of color still more difficult. Nevertheless, with care in the choice of words and judicious use of familiar objects as examples for color, a lot of color sense can be expressed and understood.

comedo [kŏm′ē-dō, -ə-dō] means a glutton in Latin and derives from a verb meaning to eat. Conjecture has it that the ancients imagined the blackhead to be a flesh-eating maggot. Since the Latin plural is *comedones* [kŏm′ĕ-dō′nēz], some, seeing this form, make a new singular, *comedone* (by a process called, in linguistic circles, back formation); others, seeing *comedo* and not knowing the Latin plural make a new plural, *comedoes*. As a result two singular and two plural forms are heard in speech and seen in print. The word does not need so much grammatical number. The preferred singular is *comedo*; the proper classical plural is *comedones* but *comedoes* will probably win out because it is easier to pronounce and because it is in the simple convention of making plurals in English with an *s*. See *blackhead*, for a description of the clinical lesion.

"comedone" is erroneous for *comedo* (which see).

comedonicus [kŏm′ē-dō′nĭ-kəs -ə-dŏn′ĭ-kəs] is a New Latin masculine singular adjectival formation meaning related to *comedones*. It appears in the title *nevus comedonicus*.

complexion [kŏm-plĕk′shən] denotes the superficial aspect of the skin of the face with respect to color, texture and other qualities of general appearance. It is also used to denote combination of abstract qualities.

compound nevus [kŏm′pound nē′vəs] is one that has thèques of melanocytic cells in both dermo-epidermal and intracutaneous position.

condyloma [kŏn′də-, kŏn′dĭ-lō′mə] derives from Greek and Latin words that mean joint, knuckle or fist. In modern usage, something knobby is suggested.

condyloma acuminatum [ə-kū′mĭ-nā′təm] names a wart of the type that occurs on the genitalia or in the genito-anal region. *Acuminate wart, venereal wart* and *verruca acuminata* are synonymous terms that describe other qualities with specifications not entirely in accord with reality, that is to say, neither so pointed (*acuminatum*), nor particularly venereal. The plural is *condylomata acuminata* (Greek and Latin for the first word, Latin for the second).

condyloma latum [lā′təm, lä′təm, -tŭm, -tōōm] names the lesions of secondary syphilis that appear around the inguinal, intercrural, perineal and general genito-anal region in the form of flat, broad (*latum*) papules and plaques.

congelation [kŏn′jə-lā′shən] derives from Latin *congelatio*, a freezing. Just as *burn* is heard more often than *combustion*, so *frostbite* is more commonly heard than *congelation*. Nevertheless there are erudite contexts where *congelation* is better applied.

congenita [kŏn-jĕn′ĭ-tə, -ə-tə], **congenitale** [kŏn-jĕn′ĭ-tā′lĕ, -tä′lĕ, -tăl′ē], **congenitalis** [kŏn-jĕn′ĭ-tā′lĭs, -tä′lĭs, -tăl′ĭs], **congenitum** [kŏn-jĕn′ĭ-təm, -ə-təm] are derived from Latin word elements meaning born (*-genit-*) together (*con-*), and therefore mean congenital, existing at or from birth. *Congenita* and *congenitum* are classical Latin feminine and neuter singular forms respectively, whereas *congenitalis* and *congenitale*, though corresponding to them in gender, are New Latin formations from the classical adjective *genitalis*, meaning belonging to or pertaining (*-alis*) to birth. These words appear in titles like *pachonychia congenita, erythroderma ichthyosiforme congenitale*, or *congenitum*, and *erythrodermia ichthyosiformis congenitalis* (in feminine forms as an alternate of the title immediately preceding).

congenital [kən-jĕn′ə-təl, -t′l] derives from Latin elements that mean relating to (*-al*) the incident of (*con-*, with) birth (*-genit-*). The word is sometimes confused with *hereditary*. Some hereditary phenomena appear congenitally, but congenital phenomena need not be gene-determined. See *congenita*.

congenital ectodermal defects [ĕk′tō-dûr-məl dē′fĕkt(s), dĭ-, də-fĕkt(s)′] is a title for conditions in which variable underdevelopment of skin, its adnexa and appendages and other structures of ectodermal embryogenesis is present. Wispy hair, thin, dry skin, onychial and dental dysplasia and a characteristic facies (exaggeration of frontal bones, depressed bridge of nose) are common signs. Intolerance to environmental heat is a prominent complaint.

congenital erythropoietic porphyria (Günther's disease) is an erythropoietic porphyria which causes extreme photosensitivity with resulting mutilating skin damage. An extremely rare disease. Due to overproduction of uroporphyrin and also of coproporphyrins. (Bissell)

congenital ichthyosiform erythroderma [ĭk′thī-ō′sĭ-fôrm, -ŏs′ĭ-fôrm ĕ-rĭth′rō-dûr′mə] names a condition in which the skin is red (*erythroderma*) and hyperkeratotic. The fish-skin allusion (*ichthyosiform*) is less apt than for the common varieties of ichthyosis. Bullae may be part of the process.

congenital syphilis [sĭf′ĭ-lĭs, -ə-lĭs] describes syphilitic process present at birth or if manifesting itself later still clearly caused by intrauterine infection with the *Treponema pallidum*.

congenitale, congenitalis. See *congenita*.

conglobata, acne, or **conglobate acne.** See *acne conglobata.*

connective-tissue disease [kə-nĕk′tĭv tĭsh′ōō dĭ-, də-zēz′] is used like *collagen disease*, in connection with dermatomyositis, lupus erythematosus and scleroderma.

connective-tissue nevus [nē′vəs] is hamartomatous over- or maldevelopment of the parenchymal elements of connective tissue.

Conradi's disease. Chondrodystrophica congenita punctata.

contactant [kən-, kŏn-tăk′tənt, kən′-, kŏn′tăk-tənt] is new coinage for a substance that approaches the skin from without and induces immunological changes.

contact dermatitis [kŏn′tăkt dûr′mə-tī-tĭs, -tē′tĭs] usually a type IV delayed or T cell mediated hypersensitivity. May be acute, subacute or chronic. Period of sensitization may be from a few days to a prolonged time. This can also be a primary irritant dermatitis. There is inflammation of both the epidermis and the dermis. Clinically this is often quite a sharply marginated condition and in poison ivy, linear or streaked lesions help to establish the diagnosis. (Fitzpatrick et al., *Atlas of Skin Disease*, McGraw-Hill)

contagiosa [kŏn-tā′jĭ-ō′sə, -jē-ō′sə], **contagiosum** [kŏn-tā′jĭ-ō′səm, -jē-ō′səm] and **contagious** [kŏn-tā′jəs] are respectively the feminine singular and neuter singular of the Late Latin adjective *contagiosus* and an English adjective, all of which signify easy communicability of infection. The Latin adjective was used only by the writer Vegetius (fourth century A.D.). The Latin forms appear in titles like *impetigo contagiosa* and *molluscum contagiosum.*

contagious. See *contagiosa.*

contusiforme [kŏn-tū′sĭ-fôr′mē] is a New Latin formation, meaning in the manner of shape (*-forme*) of a bruise or bruising (*contusi-*). It appears in the title *erythema contusiforme*, which could apply to erythema nodosum and tuberculosis cutis indurata (erythema induratum, Bazin's disease). The word is aptly descriptive of the early clinical appearance of these highly characteristic processes on the legs.

contusion [kŏn-tū′zhən] derives from a Latin word (*contusio*) that means a bruising or crushing. In ancient medical Latin *contusio*, meaning a bruise, was used much as *contusion* is used today.

copra itch [kŏp′rə, kō′prə ĭch] is an acariasis caused by infestation with *Pyemotes* (*Pediculoides*) *ventricosus*. The name is presumed to come from the handling of copra, dried coconut meat, which is infested by the mites. See also *grain itch, grocer's itch* and *vanillism.*

corium [kōʹrĭ-əm, kôrʹĭ-əm, -ē-əm] is the classical Latin word for skin, hide, shell, leather and bark. We now apply the word to that portion of the skin, in situ or excised, that is below the epidermis. *Cutis vera,* or *true skin, derma* and *dermis* are used interchangeably with *corium.*

corn [kôrn] derives from Latin *cornu,* horn. The word is applied particularly to the characteristic hyperkeratoses that form over interphalangeal joints, especially of the toes. See *callositas, callosity, callus* and *clavus.*

corn, soft, describes macerated hyperkeratosis at points of friction and pressure in intertriginous places. The sides of the last and penultimate toes are most common sites for the formation.

corneum [kôrʹnē-əm] and **corneus** [-əs] are respectively the neuter and the masculine singular of the Latin adjective *corneus,* meaning horny. They are found in titles like *stratum corneum,* the horny layer, and *lichen corneus hypertrophicus.*

cornification [kôrʹnĭ-fĭ-kāʹshən, -nə-fĭ-kāʹshən] is alternate for *keratinization,* meaning a conversion into horn or horny tissue.

cornoid lamella [kôrʹnoid lə-mĕlʹə] is the English translation of Mibelli's Italian term for the plate (*lamella*) of faulty horn or keratin (*cornoid*) that one sees in the histopathology of porokeratosis. There is a tendency to misread the first word of the term as "coronoid," which would mean "like a crown." That, however, was not intended by Mibelli, although it could have been so coined to designate the clinical lesion as a crownlike plate, which fits the fact somewhat.

cornu cutaneum [kôrʹnū, -nōō kū-tāʹnē-əm]. *Cornu* is the Latin word for horn, horny skin and excrescence. *Cornu cutaneum* describes and names a type of hyperkeratosis that takes the shape of a miniature horn. The well-developed process may be developed upon a precancerosis or be a horny formation upon an already established squamous-cell epithelioma.

corona veneris [kə-, kō-rōʹnə vĕnʹĕr-, vēʹnə-rĭs] means crown (*corona*) of sexual lust (*veneris*). The term has been picturesquely applied to syphilitic lesions that are seated on the brow and seem to circle it. Such an effect is said to occur sometimes in Moslems who are infected with syphilis. The likely reason for it is interesting. Moslems pound their heads on the ground in prayer toward Mecca. Should they do this during a stage of spirochetemia, the practice results in crush or rupture of fine blood vessels in the skin of the brow, release of treponemata into the tissues and thence development of clinical lesions. The event is an interesting illustration of the Koebner phenomenon within a situation of known cause and known injury.

corporis [kôr'pō-rĭs, -pô-rĭs, -pə-rĭs] is the genitive singular of Latin *corpus*, body, and means of the body. It appears in a title like *tinea corporis*.

corps rond [kôr' rông'] is a French term meaning round body. *Corps ronds* are degenerated epithelial cells found in keratosis follicularis that have lost their prickles, become rounded, have developed what appears to be a membrane and contain cytoplasm that is clear or peppered with keratohyalin granules.

corymbiform [kə-rĭm', kŏr-, kŏr-ĭm'bĭ-fôrm] is a word used to describe a group of lesions that looks like (*-form*) a cluster of flowers (*corymbi-*). The appearance is seen in syphilis and diseases of that class.

cosmetic [kŏz-mĕt'ĭk], derived from a Greek word meaning skilled in adornment or arrangement, means, when used as an adjective, pertaining or relating to qualities of beauty. When used as a noun, it denotes a material used for beautification.

cosmetologist [kŏz'mə-tŏl'ə-jĭst] designates an artisan who practices "beauty" treatments. *Beautician* (coined on analogy with *physician*) is an alternate word. Another related word is *cosmetician* (also formed on analogy with *physician*), one who is skilled in the use of cosmetics and practices make-up treatments.

cosmetology [kŏz'mə-tŏl'ə-jē] means the study of the body beautiful and practices thereto appertaining. The word derives from Greek *kosmetos*, well-arranged, ultimately from *kosmos*, order, harmony, the world, the universe. From so lofty an origin, as a practical matter, it comes down to the art of painting, powdering and perfuming skin, manicuring and painting nails, cutting and arranging scalp hair and performing other activities that sometimes verge on the frivolous. In modern dermatology and plastic surgery, correction of scars, removal of unsightly benign excrescences, liposuction, transplantation of scalp hair and epilation of coarse facial hairs of women are reasonable and feasible cosmetic practices.

Cowden's disease (multiple hamartoma syndrome) autosomal dominant. Very striking facial papules, trichilemmomas, nodules, thyroid goiter and acral keratoses. More than one-third of the patients develop malignancies. Breast and thyroid cancer are well documented.

cowpox [kou′pŏks′] is the lay term for *vaccinia*. *Pox* derives from Middle English where it had the meaning of bag, pouch or puffed cheek. *Cowpox* as a word probably arose because of its contagiosity from cows rather than from essential similarity to the cattle form of the disease.

crab louse [krăb, krâb lous] is a vernacular designation for *Phthir* (*i*) *us pubis*, the cause of phthiriasis (crabs).

crabs [krăbs, krâbs] is vernacular for *phthiriasis*, or *pediculosis pubis*, the infestation with *Phthir* (*i*) *us pubis* (crab louse). The physical appearance of this louse is like that of a miniature crab.

cradle cap [krā′d'l kăp] is vernacular for *seborrhea capitis* or *seborrheic dermatitis of the scalp* as seen in newborns and infants. The collection of inspissated sebum and scale gives the impression of a cap upon an inflamed scalp.

craquelé [krăklā′] is the past participle of a French verb that means to crack. *Craquelé*, meaning marred with cracks, is used to describe the appearance of a superficial inflammatory dermatosis that is marked on its scaling surface with cracks such as form in old china and ceramic tiles. It appears in the title *eczema craquelé*.

cream, as a pharmaceutical form, designates a topical preparation that "vanishes." For cosmetic use, see *cold cream*. In more sensible use, small percentages of highly active ingredients, e.g., adrenocorticosteroids, are incorporated in creams, which may be formulated from carbowaxes, dispersed mineral oil or cholesterolized petrolatum.

creeping eruption [ē-rŭp′shən] is vernacular for *larva migrans*, a cutaneous helminthiasis in which a larva (usually of *Ancylostoma brasiliense*) burrows in a channel within the epidermis and gets nowhere, to the great discomfort of the host.

crines. See *crinis*.

crinis [krī′nĭs, krĭn′ĭs] is a Latin word meaning the hair (any hair) collectively. Rarely was *crinis* used to denote a single hair, unlike the English word *hair*, which can refer to one hair or the hair collectively. *Crines* [krī′nēz, krĭn′ēz] the nominative plural of *crinis*, and *crinium* [krī′nĭ-əm, krĭn′ē-əm], genitive plural, meaning of the hair, also have a collective force. Thus, there exist the terms *crinis capitis* (hair of the head), *crinis pubis* (hair of the pubes), and *fragilitas crinium* (brittleness of the hair).

Other Latin words for *hair* used in medical terms are *capilli*, genitive singular and nominative plural of *capilus*, *capillitii*, genitive singular of *capillitium*, a Late Latin word meaning the hair collectively, and *pili* and *pilorum*, the genitive singular (also nominative plural) and genitive plural respectively of *pilus*, a hair. *Capillus* refers only to the hair of the head, whereas *pilus*, like *crinis*, refers to any hair. Moreover, only *pilus* was commonly used to denote a single hair and both the singular and plural of *pilus* and *capillus* were used collectively.

crinium. See *crinis.*

Cronkhite-Canada syndrome [krŏnk′hīt; kăn′ə-də]. Diffuse gastrointestinal polyposis associated with onychodystrophy, alopecia, and hyperpigmentation of the skin.

cross sensitization [krŏs sĕn′sĭ-tĭ-zā′shən, -tĭ-zā′shən] refers to the phenomena of immunologic response to several chemically or immunologically related substances after sensitization has been established to any one of them. Apparently the phenomenon depends on antibody direction to a radical fraction common to several antigens.

CRST syndrome [sĭn′drōm]. It is intended to be descriptive and mnemonic of a melange of findings in some cases that would otherwise be designated *acrosclerosis* or *scleroderma*. The capital letters stand for the histologic finding of **c**alcification and the clinical signs of **R**aynaud's phenomenon, **s**cleroderma and **t**elangiectasis. The combination of letters cannot be pronounced as a word unless, practicing epenthesis, one voices it as *crest.*

crud, the crud [krŭd] sound as if they were respectively a slang word and term of recent coinage. Actually, *crud* is labeled dialectal and substandard, but it is believed to go back to Middle English *curd,* the partner of *whey* in cheese making. As it is bandied about today, the word *crud* has come to be applied to filth, refuse, something unwanted, and also to indispositions that are vague or difficult to designate exactly—a usage that has come in particularly around World War II. (There is also ground for believing that the word is merely army slang, without accountable origin. Another theory is that it is derived from Welsh *kryd,* meaning a fever or plague. All in all, it is difficult to see the relation of the present meanings of *crud* to *curd,* the coagulated part of milk.)

In dermatologic "slanguage," pyodermas and fungous infections, particularly in intertriginous spaces, are frequently referred to as *crud* by racy young folk who are equally apt to tell the doctor, "Never mind all that jazz, man, just get with it and let's go, man." Interns and residents are also likely to use the word to designate symptoms and signs of any organ that are full of portent but will likely come to nothing. In short *crud* comes to some tongues like the word *junk* and some other even more indelicate four-letter words to express hopefully trivial or minor, but irksome, conditions, that are "full of sound and fury, signifying nothing."

cruris [kroō'rĭs] is the genitive of the Latin word *crus*, the leg or shank. In dermatologic terminology it means of the thigh, particularly the upper portion of the thigh. It appears in the type of title that specifies location, e.g., *tinea cruris.*

crust [krŭst] derives from Latin *crusta*, bark, shell, hard surface of a body. In descriptive dermatology the word is applied to inspissated serum on the surface of a lesion. Compare *scab* and *scale.*

cryo- [krī'ō] is a combining form from Greek meaning cold.

cryoglobulin [krī'ō-glŏb'ū-lĭn] refers to abnormal serum globulins that precipitate upon chilling to temperatures that do not precipitate normal globulins.

cryoglobulinemia [krī'ō-glŏb'ū-lĭ-nē'mē-ə, -mĭ-ə] designates the condition (*-ia*) in which cryoglobulin is present in the blood (*-em-*).

cryotherapy [krī'ō-thĕr'ə-pē, -pī] designates treatment (*-therapy*) by refrigerants or refrigeration (*cryo-*). Ordinary ice, liquid ethyl chloride, liquid nitrogen, dichlorofluoromethane (Freon) and solid carbon dioxide are common agents; contact application and spraying are the usual methods of use.

cryptococcosis [krĭp'tō-kŏ-kō'sĭs] designates the condition (*-osis*) of infection with cryptococcus (ordinarily *C. neoformans*). *Torulosis* and *European blastomycosis* are alternate terms.

A systemic mycosis due to cryptococcus neoformans. A great majority of cases are pulmonary due to inhalation of the spores. It sometimes hematologically disseminates to the skin. Skin lesions may be in almost any form, ulcers, nodules, papules, acneform, herpetic-like or pyodermatitis.

For diagnosis india ink preparations will show the distinctive capsule, culture, latex agglutination test or animal inoculation.

Ketoconazole and amphotericin B are the drugs of choice. (Tomecki et al)

Cryptococcus [krĭp'tō-kŏk'əs] is a genus of fungi. The word itself, a New Latin formation from Greek word elements, means hidden (*crypto-*) grain, seed or berry (*-coccus*). The plural of *coccus* is *cocci*, which is pronounced kŏk'sī in the English manner or, by those who prefer the Latin way, kŏk'ē, and by still others, who take a squint-eyed view of these matters, kŏk'ī. See comments under *flaccid.*

Cryptococcus neoformans [nē′ō-fôr′mănz] is a pathogenic species of *Cryptococcus* that causes a severe infection of skin, lungs and meninges that is also designated as *European blastomycosis*. *Neoformans* is a New Latin present participle used as an adjective and literally meaning new- (*neo-*) -shaping or -forming (*-formans*). The word may also mean forming (something) new. See *neoformans*.

cryptotrichotillomania [krĭp′tō-trĭk′ō-tĭl′ō-mā′nē-ə, -nĭ-ə, -nyə] designates the psychopathy (*-mania*) in which hairs (*-tricho-*) are plucked (*-tillo-*) and swallowed (*crypto-*, hidden). Trichobezoars (hair balls) could be a complication.

culicosis [kū′lĭ-kō′sĭs] designates the condition (*-osis*) caused by bites of mosquitoes (*culic-*, from Latin *culex*, gnat).

cuniculus [kū-nĭk′ū-ləs] in Latin means a rabbit or its burrow. In dermatology, the housing in the stratum corneum of a scabietic mite and possibly that of a migrating larva (e.g., *Ancylostoma brasiliense*) is called a cuniculus. *Burrow*, *channel* and *gallery* are alternate words.

curet, curette, curettage [kū′rĕt′; kū′rə-täzh′, kū̄ rĕt′ĭj] are words derived from a French verb (*curer*) meaning to clean. *Curette*, or the shortened English form *curet*, then literally means a cleanser, and *curettage* means a cleansing, or a cleansing operation. Medically, a curet(te) is the common instrument that scrapes away tissue, and curettage is the operation so performed.

Cushingoid facies [kōōsh′ĭn-goid]. The mooning of the face in Cushing's disease and in adrenocorticosteroid therapy when dosage is high.

Cushing's disease [kōōsh′ĭng]. Hyperpituitarism and hyperadrenalism caused by functioning adenomas of the glands.

Cushing's syndrome due to overproduction of adrenocortical hormone cortisol. May be due to hyperplasia of the adrenal cortex and/or tumor. Clinical features are round or moon face, buffalo hump, acne, abdominal striae, hypertension, hirsutism in females, amenorrhea and psychic disturbances.

cutanea [kū-tā′nē-ə], **cutaneum** [kū-tā′nē-əm] and **cutaneus** [kū-tā′nē-əs] are respectively the feminine, neuter and masculine singular forms of a Medieval Latin adjective meaning of or pertaining to the skin. The words appear in the titles *porphyria cutanea tarda*, *cornu cutaneum* and *nodulus cutaneus*.

cutaneous [kū-tā′nē-əs] is the English adjective derived from *cutaneus* and means of or pertaining to the skin.

cutaneous horn is a title for a characteristic hyperkeratosis shaped to a reasonable facsimile of a miniature horn. See *cornu cutaneum.*

cutaneous nodule [nŏd′ūl, nōj′ool] is a title for a collection of histiocytes in the skin that results in a characteristic hard papule of pea-size or thereabouts. The arms and legs are common sites for the process. *Dermatofibroma, histiocytoma* and *nodulus cutaneus* are alternate designations.

cutaneous tag. See *acrochordon.*

cutem [kū′tĕm] is the Latin accusative (corresponding to the English objective) singular of *cutis.* The word appears in the title *hyperkeratosis follicularis et parafollicularis in cutem penetrans.*

cuticle [kū′tĭ-k′l] means a little (-*cle*, diminutive) skin (*cuti-*), i.e., a thin, fine, slight or tiny integument. In dermatology and in lay talk, the eponychium is referred to by the word.

cutis [kū′tĭs] is taken directly from Latin. In itself the word should mean the entire skin, but it is frequently used interchangeably with *corium, derma* and *dermis*, especially as *cutis vera* (true skin), to refer to skin devoid of epidermis. The genitive singular of the word is the same and appears in titles like *tuberculosis cutis.*

cutis anserina [ăn′sə-, ăn′sēr-ī′nə, ăn′sĕ-rī′nə]. See *gooseflesh.*

cutis laxa [lăk′sə] describes skin that is redundant or excessive so that it hangs loosely rather than fits tightly.

Also known by **dermatochalasis** and **elastolysis,** or **dermatomegaly,** it results in loose hanging skin and may be either congenital or acquired. Due to defective elastic fibers. May also affect internal organs, resulting in severe medical problems, e.g., diverticulosis and emphysema.

cutis marmorata [mär′mō-rā′tə, -rä′tə] describes skin that looks like marble (*marmorata*) in its mottling of normal color, conspicuous veining and dilatation of small vessels.

cutis rhomboidalis nuchae [rŏm′boi-dā′lĭs, -dä′lĭs, -dăl′ĭs noo′-, nū′kē] describes a condition on the posterior aspect of the neck (*nuchae*) in which the skin, seemingly hypertrophied, is traversed by deep grooves that form roughly drawn rhomboids and other irregular geometric figures as they crisscross. It is an aspect of degenerative change as occurs with aging and actinism.

cutis vera [vē′rə] means true skin. See *corium.*

cutis verticis gyrata [vûr′tĭ-sĭs jī-, jĭ-rā′tə, -rä′tə] describes a condition of the skin on the vertex of the scalp and thereabouts in which markedly hypertrophied skin is thrown into folds and turns (*gyrata*) giving the appearance of cerebral convolutions or the puzzled expression of a bulldog's pate.

cyan(h)idrosis [sī′ăn-(h)ĭ-drō′sĭs], **cyanohidrosis** [sī′ə-nō-hĭ-drō′sĭs] describe the condition (-*osis*) in which sweat is colored dark blue or purple (*cyano-*).

cyanosis [sī′ə-nō′sĭs] describes a condition (-*osis*) of the skin or any other organ that is dark blue or purple (*cyan-*) from venous congestion.

cylindroma [sĭl′ĭn-drō′mə] is applied to a characteristic neoplasia of epidermal (adnexal) elements, usually on the scalp, that gives appearances that have been picturesquely dubbed *turban* or *tomato tumors*. The cylindric idea derives from the circle of hyalinization seen around masses of epithelial proliferation in histologic preparations.

A tumor in which differentiation probably is in the direction of apocrine structures.

cyst [sĭst] derives from Greek through New Latin from words that mean a sac or bladder. A circumscribed, walled process that is not inflamed and that contains air, fluid or solid matter is a cyst.

cyst, dermoid [dûr′moid]. See *dermoid.*

cyst, desmoid [dĕz-, dĕs′moid]. See *desmoid.*

cyst, epidermal [ĕp′ĭ-dûr′məl, -m′l]. See *epidermal.*

cyst, epidermoid [ĕp′ĭ-dûr′moid]. See *epidermoid.*

cyst, myxoid [mĭk′soid]. See *myxoid.*

cyst, sebaceous [sē-, sə-bā′shəs]. See *sebaceous.*

cystic [sĭs′tĭk], **cystica** [sĭs′tĭ-kə] and **cysticum** [sĭs′tĭ-kəm] are respectively an English adjective and the feminine and neuter singular of a New Latin adjective meaning relating to a cyst. The classicized forms appear in terms like *acne cystica* and *epithelioma adenoides cysticum.*

-cyte [sīt] and **cyto-** [sī′tō] are combining forms from a Greek word for cell. The first appears in words like *leukocyte* and the second in the following entry.

cytodiagnosis [sī′tō-dī′əg-nō′sĭs, -ăg-nō′sĭs] designates a procedure of diagnosis by examination of smears of shed or loosened cells. In dermatology the name of Tzanck (Tzanck test) is associated with a method of obtaining cells from blisters (of viral diseases, pemphigus and other bullous conditions), staining them in a simple manner and reading for distinctive characteristics. In oncology the name of Papanicolaou (Pap test) is attached to the reading for malignancy of cells shed from mucous surfaces. In special laboratory procedures like the study of bone marrow, and in general pathology, readings restricted to cellular qualities could be designated by the word.

D

D. The capital letter is sometimes used as an identifier, e.g., vitamin D.

dacto-, dactyl(o)- [dăk′tō, dăk′tĭ-lō] are combining forms from Greek specifying a digit (finger or toe). General medical dictionaries carry a large number of words in a needless duplication with both forms; *dactyl(o)*- should be preferred because it, not *dacto*-, contains the full stem of the source word. Two formations, common and useful in dermatology, are *dactylitis* and *dactyloylsis spontanea*.

dactylitis [dăk′tĭ-lī′tĭs] means inflammation (*-itis*) of a digit (*dactyl-*). Precession by a modifying word like *septic, syphilitic, tuberculous,* etc. is additionally informative when cause is known.

dander [dăn′dēr] is old dialectal English for scurf (scales) of the scalp. This word is not related to another *dander*, which is of uncertain, colloquial origin and means anger, as in "getting one's dander up."

dandruff [dăn′drəf] seems to be a dialectal combination of *dander* (scurf) and an old Norse word (*hrufa*) for a crust, scab or scale. It is not a good word for dermatologic terminology unless one wishes to limit its meaning merely to visible scaling that is not associated with disease. The laity uses the word for any degree of scaling of the scalp that is appreciable in the mirror, on the comb or on the clothes, and judges scaling of this sort as abnormal. The commercially motivated exaggeration of advertising matter promotes such misimpression. The "finger-nail test" (matter scratched off the scalp) is positive in everyone because the scalp has a naturally thick stratum corneum to yield scale when scratched. A certain amount of scaling from the scalp is normal, as it is from the rest of the body surface; the hair of the scalp, especially a lot of it, as on women, mechanically retains scale. Even seemingly excessive scaling (pityriasis or seborrhea sicca) may be normal for some persons. Scaling of the scalp can hardly be judged abnormal unless redness (inflammation) or other changes of skin or hair and possibly itching accompany the scaling. In the latter instances, seborrheic dermatitis, psoriasis and tineas enter into differential diagnoses.

Darier's disease [dăryāz′ dĭ-, də-zēz′]. See *keratosis follicularis*.

Darier's disease, sign [däryä′]. The diseases are several: keratosis follicularis, erythema annulare centrifugum, pseudoxanthoma elasticum; the sign is whealing of a lesion of urticaria pigmentosa upon rubbing of it.

Darier's sign is urtication of the skin or whealing from rubbing darkened lesions of urticaria pigmentosa.

Darier-Roussy sarcoid [däryä; roosē′]. Sarcoidosis of subcutaneous tissue.

darkfield microscopy. Preformed on a fresh serum specimen usually obtained by touching a glass coverslip to a chancre or suspected chancre and examining the specimen for motile "corkscrew" spirochetes, using a microscope fitted with a darkfield condenser. This is an indispensable necessity for proper immediate diagnosis of primary syphilis.

de- [dē, dĕ, də] is a prefix taken from Latin meaning from, down, reversing and away. In some words it has purely intensive force.

decalvans [dē-kăl′vănz] is a Latin present participle meaning becoming bald (-*calvans*). The prefix *de-* is intensive in this word, which appears in the title *folliculitis decalvans*.

decalvant [dē-kăl′vənt] is the English equivalent of *decalvans*. It may also be applied to an agent or agency that causes loss of hair.

decubital [dē-kū′bĭ-təl] relates to being bedded down. See *decubitus*. *Decubital ulcer* is seen in print and heard in speech less often than *decubitus ulcer*.

decubitus [dē-kū′bĭ-təs] is a New Latin noun formation from the verb *decumbere* meaning to lie down, to be bedded down or to lie ill. *Decubitus*, therefore, means the recumbent position or, as Webster's Second puts it, "an attitude assumed in lying down." See *bedsore*.

decubitus ulcer [ŭl′sēr, -sər] designates that loss of substance (skin and underlying structures) that results from prolonged or forced sojourn in bed, especially during debilitating diseases and most especially from those occasioned or accompanied by neuropathies.

degeneration [dĭ-, də-, dē-jĕn′ēr-ā′shən, -ər-ā′shən] designates the result (-*ion*) of descent (-*generat-*) from (*de-*) what is the proper state (Latin *genus, generis*, kind, race). In dermatology the greatest use of the word is in connection with histopathology where degenerations are specified as *amyloid, basophilic, colloid, fatty, fibrinous, granular, hyaline, mucinous, myxomatous*, etc.

Degos's disease [dəgōs] Malignant atrophic papulosis; Degos's original article is entitled *Dermatite papulosquameuse atrophiante* which translates as atrophying papulosquamous dermatitis.

delayed hypersensitivity, cell-mediated hypersensitivity. See *hypersensitivity reactions.*

delayed reaction [dē-lād′ rē-ăk′shən] is a term used in immunologic contexts to describe a response to a test with an allergenic or antigenic substance, or, following administration of such a substance, a clinical event that occurs within days (one to three). These are T cell mediated phenomenon.

delusion of parasitosis [dē-loo′zhən ŏv păr′ə-sĭ-tō′sĭs] is a phrase that describes a psychopathology in which there is an unwarranted conviction of infestation with metazoal parasites. *Acarophobia,* which literally means fear of (infestation with) mites, is used synonymously and with the extended sense of infestation with any "animal" parasite.

   A psychopathological condition in which there is an unwarranted conviction of infestation with parasites. A "monosymptomatic hypochondriasis occurring in an obsessional personality." (Tullett)

d'emblée [dängblā′] is an involved French adverbial phrase with meanings like at once, then and there, right off, straightaway. It is attached to the titles of processes that appear, or are recognized, with unexpected suddenness when the normal expectation is that such processes will appear slowly, or be recognized only at long last, e.g., *syphilis d'emblée, mycosis fungoides d'emblée.*

demodectic [děm′ə-, děm′ō-děk′tĭk] is an adjective meaning related to or pertaining to the genus of mites named *Demodex.*

demodectic mange [mānj] is the title for infestation of an animal with species-specific mites of the genus *Demodex,* e.g., *canis,* of the dog; *equi,* of the horse. Infestation of human beings to a symptomatic degree with *Demodex folliculorum* is termed *demodicidosis.* The latter word can just as well be applied to demodectic infestation of animals "lower" than man. *Mange* derives from an Old French word, *mangeue,* an itch, and ultimately from *manger,* to eat.

Demodex [děm′-, děm′ō-děks] names a genus of ticks or mites. From its Greek word elements the word means "fat worm."

Demodex folliculorum [fŏl-ĭk′-, fə-, fō-lĭk′ū-lō′rəm, -lôr′əm] names the mite that obligatorily infests the pilosebaceous follicle of human beings, usually harmlessly.

demodicidosis [dĕm′ō-dĭs′ĭ-dō′sĭs] and **demodicosis** [dĕm′ō-dĭ-kō′sĭs] are equal titles that designate infestation of pilosebaceous follicles of human beings with *Demodex folliculorum* in a manner that gives rise to signs (of inflammation) and symptoms (of itching or pain). Asymptomatic infestation, which is common enough, if not inevitable, is not, but could literally, be so designated. See *demodectic mange* and *mite infestations.*

Dennie-Morgan sign [dā′nā; môr′g'n] A characteristic groove in the lower lids of individuals with atopic dermatitis.

dental fistula [dĕn′t'l fĭs′tū-lə] and **dental sinus** [sī′nəs] are terms applied to that event in which an infectious process about a tooth channels to the outside, usually through the skin over the mandible. The appearance of the skin over the direction of travel is that of an inflammatory papule or tumor, or if a point of exit has already occurred, then of a pustule, an abscess with intermittent discharge or granulation tissue raggedly epithelized. Pyogenic bacteria are the usual micro-organisms that cause the phenomena. Actinomycosis as it appears on the skin from an internal focus, especially around teeth (lumpy jaw), and tuberculosis cutis colliquativa (scrofuloderma) are comparable processes. The terms *dental fistula* and *dental sinus* are not precisely apt because the tooth location and the pathway are but incidental; any abscess interiorly located tends to force an exit by creating a channel. Then the patency of the path and the nature of the infecting micro-organism decide the developing clinical appearance and the outcome of the event.

A cutaneous draining sinus tract involving the lower jaw due to an odontogenic etiology.

denudation [dĕn′ū-, dē′nū-dā′shən], as a general word, means the act or result (*-ion*) of making utterly (*de-*, intensive) bare or naked (*-nudat-*). With reference to the skin itself, total removal of the epidermis and exposure of the corium comes to a denudation; for the body, removal of the entire skin (integument) is described in the same way. The applicability of the word stems from the concept of the skin as an investiture.

deodorant [dē-ō′dĕr-ənt] as an adjective means removing of odor, and as a noun an agent that removes odor.

depigmentation [dē-pĭg′mĕn-tā′shən] as a general word means the act or result (*-ion*) of removing (*de-*) color (*-pigmentat-* from Latin *pigmentatus*, painted, related to *pigmentum*, paint). In dermatologic application, melanin is almost always the pigment implied because it is the principal natural pigment. However, there is nothing in the word that restricts it to melanin; removal of other pigments (bile salts, iron, carotin and tattoo materials) can be designated by the word.

depilate, depilation, depilatory [dĕp′ə-lāt; dĕp′ə-lā′shən; dē-pĭl′ə-tôr′ē, -ĭ, -tĕr-ē, -ĭ] are words relating to removal (*de-*) of hair (*-pil-*). There is nothing in the words to suggest means or manners of removal. There is a tendency to read into them chemical agents applied externally, but mechanical means, as well as internally administered, pilo-toxic agents, can depilate, cause depilation or be depilatory and depilatories. See *epilate, epilation, epilatory.*

Dercum's disease (adiposis dolorosa) [dĕr′kəm] soft subcutaneous rounded doughy growths, multiple lipomas composed of mature fat cells, which arise in adult life.

derm-, dermo- [dûrm; dûr′mō] are combining forms from the Greek word *derma*, skin (originally, hide). See *dermat-.*

derma [dĕr′-, dər′-, dûr′mə] derives from Greek and literally means the result of the action (*-ma*) of flaying (*der-*). It was originally applied to hide, i.e., the product resulting from flaying a dead animal.

-derma [dĕr′-, dər′-, dûr′mə], as an element of compound words like *anetoderma, erythroderma, pyoderma, scleroderma* and *xeroderma,* assumes the meaning of "an abnormal condition of the skin," the abnormality being defined by what precedes it, e.g., *aneto-*, slack; *erythro-*, red; *pyo-*, purulent; *sclero-*, hard; *xero-*, dry. French and German retain the more elaborate New Latin form *-dermia* (see below) or its modification, *-dermie.* British writers also show preference for *-dermia.* In any event *-derma* takes neuter singular Latin adjectives, e.g., *xeroderma pigmentosum,* whereas *-dermia* takes feminine forms, e.g., *erythrodermia desquamativa.*

dermabrasion [dûr′mə-brā′zhən] is new coinage for modern procedures in which skin (particularly epidermis) is removed in variable amounts or to variable depths by mechanical means (rapidly revolving wire brushes, diamond fraises and sandpaper). The word is an obvious wedding or blending of *derma* and *abrasion.*

Dermacentor [dûr′mə-sĕn′tər] is New Latin deriving from Greek elements meaning goader (*-centor*) of the skin (*derma-*). The word names a genus of ticks, members of which may cause an acariasis. While attached to skin and feeding upon tissue juices, species (such as *D. andersoni, variabilis* and *occidentalis*) of the genus are capable of transmitting, if they are carriers, the agent of Rocky Mountain spotted fever (*Rickettsia rickettsii*) and of tularemia (*Pasteurella tularensis*) and of causing the syndromes that are known as *tick* *paralysis* and *tick pyrexia*, probably by mechanisms of sensitization to products of their bodies.

dermal [dûr′məl] is an adjective from *derma* and means pertaining to skin. See *dermic*.

dermal-epidermal, or **dermo-epidermal, junction** [jŭnk′shən] refers to the line of meeting of epidermis and dermis.

Dermanyssus [dûr′mə-nĭs′əs] is a New Latin formation from Greek word elements meaning pricker (*-nyssus*) of the skin (*derma-*). The word names a genus of ticks, members of which are facultatively pathogenic to humans, e.g., *D. gallinae* (of fowl) may cause a human infestation that is called *gamasoidosis* (which see).

dermat-, dermato- [dûr′mət; dûr′mə-tō, dĕr-măt′ō-] are combining forms from the stem of the Greek word *derma*, skin, *dermatos*, of the skin. See *derm-*. The two forms, *derm*(*o*)- and *dermat*(*o*)-, give rise to a large number of words, frequently in useless synonymy, about which one is helpless.

dermatiaceous fungi are fungi which produce intrinsic melanin-like pigmentation, i.e., primarily chromoblastomycosis and phaeohyphomycosis. (Drutz)

dermatite [dârmătēt′] is the French word for *dermatitis*. The ending *-ite* is a French equivalent of *-itis*, as in *arthrite, bronchite*, etc.

dermatitic [dûr′mə-tĭt′ĭk] is a coined adjective recorded in Webster's Third New International Dictionary as meaning pertaining or relating to dermatitis.

dermatitides [dûr′mə-tī′tĭ-dēz, -tə-dēz] is the plural of *dermatitis*.

dermatitidis [dûr′mə-tī′tĭ-dĭs, -tə-dĭs] is the genitive in classical form of *dermatitis* derived by analogy with the declension of similar nouns taken into Latin from Greek. It thus means of dermatitis, and appears in the name of a fungus, to wit, *Blastomyces dermatitidis*.

dermatitis [dûr′mə-tī′tĭs, -tē′tĭs], if it had been an ancient Greek word, would have been an adjective and would have had the meaning, of the skin, i.e., cutaneous. It was not, however, an ancient Greek word but was coined later by analogy with those Greek words that are now transliterated as *arthritis, nephritis, pleuritis* and *r*(*h*)*achitis*, which were indeed ancient Greek adjectives meaning respectively, of the joints, of the kidneys, of the pleura and of the spine.

dermatitis artefacta [är′tə-, är′tē-făk′tə], or **factitia** [făk-tĭsh′ə], names the condition in which the skin is injured by mechanical, physical or chemical means (scratching with fingernails or instruments, applications of chemicals, etc.). *Artefacta* and *factitia* carry ideas of "man-made" for a purpose; in this instance, an unworthy purpose. There is an implication of psychopathic motivation (masochism, malingering) in the common use of the terms. They may be used to specify ordinary injuries of the skin if the implication of psychopathy is disavowed by context.

dermatitis exfoliativa neonatorum [ĕks'fō-lĭ-ə-tī'və nē'ō-nə-tō'rəm] names a scaly (*exfoliativa*) inflammatory condition of the skin (*dermatitis*) of infants (*neonatorum*) that is thought by some to be a severe pyoderma.

dermatitisfacitia. See *dermatitis artefacta.*

dermatitis herpetiformis [hər-, hûr'pĕt-ĭ-fôr'mĭs] names a condition which is characterized by, among other things, grouped vesicles that resemble (*-formis*) the vesicular clusters of herpes simplex (*herpeti-*). Those other things are severe pruritus as a symptom, other lesions that are edematous plaques, sites of predilection like the scalp, shoulders, small of the back and extensor aspects of the arms, and a course of great chronicity. Often associated with a gluten-sensitive enteropathy. Dietary restrictions may make a remarkable improvement in the disease. Treated with dapsone or sulfapyridine. IgA in a granular pattern in the dermal papillae in normal skin is specific and pathognomonic for dermatitis herpetiformis.

dermatitis medicamentosa [mĕd'ĭk-ə-mĕn-tō'sə] is still heard but is being displaced by *drug eruption.* The number of drugs that can cause skin changes, the variety of clinical appearances that can occur from drug causes, the complex mechanisms of such dermatoses and the extensive study these phenomena are now receiving make *dermatitis medicamentosa* a little too simple or quaint as a title.

Better known as drug eruption or drug hypersensitivity. This is a very common finding usually presenting as a generalized maculopapular, morbilliform or urticarial eruption. The causes are legion. A detailed drug history with dates given and date of rash onset are imperative in arriving at a correct determination of the offending drug or agent.

dermatitis papillaris capillitii [păp'ĭ-lā'rĭs, -lä'rĭs, -lär'ĭs kăp'ə-lĭsh'ĭ-ī] names a characteristic dermatosis on the nape of the neck that is marked by inflammation and by keloidal papules (*papillaris*, of the nature of little swellings) that seem to form around hairs (*capillitii*, of the hair, the hairy coat). *Folliculitis keloidalis* and *keloid acne* are used as alternate titles.

dermatitis, primary irritant [prī'mə-rē, -mĕr-ē, -ĭ ĭr'ĭ-tənt, -ə-tənt], adequately describes an inflammatory condition of the skin whose cause is clearly a noxum that is inherently and indubitably injurious because of its physical or chemical properties.

This is an inflammatory condition of the skin not immunologically mediated but which results from direct injury of the skin due to the physical or chemical properties of the agent that comes in contact with the skin.

dermatitis repens [rē′pĕnz, rĕp′ənz] from Latin **repens, repentis,** past participle of **repo,** to creep **(acrodermatitis continua)** literally means a creeping (*repens*) dermatitis. It has been applied to some of the appearances that are within the scope of "racalcitrant pustular eruptions," particularly on hands and feet. Acrodermatitis continua, pustular psoriasis and atypical, persistent pyodermas enter into diagnostic consideration. In all respects, a condition that would be labeled *dermatitis repens* by some would be termed something else by others.

A crusty, eczematous exudative dermatitis seen on the fingers or toes, it starts as a small ulcer or paronychia and spreads. It has palmoplantar pustulosis and may involve the mouth. It appears to be closely associated with psoriasis.

dermatitis vegetans [vĕj′ə-, vĕj′ē-tănz] names a dermatitis that is tumid, lush or exuberant (*vegetans*). It is seen in intertriginous places and seems to be caused by mixed micro-organisms of obligatory or facultative pathogenicity. Pemphigus vegetans is always a differential diagnostic problem and is not to be confused with dermatitis vegetans.

dermatitis venenata [vĕn′ə, vĕn′ē-nā′tə, -nä′tə] is another old title that is fast becoming passé and justifiably so. The incorrect implication of inflammation of the skin caused by poisons or poisoning (*venenata*) is what is so bad about the designation. Dermatitis truly caused by poisons or primary irritants like strong acids, alkalies and organic toxins (snake and bee venoms, bacterial toxins) is not designated by this title; rather allergic eczematous contact dermatitis caused by sensitization to and provocation by simple chemicals that are not inherently poisonous or toxic has long been referred to as *dermatitis venenata*.

dermato-. See *dermat-*.

dermatocele [dûr′mə-tō-sēl′, dēr-măt′ō-sēl] literally means hernia or herniation (*-cele*) of the skin (*dermato-*). It is a rarely used word that may be employed to designate the appearance and feel of skin affected by some forms of atrophy, especially those designated *anetoderma*, a word which means slack skin and also carries the idea of hernia. *Dermatolysis* and *dermatochalasia* (*-chalasis*) are still other words that have somewhat synonymous sense.

dermatochalasia, -chalasis [dûr′mǝ-tō-kǝ-lā′zhē-ǝ, -zē-ǝ, -zhǝ; -kăl′ǝ-sĭs] means abnormal looseness or relaxation (*-chalasia, -sis*) of the skin (*dermato-*). The words are applied to the appearance of skin that hangs in folds as it does in cutis laxa and sometimes in neurofibromatosis. *Dermatolysis* and *dermatocele* are words with related meaning.

dermatofibroma [dûr′mǝ-tō-fĭ-brō′mǝ] is a hard tumor (*-fibroma*) of the skin. The word is used alternately with *cutaneous nodule, histiocytoma* and *nodulus cutaneus*.

dermatofibrosarcoma protuberans [dûr′mǝ-tō-fĭ-brō-mǝ-sär-kō′mǝ prō-tōō′-, prō-tū′bĕr-ănz, -bĕr-ănz, -bǝ-rănz] is a title for a malignant process in the skin which consists of the forming (*-ans*) of tough (*-fibro-*), fleshy (*-sarco-*) masses (*-tuber-*, a swelling, lump) that stick out (*pro-*, forward). A generous biopsy is required for correct diagnosis. Often difficult to eradicate.

dermatofibrosis lenticularis disseminata [dûr′mǝ-tǒ-fĭ-brō′sĭs lĕn-tik′ū-lā′rĭs dĭ-sĕm′ĭ-nā′tǝ] describes a rare cutaneous (*dermato-*) condition as consisting of widespread (*disseminata*) lenticular (*lenticularis*) papules that show fibrous thickening (*-fibrosis*) microscopically.

dermatoglyph, dermatoglyphic(s) [dûr′mǝ-tō-glĭf; -glĭf′ĭk(s)]. The word element *-glyph* - derives from a Greek verb meaning to carve. *Hieroglyphics* refers to the sacred writing of the ancient Egyptians that was literally carved on stone; *glyph* itself appears as a distinct word meaning a character or symbol incised or carved. In English the primary meaning of the word element is a channel or groove. A dermatoglyph, then, is a natural "carving" in the skin, i.e., a furrow or fold. All together, dermatoglyphics is the study of the surface characteristics of the skin with respect to its furrows, folds, wrinkles and ridges, or, in other words, its fine sculpturing, which is individually fixed. The adjective *dermatoglyphic*, a back-formation from *dermatoglyphics*, means pertaining or relating to dermatoglyphics. As a practical matter the business of fingerprints is the main interest of dermatoglyphics. Lately, the medical significance of dermatoglyphics has aroused a great deal of interest.

derma(at)ographia, derm(at)ographism [dûr′mǝ-tō-grăf′ē-ǝ, dûr′mō-grăf′ē-ǝ; dûr′mǝ-tǒg′rǝ-fĭz′m, dûr′mō-grăf′ĭz′m] are words that literally mean a writing (*-graphia, -graphism*) on the skin (*dermato-, dermo-*).

derm(at)ographia (-ism), black. *Black derm(at)ographia (-ism)* refers to the phenomenon in which blackish (gray-, green-black) streaks appear on skin that has been powdered and has metal (jewelry, clothing clasps) riding on it. Such streaks consist of metallic particles that are rubbed off and deposited on the skin when the metal is softer than the powders abrading it. One can draw up lists of powders (talcum, zinc oxide, titanium oxide, magnesium carbonate, etc.) and metals (gold, silver, copper, nickel, iron, platinum, etc.) according to a scale of hardness (in the physicist's sense of power to abrade) and predict which combination of powders and metals in abrasive position will produce black dermatographia (-ism).

derm(at)ographia (-ism), urticarial [ûr′tĭ-kâr′ē-əl]. *Urticarial derm(at)ographia (-ism)* designates the phenomenon of whealing in the precise form of application of moderate stroke, pressure or friction on the skin. A whiplash produces the effect, but the term is reserved for the abnormality of whealing upon physical force of a degree less than that which normally produces whealing.

derm(at)ographia (-ism), white. *White derm(at)ographia (-ism)* refers to the blanching that occurs upon stroke of skin affected atopic dermatitis when the process is erythematous and lichenified. It is particularly elicitable on the affected brow of patients in the adult phase of atopic dermatitis.

dermatohistopathology [dûr′mə-tō-hĭs′tō-pə-thŏl′ə-jē, -jĭ] is pretty obvious in its statement of study (*-logy*) of abnormal (*-patho-*) tissue (*histo-*) structure of the skin (*dermato-*). Histology, by traditional understanding, relates to fine (microscopic) structure since gross examination of tissue reveals so relatively little.

dermatologic(al) [dûr′mə-tō-lŏj′ĭk; (-əl)]. The interest of the two adjectival forms resides in the fine meaning of the suffixes *-ic* and *-ical*. In some words the suffixes make for sharply distinct meanings, e.g., *historic* and *historical, politic* and *political, economic* and *economical*, etc. If there is reason for two adjectival forms of nouns that end in *-logy*, then it must be in agreement that *-ic* relates matter specified by the root more closely, and *-ical* relates such matter more loosely or more remotely.

dermatologist [dûr′mə-tŏl′ə-jĭst] means one versed in matters relating to the skin.

dermatology [dûr′mə-tŏl′ə-jē] is the field of study (*-logy*) of everything that relates to the skin (*dermato-*) in health and disease. There is a growing tendency to use the word *dermatology* as an adjective in terms like *dermatology department, dermatology research.*

What is the good of it? There is a formal adjective *dermatologic* which has everything to recommend it.

dermatolysis [dûr′mə-tŏl′ĭ-sĭs, -ə-sĭs] literally means separation (*-lysis*) of the skin (*dermato-*), but what is meant is looseness or relaxation of the skin. *Dermatolysis* could also describe avulsion of a piece of skin or slough from a burn or from an infection, but is not used that way. See *dermatocele* and *dermatochalasia* for alternate words.

dermatome [dûr′mə-tōm] has two disparate meanings. In one sense, it names a machine for cutting (*-tome*) fine slivers of skin (*derma-*) such as are used in dermatohistopathology, plastic surgery and possibly tissue culture. In another sense, the word means a section, segment or cut (*-tome*) of skin (*derma-*) in terms of a part innervated by definable peripheral nerves.

dermatomycosis [dûr′mə-tō-mī-kō′sĭs] means a fungous infection (*-mycosis*) of the skin (*dermato-*). The word is exceedingly general; any fungous infection, superficial, deep and of any fungal cause, is so designated.

dermatomyositis [dûr′mə-tō-mī-ō-sī′tĭs] is the title of a condition in which the skin (*dermato-*), of the face particularly, and frequently of the neck and upper portion of the trunk, and the muscles (*-myos-*, genitive singular of *mys*, used in this word formation instead of the usual combining form *myo-*, probably for the sake of euphony) of the regions are inflamed (*-itis*). The precise cause and mechanism of the phenomenon are not known. An association with cancer in internal organs is common (50% or more) excepting the childhood variant where that does not hold. Proximal muscle weakness is characteristic as is periorbital swelling and purplish discoloration of the skin about the eyes known as a heliotrope.

dermatopathia pigmentosa reticularis is a pigmentary disorder. At about two years of age, fine pigmented macules develop and spread over the body in a net-like pattern. Histopathology: localized pigmentary incontinence in the dermis with clumps of melanin-laden macrophages are separated by pigment-free zones. (Rycroft et al)

dermatopathic lymphadenopathy [dĕr-măt′ō-, dûr′mə-tō-păth′ĭk lĭm-fad′ə-nŏp′ə-thē, -thĭ] literally means abnormality in the skin. The term is applied to enlargement of superficial lymph nodes in the groins, axillae and neck that frequently attends long enduring erythroderma.

dermatophyte [dĕr-măt′ō-, dûr′mə-tō-fīt′] designates a plant (*-phyte*) that is capable of infecting the skin (*dermato-*). The word is generally applied to those fungi that infect the skin exclusively and superficially, but there is nothing in the word to limit it that way.

dermatophyte test medium is a commercially available Sabouraud's agar with a dye that becomes activated, changing the color of the media, when dermatophytic fungi start to grow. Its use is not recommended. (RLC)

dermatophytid(e) [dēr-măt′ō-, dûr′mə-tō-fīt′ĭd, -ēd]. Many -*id*(*e*) words present philologic problems. Literally, the suffix (which see) relates things to a family or class. In the matter of *dermatophytid*(*e*), the word is incorrectly formed for the meaning it has. As it is, it should mean a member of the botanical class of dermatophytes; for what was intended, it should have been formed as *dermatophytosid*(*e*), i.e., comprehensive of any lesion of the skin within the capability of a superficial fungous infection. However, *dermatophytid*(*e*) is ingrained with the latter meaning and perhaps mycologists could yield it that way. Then, additionally, the common practice of dermatologic jargon is to reserve it for mycotic lesions that are "secondary," i.e., following upon a primary or persistent focus of fungal infection. Finally, an ascription of allergic mechanism attaches to the word, as though primary infection were not based on immunologic developments. Such are the vagaries of language.

dermatophytosis [dûr′mə-tō-fī-tō′sĭs], like *dermatomycosis*, names any fungous infection (-*phytosis*) of the skin (*dermato-*). There is a strong tendency to reserve the word for superficial fungous infections of the feet and hands. There is, however, nothing in the word to limit it that way. Fungous infections of the scalp and body generally are also properly designated *dermatophytoses*.

dermatopolyneuritis [dûr′mə-tō-pŏl′ē-nū-rī′tĭs, -rē′tĭs] is alternate for *acrodynia. Erythredema* and *pink disease* are synonymous titles. Each title tells something of the appearance of the condition, namely, a painful, reddish, swollen skin over acral areas.

dermatorrhexis [dēr-măt′ō-, dûr′mə-tō-rĕk′sĭs] literally means rupture (-*rrhexis*) of the skin (*dermato-*). The word might be used to describe fragility and scarring of the skin as it occurs in the Ehlers-Danlos syndrome, the process of formation of striae distensae and any other phenomenon in which the skin scars because it parts easily.

dermatoscopy [dûr′mə-tŏs′kō-pē, -kə-pē] simply means gross inspection or examination (-*scopy*) of the skin (*dermato-*) by eye.

dermatosis [dûr′mə-tō′sĭs] is a most generic word meaning a pathologic condition (-*osis*) of the skin (*dermat-*). It is also used in titles with modifying adjectives. One example follows:

dermatosis papulosa nigra [păp′ū-lō′sə nī′grə] names that condition in Blacks that consists of darker colored (*nigra*, black) conglomerates of papules (*papulosa*) on the nose and adjacent areas of the face. The papular units are composed of acanthotic epidermal proliferation with more melanin and some disordered over-development of pilosebaceous structures resembling seborrheic keratoses.

dermatosis, subcorneal pustular a mild form of generalized pustular psoriasis appears in middle-aged women and is characterized by superficial (subcorneal) pustules that form arcuate configurations on the skin surface (Patterson & Blaylock)

dermatothlasia (-sis) [dĕr-măt′ō-, dûr′mə-tō-thlā′zhē-ə, -zē-ə, -zhə; (-sĭs)] is a rare word that designates the compulsion and action of pinching or bruising (-*thlasia*) the skin (*dermato-*).

dermatotropic [dĕr-măt′ō-, dûr′mə-tō-trŏp′ĭk] literally means turning to or toward, attracted to or stimulating (-*trop-*) the skin (*dermato-*). The word is used to designate micro-organisms (viruses, fungi) that are particularly "attracted to" the skin in the sense of preferring to infect it rather than other organs. See *troph(o)-* and *trop(o)-* for fine distinctions.

-dermia [-dûr′mē-ə] is somewhat better, puristically, than -*derma* (which see) in compound words like *anetoderm(i)a, erythroderm-(i)a, pyoderm(i)a, scleroderm(i)a* and *xeroderm(i)a*. -*Dermia* clearly means a (pathologic) state or condition (-*ia*) of the skin (-*derm-*) and is widely used just so in England; in France and Germany it is also used as such or transliterated to -*dermie*. However, American practice favors -*derma* and that practice will probably become standard in time even in other lands. When modified by Latin adjectives, words ending in -*dermia* take the feminine singular form, e.g., *erythrodermia exfoliativa*, whereas words ending in -*derma* take the neuter singular form, e.g., *xeroderma pigmentosum*.

dermic [dûr′mĭk] is an adjective from *derma* and means relating to the skin.

dermis [dûr′mĭs] in Greek was a combining form only but came to be a word by itself in New Latin. In present-day common use, *dermis* refers to the corium alone; what is above or on it is distinctively named *epidermis*, which illustrates the ancient Greek use of -*dermis* as a combining form.

dermite [dârmēt'] is a French formation from *derm-* as a combining form meaning skin and with *-ite* as an element having an extended meaning of inflammation. It is odd that such a coinage was made and persists when *dermatite* is so much more current and better-known.

dermitis [dēr-, dûr-mī'tĭs, -mē'tĭs] is found in English medical and large general dictionaries as a synonym for *dermatitis*, but that's about all. Who ever utters it?

dermo-. See *derm-*.

dermo-epidermal junction [dûr'mō-ĕp'ĭ-dûr'məl jŭnk'shən] specifies the line of joining of *dermis* and *epidermis*. See *dermal-epidermal junction*.

dermographia (-ism) [dûr'mō-grăf'ē-ə, dēr-, dûr-mŏg'rə-fĭz'm]. See *derm(at)ographia (-ism)*.

dermoid [dûr'moid] means like (*-oid*) skin (*derm-*). The word is used in the following title.

dermoid cyst [sĭst] describes an encapsulated mass that contains ectodermal structures of epithelial, pilary, dental, neural and glandular elements in disorganized arrangement and incomplete formation. Admixed with mesodermal and endodermal elements, a frustration of twinning is conceivable.

dermopathy [dər-, dēr, dûr-mŏp'ə-thē] means a condition (*-y*) of fault or abnormality (*-path-*) in the skin (*dermo-*).

dermopathy, diabetic [dī'-ə-bē'tĭk, -bĕt'ĭk] is a concept developed to encompass lesions in diabetics that start clinically as multiple, small, round or oval, discrete macules or papules on the extensor surface of the extremities and progress through ulceration to pigmented scars or atrophic spots. Histologically, angiopathy of small vessels is seen.

dermotropic [dûr'mō-trŏp'ĭk]. See *dermatotropic*.

DeSanctis-Cacchione syndrome [dē-sănk'tĭs, cătch'ĭ-ō'ne]. Xeroderma pigmentosum with mental retardation, severe neuropathies, stunted growth, and other physical and functional anomalies. Xerodermic idiocy.

desensitize, desensitization [dē-sĕn'sĭ-tīz, -sə-tīz; dē-sĕn'sə- tī-zā'shən, -tī-zā'shən] refer to and denote the process and result of reducing sensitivity or rendering insensitive. The ready implication is restoration to original or natural insensitivity, a circumstance which probably never is the case.

desert sore [dĕz'ĕrt sôr]. See *Barcoo disease.*

desiccation [dĕs'ĭ-kā'shən] means a thorough (*de-*, intensive) drying out (*-siccation*). Aside from general uses, the word finds use in dermatology in connection with that electrosurgical procedure in which tissue is burned up to the point of carbonization by means of an instrument that operates on a high frequency, unidirectional current (Oudin) and yields concentrated heat in the form of a fine, controllable spark. The effect is a rapid boiling off of water and then oxidation of organic materials as in any conflagration.

desmo- [dĕz'-, dĕs'mō] is a combining form from a Greek word meaning to bind. It is used in medical terminology for things like ligamentous or fibrous structures that bind firmly, and consequently, it has acquired senses of toughness or hardness.

desmoid [dĕz'-, dĕs'moid] is applied to what is ligamentous, fibrous, tough or hard in quality.

desmoid cyst, or **tumor,** is sometimes applied to particularly hard fibromas.

desmolysis [dĕz-, dĕs-mŏl'ĭ-sĭs, -ə-sĭs] means dissolution (*-lysis*) of binding (*desmo-*) elements. The word is used to describe the melting away of intercellular bridges of prickle cells in processes like herpes and varicella.

desmorrhexis [dĕz'-, dĕs'mō-rĕk'sĭs] means rupture (*-rrhexis*) of binding (*desmo-*) elements. The word is used to describe disruption of intercellular bridges of prickle cells in processes that cause intra-epidermal bullae, particularly in pemphigus.

desmosome [dĕz'-, dĕs'mō-sōm], meaning a binding (*desmo-*) body (*-some*), names a point of multiple attachment of tonofibrils and intercellular bridges on epidermal cells.

desquamate, desquamation [dĕs'kwə-māt; -mā'shən] are respectively a verb and a noun relating to scales (*-squam-*), especially loose scales peeling away (*de-*), and mean to peel off and the act of peeling off. See *desquamativa.*

desquamativa, desquamativum [dē-skwăm'ə-tī'və; -vəm] are the feminine singular and the neuter singular respectively of a New Latin adjective formed from the past participle, *desquamatus*, of the Latin verb *desquamare*, to scale (*-squama-*) off (*de-*). The two forms, which therefore mean causing or attended by peeling, or scaling off, appear in the titles *erythrodermia desquamativa*, or *erythroderma desquamativum* (Leiner's disease).

desquamative [də-skwăm′ə-tĭv, dĕs′kwə-māt′ĭv], meaning causing or attended by peeling, is the English adjective corresponding to *desquamativa, -tivum.*

detergent [dĭ-, dē-tûr′jənt] is a word that is being sadly vitiated these days. Literally and as an adjective it means rubbing or wiping (*-tergent*) away (*de-*); as a noun it means an agent that does the job. It is thus a general word for a cleanser and encompasses water, ordinary soap, sandpaper and anything else that cleans by any means. Nowadays nearly everyone has been corrupted by advertising and uses the word to mean a cleanser of the order of the lauryl sulfates, and in a manner that excludes ordinary soap. It is becoming impossible to use *detergent* in its original or general senses.

detritus [dĭ-, də-, dē-trī′təs] is a direct borrowing of a Latin noun whose elements mean that which is rubbed (*-tritus*) off (*de-*). Thus scales, crusts, scabs, exudation and adventitious matter on the skin are *detritus* (the plural is the same form as the singular with a lengthening of the *u* in Latin).

DF2 septicemia is caused by the Gram-negative rod DF2 after a dog bite. A necrotic escar at the site of the bite is a prominent finding. These patients are gravely ill with severe septicemia. DIC (disseminated intravascular coagulation) and gangrene may supervene. Parenteral antibiotics are required for treatment. (Kalb R, et al., Am J Med 1985)

di-, dis- [dĭ, dī; dĭs, dĭz] are prefixes of Greek and Latin origin termed inseparable because they appear in combinations only. When of Greek origin, *di-* and *dis-* mean two, twice or double, e.g., *dimorphous*, of two forms; *dichromatic*, of two colors; *distichia*, double-rowed. When of Latin origin, these prefixes denote separation, negation, deprivation, opposite of, absence of, e.g., *divulse*, to pull apart, *dissect*, to cut apart, *dishonest*, not honest.

diabetic dermopathy. See *dermopathy, diabetic.*

diabeticorum [dī′ə-bĕt′ĭ-kō′rəm, -bē′tĭ-kôr′əm] means of diabetics. It occurs in the titles *necrobiosis lipoidica diabeticorum* and *xanthoma diabeticorum.*

diabetic ulcer [dī′ə-bĕt′ĭk, -bē′tĭk ŭl′sĕr, -sər] designates an ulcer in a person afflicted with diabetes and attributable to factors like vasculitis, arteriosclerosis, easy infectability operating in the disease and diabetic neuropathy.

diaper [dī′ə-pĕr, dī′pər] **dermatitis,** or **rash,** is another of those unsatisfactory titles like *athlete's foot, barber's itch* and *baker's dermatitis* that mislead more than inform. The condition is an intertrigo that has more to do with wetness, warmth and friction than with the diaper material per se. Comparable effects occur in the undiapered given enough provocation of the same mechanical and physical factors.

diascope [dī′ə-skōp] designates an instrument through (*dia-*) which to look, see or examine (*-scope*). In examination of the skin (dermatoscopy) any piece of firm, translucent material (glass, clear plastic) may be used to view the skin upon which it is pressed. Lesions that are obscured by erythema are then better seen in a momentarily dehematized condition; lesions that consist of functioning blood vessels may thus be made largely to disappear, whereas hemorrhages, pigmentations and cellular infiltrates persist.

diascopy [dī-ăs′kō-pē, -kə-pē, -pī] is the procedure of viewing the skin through a diascope.

diffusion of the lunula [dĭ-fū′zhən ŏv thə lōō′nyə-lə, lōō′nū- lə] describes a color change in a nail plate which leads to an obscuring of the sharp definition of the lunula. The effect is to make it appear as if the lunula has spread toward the free edge of the nail. The condition occurs in many onychodystrophies, particularly that one which occurs in leprosy.

diffusum [dĭ-fū′səm] is the neuter singular of a Latin adjective meaning widespread. It occurs in the title *angiokeratoma corporis diffusum*. (Fabry's disease).

DiGeorge syndrome. See *thymic hypoplasia*.

digitate [dĭj′ə-, dĭj′ī tāt], derived from Latin, means made into or shaped like (*-ate*) a finger (*digit-*).

digitate warts [wôrts] is descriptive of common warts as they appear on the face and other relatively protected places where they grow or develop finger-like shapes. *Filiform warts* is an alternate descriptive term. See *verruca digitata* and *verruca filiformis*.

dimorphous [dī-môr′fəs] derived from Greek, means of two (*di-*) forms (*-morph-*).

dimorphous leprosy [lĕp′rə-sē, - sī] is that type of leprosy that consists of clinical and histologic lepromatous and tuberculoid process simultaneously or concurrently in the same patient. *Borderline* and *intermediate* are alternate to *dimorphous*.

dimple [dĭm′p′l], a word of uncertain origin, is said to be perhaps a nasalized derivative of *dip*. Whatever its source, it is a common word for a small depression anywhere or of anything. Anatomically, the well-known depressions in the chin or cheeks of some individuals are dimples created by the pull of small bundles of striated muscles vertically oriented from the skin to some point of attachment subcutaneously.

diphtheria cutis [dĭp-, dĭf-thēr′ē-ə, -thĭr′ē-ə kūt′tĭs] is the title in classical form for diphtheritic infection of the skin. The process is an ulcer that contains *Corynebacterium diphtheriae*, the micro-organism of diphtheria (more abundantly early than later), and special characteristics in the form of a rolled edge, a dirty base, a tendency to bulla formation beyond the lesion, painfulness in the beginning and local hypesthesia later on.

dis-. See *di-, dis-.*

disciform [dĭs′kə-, dĭs′ĭ-fôrm] and **disciformis** [dĭs′kĭ-, dĭs′ĭ-fôr′mĭs] are an English and a New Latin adjective respectively, meaning flattish. The latter occurs in the title *granulomatosis disciformis et progressiva.*

discoid [dĭs′koid] means like (-*oid*) a disc. The word is widely used to describe lesions that are solid, round and moderately raised. It is also used in titles like *chronic discoid lupus erythematosus* and *distinctive exudative discoid* and *lichenoid chronic dermatosis.*

dissecting cellulitis [dĭ-, də-, dī-sĕkt′ĭng sĕl′ū-lī′tĭs, -lē′tĭs] **of the scalp** is an alternate title for *folliculitis et perifolliculitis abscedens et suffodiens.* In the entry title, ideas of diffuse inflammation (*cellulitis*) and undercutting (*dissecting*) are conveyed; in the other title, location (follicular and perifollicular), discharge (*abscedens*) and undermining (*suffodiens*, digging under) are told.

disseminated [dĭ-sĕm′ə-nāt′ĕd] means seeded (-*semin-*) afar (*dis-*, apart) and carries the idea of dispersion or widespread distribution.

disseminated intravascular coagulation. Also called consumption coagulopathy or defibrination syndrome, it represents complications in which the intrinsic and extrinsic coagulation systems are activated with resulting local and general escape of thrombin into the circulatory system. Fibrinogen is depleted and platelets are activated and deposited in the microcirculation leading to thrombocytopenia. The initial thrombotic phase is followed by a hemorrhagic disorder due to depletion of platelets and coagulation factors. Hemorrhage into skin and mucous membranes is followed by bleeding in other tissues and organs. Fibrinolysis ensues and degradation products formed by the action of plasmin appear as a secondary complication. (Aaron J. Marcus, *Cecil Textbook of Medicine*, 18th Edition, Wyngaarden & Smith, Editors, Saunders)

disseminated lupus erythematosus [lōō′pəs ĕr′ĭ-thĕm′ə-tō′səs, -thē′mə-tō′səs] describes lupus erythematosus in the form of new, dispersed lesions of the chronic, discoid variety. Under this predication, the title may mean merely more of chronic discoid lupus erythematosus or graduation into subacute, acute or systemic lupus erythematosus with all the added signs and symptoms within the possibilities of lupus erythematosus.

disseminated neurodermatitis [nū′rō-dûr′mə-tī′tĭs, -tē′tĭs] is a term used by some for widespread atopic dermatitis, especially the eczematized and lichenified form in the adult. Others use it for any eczematized and lichenified dermatitis that is widespread, chronic and of unknown cause. It is not a good title. See strictures under *neurodermatitis*.

disseminated superficial actinic porokeratosis [dĭ-sĕm′ə-nāt′ĕd sōō′pēr-fĭsh′əl pō′rō-kĕr′ə-tō′sĭs] describes a clinical and histologic appearance that is similar to Mibelli's porokeratosis, but related in cause to ultraviolet light. Multiplicity, widespread dispersion, and superficiality of lesions are also specified.

The most common form of four clinical variants of porokeratosis, it is characterized by multiple small lesions that appear on sun-exposed areas of the body during the third or fourth decades of life. It rarely occurs on the face. This condition frequently expresses itself in occupants of regions with intense doses of sun exposure and is commonly mistaken for solar keratosis. (Shumack and Commens, Disseminated superficial actinic porokeratosis: A clinical Study, JAAD, June 1989; 20:1015-1021).

disseminatum [dĭ-sĕm′ĭ-nā′təm, -nä′təm, -tŭm, -tōōm] and **disseminatus** [-təs, -tŭs, -tōōs] are respectively the neuter singular and the masculine singular of the perfect passive participle of the Latin verb *disseminare*, to scatter seed, to sow, and used as an adjective it means disseminated (which see). The neuter form appears in the title *xanthoma disseminatum*, the masculine, in *lupus miliaris disseminatus faciei*.

distichia, distichiasis [dĭs-tĭk′ē-ə, -ĭ-ə; -ĭ′ə-sĭs] designate an anomalous condition (-*ia*, -*iasis*) of eyelashes in which there is a double (*di-*) row (-*stich-*) of hairs on the eyelids. What makes the condition so special to name so distinctively is that one or both rows tend to turn toward the eyeballs with obvious serious consequences.

distinctive exudative discoid and **lichenoid chronic dermatosis** is the kind of title that forces an eponym or some other form of curtailment that is mnemonic. In this case, the eponym is *Sulzberger-*

Garbe disease and the mnemonic device is *oid-oid*. The clinical characteristics are severe pruritus, discoid lesions that tend to exude and lichenoid lesions that are of great chronicity. A penile lesion is common. Men are by far more commonly affected, and patients afflicted are commonly of a neurotic habitus.

diutinum [dī-, dǐ-ōō′-, dǐ-ū′tǐ-nəm] is the neuter singular of a Latin adjective meaning lasting for a long time. It occurs in the title *erythema elevatum diutinum*.

dolens [dō′lĕnz] is a Latin present participle meaning feeling pain, aching. It appears in the title *phlegmasia alba dolens*.

dolor [dō′lôr, -lēr, -lər] and **dolorosa** [dŏl′ə-, dō′lō-rō′sə], are respectively a Latin noun meaning pain, sorrow, and the feminine singular of a Latin adjective meaning literally full of (*-osa*) pain, and sorrowful. The adjective appears in the title *adiposis dolorosa*.

The word *dolorosa* has long been familiar through its appearance in two expressions, *Mater Dolorosa* (The Sorrowful Mother), which is found in the first line of one of the greatest of all medieval hymns, *Stabat Mater*, and *Via Dolorosa* (The Sorrowful Road). The former expression refers, of course, to Mary, and the latter to the journey of Christ from the judgment-seat of Pontius Pilate to be crucified at Golgotha. As an everyday phrase, *via dolorosa* refers to a painful and difficult task, e.g., the compiling of a lexicon—even like this one.

DOPA (3,4-dihydroxyphenylalanine) stains the melanocytes in suitable preparations of skin, i.e., not stored in formalin, or fresh skin, black due to the action of their dopa oxidase enzymes on clear DOPA. The DOPA reaction.

dopa [dō′pə] is an acronym for **d**ihydr**o**xy**p**henyl**a**lanine.

dopa-oxidase [ŏk′sə-, ŏk′sǐ-dā] is an enzyme that oxidizes dopa.

dopa reaction [rē-ăk′shən] is the artifice by which dopa oxidase is brought to bear upon dopa. If positive, the result is melanogenesis; if negative, the result is status quo.

Dowling-Degos disease is a reticulate pigmented anomaly of the flexures, much like acanthosis nigricans but it does not become warty or raised. Not associated with internal malignancy. Has been called "dark dot" disease. Not to be confused with acanthosis nigricans.

Down's syndrome [doun]. Mongolism (trisomy 21 or 22).

dracontiasis [drăk′ən-tī′ə-sǐs] is a title for the condition (*-iasis*) of infestation with *Dracunculus medinensis*. The infestation is highly characteristic. Within an excavation, most usually on a foot or leg, the organism nidates, grows and reproduces. To cure the infestation, an effective trick of knowledgeable natives of regions where the infestation is endemic is to locate the end of the worm, attach it to a stick and then gently and slowly (over hours or days) wind it out of its housing until the several feet or yards of it are completely extricated.

dracunculiasis, dracunculosis [drā-kŭng′kū-lī′ə-sĭs; -lō′sĭs] are additional titles for the condition (-*iasis*, -*osis*) of infestation with *Dracunculus medinensis*. See *dracontiasis*.

Dracunculus medinensis [drā-kŭng′kū-ləs mĕd′ĭ-nĕn′sĭs] literally means the little (-*unculus*) dragon (*drac-*) of Medine (Western Africa). Also known as the Guinea worm, *D. medinensis* is a filarial nematode that is capable of infesting the skin. See *dracontiasis*.

drug eruption [drŭg ē-rŭp′shən] is a general term for a dermatosis caused by a drug. Drug eruptions may take clinical forms that span the spectrum of dermatologic conditions from acne to zona and may be based on mechanisms from delayed hypersensitivity to graft vs. host disease.

drug hypersensitivity. "Allergic" drug reactions probably result from the drug or a reactive metabolite combining with a protein to form an antigenic drug-protein complex that stimulates the immune response. Without such a reaction, most drugs, which have a molecular weight less than 1,000, would not be able to elicit an immunologic response. Drug hypersensitivity can produce mediator release, initiate cell lysis, activate the complement system, or activate cellular hypersensitivity reactions. (Nies)

dry ice is a popular term for solid carbon dioxide.

Dubreuilh's circumscribed precancerous melanosis [do͞obrûy′]. Hutchinson's freckle.

duct [dŭkt] derives from the Latin noun *ductus*, a leading. A duct, then, is a structure that leads from one place to another and conducts material through it.

Duhring's disease [dū′rĭngz dĭ-, də-zēz′]. See *dermatitis herpetiformis*.

Duke's disease [dūk] Fourth disease (parascarlatina).

Dupuytren's contracture [do͞opwēträng′]. Fibrosis of the palmar or plantar fascia. May occur in children but more common in the adult patient.

durum [dōō′-, dū′rəm] is the neuter singular form of a Latin adjective meaning hard. It appears in the title *ulcus durum*.

dys- [dĭs] derives from a Greek prefix that means ill, bad, difficult and painful. It is antonymous to *eu-* (good, well). Compare *dyspeptic* and *eupeptic*. A large number of words of dermatologic interest employ this prefix, of which a number of examples follow.

dys(h)idrosis [dĭs′(h)ə-, dĭs′(h)ĭ-drō′sĭs] denotes any fault (*dys-*) of sweating (*-hidrosis*, *-idrosis*) and, restrictedly, is used to denote that vesicular condition of the hands (and sometimes of the feet) that was formerly called *cheiropompholyx* and now *pompholyx*, on the theory that the pathogenesis of the condition lies in a fault of sweating which modern day thinking rules out.

dyshidrotic [dĭs′hə-, dĭs′hĭ-drŏt′ĭk] is the adjective from *dyshidrosis* and means pertaining to faulty sweating. (See above entry.)

dyskeratinization [dĭs′kĕr′ə-tĭn′ĭ-zā′shən] means a fault (*dys-*) of formation (*-ization*) of keratin.

dyskeratosis [dəs′-, dĭs′kĕr′ə-tō′sĭs, -səs] means a condition (*-osis*) of faulty (*dys-*) keratin (*-kerat-*).

dyskeratotic [dĭs′kĕr′ə-tŏt′ĭk] is the adjective from *dyskeratosis* and means pertaining or relating to (*-ic*) faulty keratin.

dysplasia [dĭs-plā′zhē-ə, -zē-ə, -zhə] is a New Latin noun that means an abnormal or faulty (*dys-*) state or condition (*-ia*) of development (*-plas-*, from Greek *plasis*, a molding).

dysplastic nevi these are dysplastic (malignant melanoma prone) moles as distinguished from normal moles. The color is a mixture of tan, brown, black and red/pink. Moles on one person often look quite different from those on another. They have irregular borders and often notches and may fade into surrounding skin. They may be smooth or have a rough scaly "pebbly" appearance. These are large moles, i.e., greater than 5 to 10 mm in size. May be very numerous but not necessarily. Most often on the back but can be on the scalp, breast, buttocks and below the waist. Diagnosis is established by biopsy. (National Cancer Institute)

Dysplastic nevi may represent those melanocytic lesions that are in an active phase of radial growth.

dysplastic nevus syndrome a relatively newly recognized syndrome, widely treated in the literature, in which large, splotchy, slightly irregular appearing, often erythematous, prominent, pigmented nevi may degenerate to malignant melanoma. Diagnosis is made by having a high index of suspicion when examing the skin, with biopsy of suspicious appearing nevi.

dysproteinemias. Chronic increase in gamma globulin not caused by infection may be of two types: monoclonal or polyclonal. The latter is found in many conditions which are sometimes interpreted as being autoimmune. (Waldenström)

dystrophia [dĭs-trō'fē-ə, -fī-ə] and **dystrophy** [dĭs'trō-, dĭs'trə-fē, -fī] are respectively a New Latin noun formed from Greek elements and its English derivative, both meaning a condition (-*ia*, -*y*) in which there has been a maldevelopment through a fault (*dys-*), supposedly, of nutrition (-*troph-*).

dystrophia unguium [ŭng'gwĭ-əm] is an example of a title in classical form that designates nutritional maldevelopment (*dystrophia*) of the nails (*unguium*).

dystrophic [dĭs-trŏf'ĭk, -trō'fĭk] is the adjective from *dystrophy* and means pertaining or relating to (-*ic*) nutritional maldevelopment.

dystrophy. See *dystrophia*.

E

E. The capital letter is sometimes used as an identifier, e.g., vitamin E.

e, e- [ē, ĕ], **ex, ex-** [ĕks, ĕgz] are forms of a Latin preposition and prefix (*e-* is used only before certain consonants, never before vowels, whereas *ex-* is used before both consonants and vowels; *ex-* may change to *ef-* before the letter *f*, as in *effluvium*). The general meaning is from, out of, away from; the extended meaning is lacking in, without. In addition *e(x)-* may have an intensive force, i.e., a sense of thoroughly or completely, as in *exacerbate*.

ec- [ĕk], **ex-** [ĕks] are forms of a Greek prefix corresponding in meaning (except for the intensive force) to the Latin forms *e-* and *ex-*. Before consonants *ec-* is used, as in *eczema*; *ex-* appears before vowels, as in *exanthema*.

ecchymosis [ĕk′ĭ-mō′sĭs], from its Greek elements, means a condition (*-osis*) in which there has been a pouring (*-chym-*) out (*ec-*). In medical context an extravasation of blood into tissue spaces is understood, particularly a largish extravasation that shows itself in the form of a patch of purple color and that is expected to resorb shortly. Compare *hematoma, peliosis, petechia, purpura, suggillation* and *vibex* for other types of hemorrhage into tissues.

ecchymotic [ĕk′ĭ-mŏt′ĭk] is an adjective meaning related to or having the characteristics of ecchymosis.

eccrine [ĕ′krīn, -krēn, -krĭn], from its Greek word elements, literally means separated or secreted (*-crine*) out or outward (*ec-*). When set beside *holocrine* and *merocrine*, *eccrine* carries a sense of free flow as of a fluid. The word is literally equal to *exocrine* (which see) but is not used as its synonym; it has become restricted to describe the flow of ordinary sweat.

eccrine adenocarcinoma is a primary eccrine carcinoma with high incidence of metastasis.

eccrine carcinoma is a malignant neoplasia of the eccrine sweat glands which is divided into two groups: primary eccrine carcinoma, i.e., adenocarcinoma, and other types; and secondary eccrine carcinoma which may arise from benign tumors. A dermatology pathology text should be consulted for a survey of these rare and difficult to remember tumors, i.e., eccrine poroma with malignant degeneration.

eccrine gland is another term for the sweat gland.

eccrine hidrocystoma is a skin tumor with eccrine gland differentiation. In this condition usually one lesion, but occasionally a few and rarely numerous lesions are present on the face. The individual cysts are 1 to 3 mm in size, translucent, yellowish or slightly bluish in color, and tense in consistency. (Hashimoto & Lever)

eccrine poroma [pə-, pō-, pô-rō′mə] a benign neoplasia (-*oma*) of the pore (*por-*) or intraepidermal ductal portion of the eccrine gland. A papule of no distinction is the clinical mark, and disordered hyperplasia of the epithelial cells that form the ductal portion of the eccrine gland is the histologic mark of the condition. The foot is the most common site of the lesion.

ecthyma [ĕk-thī′mə], from its Greek word elements, means the result of (-*ma*) a breaking (-*thy-*) out (*ec-*). The original word was used by Hippocrates for an eruption of pimples or pustules. Nowadays the word is applied to that relatively superficial pyoderma that evolves into firm crusts or scabs composed of necrotic tissue and inspissated pus and seated upon shallow ulcers. The legs and arms are common sites of process. Minor trauma (prick wounds, insect bites) and secondary infection are the preceding events. Scarring is a characteristic sequela.

   ecthyma contagiosum [kŏn-tā′jĭ-ō′səm, -jē-ō′səm] or **infectiosum** [ĭn-fĕk′shĭ-ō′səm] is the formal classicized title for orf, a viral disease that is epizootic in sheep and is an occasional infection, as an occupational event, in humans. When the condition occurs in humans, the primary lesions are chancriform, hemorrhagic, pustular or vacciniform. The course of the process is benign and self-healing in a matter of weeks.

ect(o)- [ĕk′tō] is a combining form from Greek (derived from *ex-*) specifying what is on the outside, or external. See *ec-*.

ectoderm [ĕk′tō-dûrm], literally the external (*ecto-*) skin (*derm-*), names the outermost of the three primary layers of the developing embryo. From it arise the mature skin, the nervous system, the eye, the ear and the mucous membranes of the conjunctiva, glans penis and orifices (mouth, anus, urinary meatus).

ectodermal [ĕk′tō-dûr′məl] is an adjective meaning related to ectoderm.

ectodermal dysplasia [dĭs-plā′zhē-ə, -zē-ə, -zhə] refers to the anomaly in which there is faulty development of structures that derive from the ectoderm. See *congenital epidermal dysplasia.*

ectodermosis erosiva pluriorificialis [ĕk′tō-dûr-mō′sĭs ē′rō-sī′və plōōr′ĭ-ō′rĭ-fĭsh′ĭ-ā′lĭs, -ē-ä′lĭs, -ē-ăl′ĭs] is a title that specifies a condition (-*osis*) characterized by erosion (*erosiva*) of the mucocutaneous membranes (ectodermal derivatives) of several orifices (*pluriorificialis*). The condition is now taken to be a severe form of erythema multiforme. *Stevens-Johnson syndrome* is a current eponymic synonym for the condition.

ectothrix [ĕk′tō-thrĭks] means on the outside (*ecto-*) of hair (*-thrix*). The word is used in connection with the position of attachment or lodgment of fungal elements (spores, hyphae) on the surface of hair shafts. Compare *endothrix.*

eczema [ĕk′sə-mə, ĕk′zə-mə, ĕg-zē′mə, ĕg′zə-mə], from its Greek word elements, literally means the result of (*-ma*) boiling (*-ze-*) out or over (*ec-*). Although the word is as ancient as classical Greek, *eczema* is in constant need of restatement of definition. Its original sense was about as vague or indefinite as that of our present sense of *eruption* or *rash.* Nowadays, because it appears in so many definitive titles, *eczema* ought not to be used vaguely. Nevertheless, one still hears it used in about as generalized a meaning as *dermatitis* or with utterly uncertain connotations. Its best use is to describe a clinical process that is clearly superficial in form and that, early, is erythematous, papulo-vesicular, oozing and crusting and, later, red-purple, scaly, lichenified and possibly pigmented. The very best application of the word is in the above clinical sense plus histologic certainty of primary pathology in the epidermis in the form of intracellular edema, spongiosis (intercellular edema) or vesiculation. Such requirements are fulfilled by allergic contact dermatitis, superficial dermatitides from some primary irritants, superficial viral, fungous and pyodermatous infections and some conditions of unknown cause like nummular eczema. Following is a sampling of titles that one sees and hears with *eczema.*

eczema, atopic [ə-, ā-tŏp′ĭk]. *Atopic eczema* is frequently heard in speech and seen in print. If the definition of eczema given above is accepted, then the word is inapplicable in the *atopic* context because the cutaneous expression of atopy is not primarily an epidermal process. The locus of initial dermatitis in atopic reactivity is in the upper cutis around the papillary vessels, and that reactivity is vague edema. However, in the infantile phase of atopic dermatitis particularly, eczematization, as an event secondary to edema in an easily permeable epidermis and secondary to scratching and inevitable secondary infection, is common. Therefore, one may meaningfully say *eczematized atopic dermatitis*, but to say *atopic eczema* in place of *atopic dermatitis* reduces the word *eczema* to the old ambiguity.

eczema, contact [kŏn′tăkt]. *Contact eczema* is all right in quick talk when context has specified or is going to specify allergic or primary irritant mechanism. In itself it is not a good formal title because it is not informative enough; it merely suggests that something approaching or encroaching on the skin has caused superficial, epidermal inflammation. Minor trauma and ordinary mechanical irritation, however, are not meant; usually *allergic contact dermatitis* is what is intended to be conveyed.

eczema herpeticum [hər-, hûr-pĕt′ĭ-kəm]. A better title would be *disseminated herpes simplex*. The term is applied to that extensive infection with the virus of herpes simplex to which patients afflicted with atopic dermatitis are peculiarly susceptible. Since the process is well limited to epidermis, *eczema* is an apt designation.

eczema herpeticum and **eczema vaccinatum (Kaposi's varicelliform eruption)** is the title for widespread uncontrolled involvement of the skin by herpes virus lesions. This may be caused by either herpes virus type 1 or type 2. One of the most feared and serious dermatologic conditions. Often takes place in the clinical setting of atopic dermatitis. May lead to generalized herpes simplex. Also seen in Hailey-Hailey's disease, Darier's disease, pemphigus foliaceus, CTCL and ichthyosis vulgaris.

eczema, infantile [ĭn′făn-, ĭn′fən-tīl′]. *Infantile eczema* is a popular title among pediatricians, but is not a good title for modern dermatology. Nowadays eczematous processes in infants can be more easily differentiated as atopic dermatitis, seborrheic dermatitis, intertrigo and allergic contact dermatitis. These are the most common cutaneous conditions requiring differentiation in children.

eczema, nummular [nŭm′ū-lēr]. *Nummular eczema* is aptly named in description of an epidermal process that is in the form of a round, coin (*nummular*) shape. Otherwise, the common condition is strangely resistant to our understanding of its cause or mechanism.

eczema vaccinatum [văk′sĭ-nā′təm, -nä′tŭm]. It would be better if *eczema vaccinatum* were displaced by *disseminated vaccinia*. The term is applied to extensive infection with the virus of vaccinia (cowpox) to which patients with atopic dermatitis are peculiarly susceptible. As in eczema herpeticum, the process is epidermal, and *eczema* is an apt designation.

eczématide [ĕgzāmătēd′] is found in French dermatologic writing but is rarely seen in English. On etymologic grounds, a lesion in the family (-*ide*) of eczema is named. The French employ the word with modifying adjectives (*figurée, pityriasiforme, psoriasiforme* and *stéatoïde*) to describe lesion types of seborrheic dermatitis.

eczematize, eczematization [ĕg-zēm′-, ĕg-zĕm′ə-tīz; ĕg-zĕm′ə-tĭ-zā′shən, -tī-zā′shən] are formations from *eczema* that denote the action and result of superimposition of eczematous process upon something original. The words have applicability only to a secondary development of, or complication by, eczema, not to the primary process. For example, atopic dermatitis and psoriasis, which are not eczemas, may become eczematized.

eczematogenic, eczematogenous [ĕg-zēm′-, ĕg-zĕm′ə-tō-jĕn′ĭk; ĕg-zēm′-, ĕg-zĕm′ə-tŏj′ə-nəs] are adjectives relating to developments in eczema. One hears words ending in -*genic* and -*genous* used interchangeably. Dictionaries have been forced to accord equal meaning to the suffixes. There are situations in which a distinction between them must obtain and the distinction is that -*genic* means giving rise to, whereas -*genous* means arising from. If the distinctions were to be maintained for the words in point, *eczematogenic* should mean giving rise to eczema per se and *eczematogenous* should mean arising from eczema (as a consequence or a complication). To illustrate the usefulness of the distinction, sensitization to, say, nickel and subsequent evocation of clinical response from exposure to nickel are eczematogenic events; the discomfort of the events is eczematogenous.

eczematoid [ĕg-zēm′-, ĕg-zĕm′ə-toid] is an adjective that designates what is, looks or behaves like (-*oid*) eczema.

eczematous [ĕg-zēm′-, ĕg-zĕm′ə-təs] is an adjective meaning pertaining or relating to eczema.

edema [ĭ-, ē-, ə-dē′mə] derives from Greek word elements that mean the result of (-*ma*) swelling (-*ede*-). Swelling that is caused by retention of abnormal amounts of fluid in tissues is meant.

edema, angioneurotic. See *angioneurotic edema*.

edema neonatorum [nē-ō-nə-tō′rəm, -nä-tôr′əm] is the title for a more or less generalized pitting edema that sometimes occurs in newborn infants under conditions of prematurity, malnutrition and poor personal and environmental hygiene.

edematous [ĭ-, ē-, ə-dĕm′ə-təs] is an adjective meaning pertaining or relating to edema.

eggshell nails [ĕg′shĕl′ nālz] is moderately well descriptive in terms of a nearly universally familiar object of nail plates that have a dull gloss and are brittle, easily split or broken because they are thin or delicate. There are many more abnormal appearances of nails that are more distinctive and designated by words of Greek origin (see *hapalonychia, koilonychia, onychoschizia*). In general, however, dystrophic processes of the nails are difficult to describe well as an appearance and explain well as to cause.

Ehlers-Danlos syndrome [ā′lĕrz-dăn′lōz sĭn′drōm], cutis hyperelastica, is eponymic for a complex and systemic condition, *ten different types,* based on clinical, genetic and biochemical data, of which the major signs are hyperstretchability of the skin, hyperextensibility of joints, and fragility of skin that results in broad scars of anetodermatous quality following injury. There is a certain softness and weakness of musculature. Other tissues, even bone, have anomalous phenomena of stretchability and elasticity.

elacin [ə-, ē-lăs′ĭn, -ən] is degenerated material (*-in*) from elastic fibers.

elastic fibers [ə-, ē-lăs′tĭk fī′bĕrz, -bərz] are fibrillar proteins that bag collagen bundles in a characteristic way normally. They are made especially visible by special stains. In themselves they are not particularly stretchable but rather retard excessive stretch and contribute return to normal tightness by their resistance, position and function.

elastin [ə-, ē-lăs′tĭn] is the normal material (*-in*) of elastic fibers.

elastorrhexis [ə-lăs′tə-, ē-lăs′tō-rĕk′sĭs] describes the histologic appearance of rupture (*-rrhexis*) of elastic fibers.

elastosis [ə-, ē′lăs-tō′sĭs] means an abnormal condition (*-osis*) of elastic fibers. The histologic mark of the condition is tinctorial change in hematoxylin and eosin staining from normal pink to blue.

elastosis, actinic. See *actinic elastosis.*

elastosis perforans serpiginosa [pĕr′-, pûr′fō-rănz, -fə-rănz sûr-pĭj′ĭ-nō′sə] names a condition (*-osis*) in which abnormal elastic fibers (*elast-*) tend to perforate (*perforans*) the epidermis and in which lesions seem to progress in a creeping (*serpiginosa*) fashion.

Small hyperkeratotic patterned papules may be present on the back of the neck, face or extremities. Sometimes associated with Down's syndrome or a connective tissue disease, i.e., pseudoxanthoma elasticum or Ehlers-Danlos syndrome, etc.

elastosis, senile [sē'nĭl]. *Senile elastosis* names the appearance in aged individuals of cutaneous papulation which histologically shows the degenerative change specified by *elastosis*.

electrocautery [ē-, ə-, ē-lĕk'trō-kô'tēr-ē] specifies both the instrument and the procedure of destroying tissue by combustion from heat or sparks generated by an electrical current. See *cautery*.

electrocoagulation [ē-, ə-, ē-lĕk'trō-kō-ăg'ū-lā'shən] refers to the procedure of destroying tissue by curdling (*coagulation*) with heat generated by a bipolar electrical instrument.

electrodesiccation [ē-, ə-, ē-lĕk'trō-dĕs'ĭ-kā'shən] refers to the procedure of destroying tissue by drying it out (*desiccation*). The actual event is destruction by combustion. This electrical instrument employed is one that involves high frequency, unidirectional current that concentrates heat at a point in the form of a spark.

electrolysis [ē-lĕk'-, ə-lĕk'-, ē'lĕk-trŏl'ə-sĭs] literally means separation (-*lysis*) by means of electricity. In dermatology the process of destruction of tissue by means of dissociation or ionization of chemical arrangements, particularly destruction of hair bulbs, is described by the word. It is a carelessness to make the word unqualifiedly synonymous with *epilation* or *depilation*.

elementary lesion. See *lesion, elementary.*

elephantiasic [ĕl'ə-făn-tī'ə-sĭk] is an adjective meaning relating to, characteristic of, or affected by elephantiasis.

elephantiasis [ĕl'ə-făn-tī'ə-sĭs] is a word that occurs in ancient Greek with the meaning of a condition (-*iasis*) of enlargement of a part or region of the body, enlargement of proportions that brings to mind elephantine size. The word is usually applied to hypertrophies caused by metazoal or bacterial pathogens that cause lymphatic obstruction. Other hypertrophies, as from surgical procedures (radical mastectomy), angiomatoses and Milroy's disease, can also be designated by the bare word.

elephantiasis, filarial [fĭ-lăr'ē-əl, -lä'rē-əl]. *Filarial elephantiasis* is applied to enlargement of the scrotum and parts thereabouts resulting from long enduring lymphangitis and lymphatic obstruction caused by chronic infestation with filarial organisms, particularly *Wuchereria (Filaria) bancrofti.*

elephantiasis nostras [nŏs'trăs] literally means elephantiasis of our region (*nostras* is the nominative of a Latin word related to *noster*, our). The special implication of "our region" is that it is a place not ordinarily noted for a condition, to wit, elephantiasis, particularly not filarial elephantiasis in this instance. The entire term is applied to enlargements, particularly of legs, resulting from lymphangitis and lymphatic obstruction caused by banal infectious agents (e.g., streptococci) that abound in any region. Chronic or recurrent erysipelas-like infections are notable for promoting elephantiasic hypertrophies of this type.

elevatum [ĕl′ə-, ĕl′ē-vā′təm, -vä′təm, -tŭm, -to͞om] is the neuter singular of a Latin adjective meaning raised. It appears in the title *erythema elevatum diutinum.*

em-. See *en-.*

emollient [ə-, ē-mŏl′yənt, -ē-ənt], as an adjective means softening (-*mollient*, from present participle of Latin verb meaning to soften) up (*e-*, intensive), and as a noun it means a softening agent.

emulsion [ə-, ē-mŭl′shən], derived from *emulsio*, act of milking out, a milky liquid, a New Latin formation from the Latin verb *emulgere*, to milk out, designates a pharmaceutical preparation in which inert powders are suspended in vehicles that contain about 50% of oil. The result is a milk-like product resembling sweet cream.

en-, em- *em-* is an assimilated form of *en-* before the labials *b*, *p*, and *m*; *en-* is a versatile classical prefix that in medical and scientific words in general has the sense of "in" or "into." See also under *in.*

enanthem, enanthema [ĕn-ăn′-, ə-năn′thəm; ĕn′ăn-thē′mə], from their Greek word elements, literally mean a flowering (-*anthem*, -*anthema*) within (*en-*). A quickly or suddenly eruptive lesion or process on mucous membrane (for example, in the mouth, like Koplik's spots in measles) is an enanthem(a). Compare *exanthem, exanthema.*

en coup de sabre [äng ko͞o′ də säb′r(ə)] is a French phrase which means in the form of a sabre blow or cut. The description is applied to a form of circumscribed scleroderma that appears like a healed wound of a sabre cut. The forehead is a common site of the phenomenon in the disease; the sides of the cheeks are the commonest sites from duels—or were, in the days of The Student Prince.

end(o)- [ĕn′dō] is a combining form from the Greek adverb *endon* meaning within, inward, in, on the inside, at home. See *en-.*

endocrine [ĕn′dō-krīn, -krēn, -krĭn], from its Greek elements, means separating or secreting (-*crine*) within (*endo-*). The word is applied to the manner of dissipation of hormones by absorption into, and dispersion by, the circulation. Compare *eccrine* and *exocrine.*

endoderm [ĕn′dō-dûrm] meaning, from its Greek elements, the skin (-*derm*) within (*endo-*), is applied to the innermost of the three principal layers of the developing embryo. From it arise the internal linings of hollow viscera and enveloping structures like the peritoneum and pleura.

endothelial [ĕn′dō-thē′lē-əl, -lĭ-əl] is an adjective meaning pertaining or relating to endothelium.

endothelioma [ĕn′də-, ĕn′dō-thē-lē-ō′mə] means hypertrophy or neoplasia (-*oma*) of endothelium. As for *epithelioma*, any hypertrophy or neoplasia, benign or malignant, is designated by the word, but in loose talk or writing, malignant connotation more often attaches.

endothelium [ĕn′də-, ĕn′dō-thē′lĭ-əm, -lē-əm], from its Greek word elements, literally means nippling (-*thelium*, from *thele*, a nipple) within (*endo-*). The New Latin formation was probably occasioned by the stippled appearance (nippling in miniature) of some internal linings, particularly of the gut.

endothrix [ĕn′dō-thrĭks] designates position within (*endo-*) a hair (-*thrix*). The word is applied to fungi whose spores and hyphal elements invade the interior of hair structure. Compare *ectothrix*.

en plaque(s) [ŏng plăk′] is a French phrase meaning in the form of a plaque or plaques. It occurs in the title *parapsoriasis en plaque(s)*.

Enterobius (Oxyuris) vermicularis [ĕn′tēr-ō-bī′əs (ŏk′sē-, ŏk′sĭ-ū′rĭs, -ōō′rĭs) vûr-mĭk′ū-lā′rĭs, -lä′rĭs, -lăr′ĭs] is the highly technical name for the lowly pinworm. The words mean something like pertaining to (-*aris*) a little worm (*vermicul-*) with a sharp-pointed (*oxy-*) tail (-*uris*) living (-*bius*) in the gut (*entero-*). Infestation with the metazoa is one cause of pruritus ani.

eosin [ē′ō-sĭn, ē′ə-sən]. The common dye (dibromo-dinitro-fluorescein sodium) of histologic processing derives its name from Greek *eos*, dawn, or with a bow to Homer, "rosy-fingered dawn," "the red of the morning." Thus eosin is a material (-*in*) that makes things pink or red like dawn.

eosinophilic [ē′ō-sĭn-, ē′ə-sĭn′ō-fĭl′ĭk, -sĭ-nŏf′ə-lĭk] describes what takes the color imparted by eosin, e.g., the pink color of nuclei of eosinophilic leukocytes. The letter *o* between *eosin-* and *-philic* is a good example of a connecting insert (see *zosteriform*).

eosinophilic fasciitis (Shulman's syndrome). This diffuse fasciitis with hypergammaglobulinemia and eosinophilia appears to be a newly recognized scleroderma-like syndrome.

The fascial component of subcutaneous morphea presents with tenderness affecting several extremities but at times only one. The extremity may be tensely swollen. This is a variant of morphea. It is a self-limited disease.

eosinophilic granuloma [grăn′ū-lō′mə] refers to a collection of eosinophiles in the skin or mucous membrane. One of the histiocytoses. This is a chronic localized form.

eosinophilic granulomatosis, unifocal Langerhan cell (eosinophilic) granulomatosis, multifocal Langerhan cell (eosinophilic) granulomatosis generally presents in children, predominantly in males and often with osteolytic bone lesions. Dermal lesions may appear papulosquamous, seborrheic, eczematous, and rarely xanthomatous. Vulvar lesions with ulceration are not uncommon. (J.E. Groopman)

eosinophilic myalgia syndrome is associated with L-troptyophan ingestion, an agent contained in substances used as "sleeping pills." Causes a vague but widespread type of erythematous dermatitis in some ways resembling eosinophilic fasciitis. Etiology is not clear. May be an immunologic reaction to either the L-troptyophan or one of its toxic degradation products.

eosinophilic pustular folliculitis (Ofuji's disease) was first described in Japan. There are pruritic erythematous patches with 1 to 2 mm follicular papules and pustules. Plaques may occur. Involved areas are usually the face, trunk and arms. Especially seen in patients with AIDS. Biopsy of follicular lesions show infiltration of the entire hair follicle and sebaceous glands primarily with eosinophils and some mononuclear cells and neutrophils. Eosinophils also infiltrate the epidermis and dermis, and there may be peripheral eosinophilia.

ep-, eph-, epi- [ĕp; ĕf; ĕp′ĭ, ĕp′ə, ĕp′ē] are forms of a prefix from Greek meaning on, upon, above, over, beside and among. Before a vowel the *i* is omitted (e.g., *eponychium*); before a Greek aspirate, *eph-* is used (e.g., *ephelis*).

ephelis [ĕf′ə-, ə-fē′-, ĕf-ē′lĭs]. *Ephelis* is an ancient Greek word whose modern meaning is a macule of pigmentation, a freckle on the face, back and shoulders. The plural is *ephelides* [ĕf-ĕl′ĭ-dēz]. It is incorrect to make a new singular by removing the *s* of *ephelides* in a back-formation, a mistake also made with *comedo, comedones* and "*comedone*" and with *lentigo, lentigines* and "*lentigine*."

epi-. See *ep-. Epi* may be pronounced as ĕp′ə and ĕp′ē also in the following words that begin with this prefix.

epidermal [ĕp′ĭ-dûr′məl, -m'l]] is an adjective meaning pertaining to the epidermis.

epidermal cyst [sĭst] is a term for a keratinous mass in the skin. The cells of the sebaceous glands, gone to keratinization rather than production of sebum, or cells of other parts of the hair apparatus, seem to be the origin of epidermal cysts. *Atheroma* and *wen* are alternate terms. Milium is another species of epidermal cyst, possibly arising from sweat-gland epithelium.

epidermal nevus is a clinically very distinctive, raised, frequently verrucous growth that often appears as though superimposed on the skin. Benign tumor of the epidermis also known as nevus verrucosus and ichthyosis hystrix, if single, linear epidermal nevus. It is an important entity as it may be associated with other findings of mental retardation, epilepsy, cardiovascular abnormalities, and eye changes.

epidermis [ĕp′ĭ-dûr′mĭs] is a word that existed in classical Greek. It literally means that which is upon (*epi-*) the skin (*-dermis*). We imagine the word was formed originally to designate the part of a hide that is removed in processing skin (hide) for leather (corium).

epidermodysplasia verruciformis [ĕp′ĭ-dûr′mō-dĭs-plā′zhē-ə, -zē-ə, -zhə vĕ-rōo′sĭ-fôr′mĭs] literally means faulty (*-dys-*) growth or development (*-plasia*) of epidermis in the manner of (*-formis*) warty (*verruci-*) excrescences. The title is applied to a characteristic genodermatosis in which the hands and feet particularly develop verrucous acanthomas leading to malignant changes with HPV virus types 5 and 8; 16, 18, 31 and 33 are oncogenic in this condition.

epidermoid [ĕp′ĭ-dûr′moid] means like (*-oid*) epidermis. It appears in the following title.

epidermoid cyst [sĭst] is alternate for *epidermal cyst*.

epidermolysis [ĕp′ĭ-dûr-mŏl′ə-sĭs] means separation (*-lysis*) of the epidermis. Any blistering process, particularly where separation occurs at the dermo-epidermal junction is an epidermolysis.

epidermolysis bullosa Term for a group of blistering disorders that develop as a result of trauma, i.e. the mechanobullous diseases. Many types exist, with three important groups: epidermal, dermal and junctional. Marked difference in prognosis so type should be identified.

Most of these are genetically determined and start in infancy or childhood. There is an acquired type. These diseases are separated by their modes of inheritance, level of the "split" and associated problems. (Patterson & Blaylock, *Dermatology*. Medical Exam. Publishing Co. 1989)

epidermolysis bullosa acquisita (EBA) [bool-, bŭl-ō'sə ăk'wĭ-sī'tə, ə-kwĭz'ĭ-tə] is a blistering disease of the skin characterized by acquired chronic bullae, usually trauma induced with an acral distribution and heals with scarring and/or milia; no family history of a similar disease; subepidermal blisters with a sparse inflammatory cell infiltrate; and deposits of IgG and/or C_3 at the basement membrane zone (BMZ) in most patients and circulating BMZ antibodies in about 50% of patients. (Zhu et al. *Arch Dermatol*. Vol 126, No 2)

epidermolytic [ĕp'ĭ-dûr-mō-lĭt'ĭk] is an adjective meaning pertaining or relating to epidermolysis.

epidermolytic hyperkeratosis [ĕp'ĭ-dûr-mō-lĭt'ĭk hī'pĕr-kĕr'ə-tō'sĭs] is new coinage for a kind of ichthyotic dysplasia that has long been titled *congenital ichthyosiform erythroderma*. The intent of the new title is to emphasize the tendency to epidermolysis recognizable in the microscope at any stage, but clinically obvious only when there is excessive scaling or frank blisters.

Epidermophyton [ĕp'ĭ-dûr-mŏf'ĭ-tŏn, -ə-tən] designates a genus of dermatotropic fungi. The word literally means a plant (*-phyton*) that lives upon the epidermis.

Epidermophyton floccosum (inguinale) [flŏk-ō'səm (ĭng'gwĭ-nā'lē, -nä'lē, -năl'ē)] is a pathogenic and anthropophilic species of the genus. *Floccosum* (Latin *floccus*, a tuft of wool) describes it in a cultural characteristic as woolly, and *inguinale* (*inguin-*, from Latin *inguen*, groin) characterizes (*-ale*) it as inhabiting or infecting the groin.

epidermophytosis [ĕp'ĭ-dûr'mō-fĭ-tō'sĭs] can mean either a condition (*-osis*) of infection with any superficially infecting fungus or a specific infection with an Epidermophyton.

epidermotropic [ĕp'ĭ-dûr'mō-trŏp'ĭk, -trō'pĭk] means turning toward or attracted to (*-tropic*) the epidermis. The word is perhaps a bit more exact than *dermatotropic* to describe the avidity of the superficially infecting fungi because the latter do not reach the true skin; in fact they hardly reach beyond the stratum corneum of the epidermis.

epilate, epilation, epilatory [ĕp'ĭ-lāt; ĕp'ĭ-lā'shən; ĕ-pĭl'ĭ-tôr'ē, -tō'rē, -rĭ] mean respectively to remove, the result or process of removing and an agent that removes (*e-= ex-*, out) hair (*-pil-*).

epiloia [ĕp′ĭ-loi′ə] looks like a word properly derived from Greek. As a matter of fact it has no such formal etymology but was coined by a neurologist (Sherlock) to designate the widest expression of that condition which includes adenoma sebaceum and tuberous sclerosis as structural anomalies, and convulsions and mental retardation as symptoms. Sherlock apparently wedded part of the word *epilepsy* and *-oia* (as it appears in *anoia* and *paranoia*) in the mistaken belief that the latter fragment means a state of mind. *-Anoia* rather than *-oia* would have been correct and "epilepsanoia" would have been a better formation to convey the ideas of epilepsy plus feeblemindedness as clinical characteristics of the condition. There is no good, single word that designates comprehensively the dysplasias of many tissues that may occur in the condition.

epitheli, or **epithelio-** [ĕp′ĭ-thē′lē-ō], is the combining form from *epithelium*.

epithelial [ĕp′ĭ-thē′lē-əl] is an adjective meaning pertaining or relating to cpithelium.

epithelial cyst [sĭst] is a term used to designate keratinous mass that results from what seems to be a traumatic imbedding of a bit of epidermis into the skin or traumatic distortion of normal arrangements with subsequent internal, ectopic keratinization.

epithelioid [ĕp′ĭ-thē′lē-oid] means like or resembling (*-oid*) epithelium.

epithelioid cell is a histocyte that looks like an epithelial cell in morphology and tinctorial properties but is not, of course, derived or descended from the epithelium. Epithelioid cells are seen in granulomatous processes like tuberculosis, sarcoidosis, etc.

epithelioma [ĕp′ĭ-thē′lē-ō′mə, -lĭ-ō′mə] names neoplasia or overdevelopment (*-oma*) of epithelium. Strictly speaking, both benign and malignant processes are encompassed by the word. In most contexts the bare word is taken to signify malignant process but with care it can be used to designate relatively benign processes as well.

epithelioma adenoides cysticum [ăd′n-oi′dēz, ăd′ə-noi′dēz sĭs′tĭ-kəm] is a title for just such relatively benign epitheliomatous development as has been noted above. The condition is otherwise known as *tricho-epithelioma* and *multiple benign cystic epithelioma*. The histologic characteristics of the process may be divined from parts of its various names, namely, neoplasia of epithelium, relation to the hair apparatus (*tricho-*), cystic, and resembling gland structure (*adenoides*).

epithelioma basal-cell, squamous-cell. See *basal-cell epithelioma* and *squamous-cell epithelioma.*

epitheliomatosis [ĕp′ĭ-thē′lē-ō-mə-tō′sĭs] means a condition (*-osis*) in which there has been epitheliomatous development. It is one of those generalized words that can be applied to any quality (benign or malignant) of epithelial development just so long as it is more than normal in quantity or different from normal in quality.

epitheliomatous [ĕp′ĭ-, ĕp′ē-thē′lē-ō′mə-təs, -ŏm′ə-təs] is an adjective meaning pertaining or relating to epithelioma.

epithelium [ĕp′ē-, ĕp′ĭ-thē′lĭ-əm, -lē′əm] literally means upon (*epi-*) a nippled (*-thel-*) structure. The pars papillaris of the corium is sort of nippled. The word is applied generally to cellular linings that are present on the surface of the body structure. That surface may be toward the external world (as in the case of the skin) or toward an internal hollow (as in the case of the gut).

epithelize, epithelization [ĕp′ĭ-thē′līz; -lĭ-za′shən, -lī-zā′shən] mean respectively to produce the action (*-ize*), and the result (*-ization*), of covering with, or turning into, epithelium.

epitrichium [ĕp′ĭ-trĭk′ĭ-əm, -ē-əm] literally means something on top (*epi-*) of hair (*-trich-*). This is not what it really is. It names the outer of the two layers of the fetal epidermis. *In utero* the epitrichial layer becomes a membrane over the developing under-layer which produces the eventual epidermis and epidermal appendages of the infant. Normally, the epitrichium disappears before term everywhere but around the nails where it persists as a viable remnant in the form of eponychium and hyponychium. *Periderm* is an alternate and better word.

eponychium [ĕp′ō-nĭk′ĭ-əm, -ē-əm] literally means something on top (*epi-*) of the nail (*-onych-*). It names the vestigial remnant of epitrichium which overlies the matrix of the nail.

eponym [ĕp′ə-, ĕp′ō-nĭm]. Eponyms are designations derived from proper names of persons, families or places that come to stand for something those persons, families or places are strongly or long associated with. As a word, *eponym* means a name (*-onym*) tacked on (*ep-*, upon), in a sense, a surname. The practice of forming eponyms bothers some people. It is true that many eponyms are exceedingly parochial or ill-chosen and many are out-dated, but the practice is, nevertheless, universal, more or less useful and often necessary whenever codification, nomenclature and taxonomy are required.

epulis [ĕp-ū′lĭs, ə-pū′lĭs, -pool′ĭs] literally means something (-*is*) upon (*ep-*) the gums (-*ul-*). The word exists in ancient Greek with the meaning of a growth on the gums or a gum boil. Nowadays the word is applied to a tumor (which may be a fibroma or sarcoma) of the gingiva or of underlying bone.

equinia [ē-kwĭn′ē-ə, -ĭ-ə], a New Latin word, literally means a condition (-*ia*) of horses (*equin-*). Glanders is meant.

ergotism [ûr′-, ēr′gə-tĭz′m, -tĭz-əm] names the consequences of ingestion of ergot. The dermatologic mark of the condition is a rubor of the skin.

erosio interdigitalis blastomycetica [ē-rō′shĭ-ō, -zhĭ-ō, -shō, -shē-ō ĭn′tēr-dĭj′ĭ-tā′lĭs, -tä′lĭs, -tăl′ĭs blăs′tō-mĭ-sē′tĭ-kə, -sĕt′ĭ-kə] literally means an erosion (*erosio*) between digits (*interdigitalis*, between fingers or toes) caused by a budding fungus (*blastomycetica*). The condition actually named is a moniliasis (candidiasis) that is most characteristically seen in the webs between the third and fourth fingers of the hands.

erosion [ə-, ē-rō′zhən] derives from Latin word elements that mean severely (*e-*, intensive) gnawed (*ros-*, from past participle of *rodere*) away. In dermatologic use the word *erosion* has been itself eroded in that the sense of intensity of process has been lost and the word is applied to superficial denudation as is its Latin original in *erosio interdigitalis blastomycetica*.

erosiva [ē′rō-sī′və] is the feminine singular form of a New Latin adjective meaning worn away. It appears in the title *ectodermosis erosiva pluriorificialis*.

eruption [ē-rŭp′shən] literally means a rushing (-*ruption*) out (*e-* = *ex-*, out), from *eruptio* in classical Latin. The word has since been sadly vitiated. One sees it applied now to any old dermatosis, even the most slowly developing and sometimes, especially in the plural, to the lesions of any dermatosis. Strictly speaking—like *rash*—the word is most meaningfully applied to dermatoses that develop, or whose lesions appear, rapidly, like the viral exanthemata, urticaria, etc.

eruptiva [ē′rŭp-tī′və] and **eruptive** [ē-rŭp′tĭv] are respectively the feminine singular of a New Latin adjective and an English adjective meaning bursting (-*ruptiva*, -*ruptive*) forth or out (*e-*). The classicized form appears in the title *telangiectasia macularis eruptiva perstans*, the English word, in *eruptive xanthoma*.

erysipelas [ĕr′ə-, ĕr′ĭ-sĭp′ə-ləs, -sĭp′′l-əs] is a word that existed in classical Greek (Hippocrates, Galen). Its etymology is doubtful but the most meaningful possibility is that its elements mean red (*erysi-*) skin (*-pelas*). In any event, the word nowadays names the well-known streptococcal infection that takes the form of an acute, demarcated cellulitis attended by fever and other signs and symptoms of consititutional disturbance (malaise, weakness, anorexia, etc.). *The Rose* and *St. Anthony's fire* are lay synonyms.

erysipelas (St. Anthony's fire) consists of superficial cellulitis with lymphatic involvement. An accute infection of the skin and subcutaneous tissues. Most often due to group A streptococci and responds to penicillin. May be due to other organisms, e.g., staphylococcus aureus. There is an increased incidence of erysipelas. (Charteir & Grosshans. *International Journal of Derm.*, v. 29, Sept. 1990. p. 459.)

erysipelas-like dermatophytid [dĕr-măt′ō-, dûr′mə-tō-fīt′ĭd, -ĕd] is a type of complication that one sometimes sees in fungal infections, particularly of the feet.

erysipelatous [ĕr′ĭ-sĭ-pĕl′ə-təs] is an adjective meaning pertaining or relating to erysipelas.

erysipeloid [ĕr′ĭ-sĭp′ɔ-loid] literally means like (*-oid*) erysipelas. The word is, however, never used adjectivally, but is applied to a particular disease, namely, that cellulitis, commonly on the hands and commonly in food handlers (of flesh, fish or fowl), caused by *Erysipelothrix rhusiopathia*.

erythema [ĕr′ĭ-thē′mə] is New Latin from Greek elements that literally mean the result of the action (*-ma*) of reddening (*erythe-*). The word is used to designate the sign of redness and to form a part of titles.

erythema ab igne [ăb ĭg′nē, ĭg′nĕ]. The specification in this title is redness (*erythema*) induced by (*ab*, from) fire (*igne*).

erythema annular. See *annular erythema*.

erythema annulare centrifugum [ăn′ū-lā′rē, -lä′rē, -lar-ē sĕn-trĭf′ū-gəm, -ə-gəm] describes an appearance in which erythematous papules or plaques arise rapidly and evolve slowly by peripheral extension (*centrifugum*) into circular or ring (*annulare*) forms that show normal skin within red borders. The condition is probably in the class of erythema multiforme and urticaria. Other titles like *erythema figuratum* (*gyratum*) *perstans* are descriptive of the process of certain stages or phases and in certain shapes.

erythema contagiosum. See *erythema infectiosum* and *fifth disease*.

erythema dyschromicum perstans [ĕr′ĭ-thē′mə dīs-krōm′ĭ-kəm pĕr′stăn] is the title of an uncommon and acquired anomaly of cutaneous pigmentation that is described as discolored (*dyschromicum*) redness (*erythema*) that persists (*perstans*). The discoloration is more than of simple redness. Gray, ashy, or livid colors mingled with purple and red and are more startling in sharply delimited, linear, or round shapes that tend to enlarge. There are no consequences of the condition beyond the cosmetic. Also known as ashy dermatosis—especially seen in Latin Americans. An extensive asymptomatic eruption. Starts with disseminated macules which extend widely and run together. May be red at first or, indeed, start with the classic bluish grey color on the trunk areas and face. Cause unknown. (Lever)

erythema elevatum diutinum [ĕl′ə-, ĕl′ē-vā′təm dī-, dĭ-ōō′, dĭ-ū′tĭnəm] literally describes a redness (*erythema*) that is raised (*elevatum*) and lasts a long time (*diutinum*). Due to an immune complex vasculitis, i.e., leukocytolastic vasculitis (Katz)

erythema figuratum (gyratum) perstans [fĭg′ū-rā′təm, -rä′təm jĭ-, jĭ-rā′təm pĕr-, pûr′stănz] describes redness (*erythema*) that assumes shapes or forms roughly of something like a number or a body (*figuratum*) or that is spiraled, circular or convoluted (*gyratum*) and tends to last (*perstans*). An association with overt or covert carcinomatosis has occasionally been found. See *erythema annulare centrifugum* and *erythema multiforme*.

erythema gyratum repens is strongly associated with underlying malignant disease.

erythema induratum [ĭn′dū-rā′təm, -rä′təm], or **indurativum** [ĭn′dū-rə-tī′vəm], is another title for tuberculosis cutis indurativa or what is eponymically known as *Bazin's disease*. In any event, either form of the term means a very (*in-*, intensive) hardened (*-duratum*, *-durativum*) redness (*erythema*). One has to have in mind a varying scale of relative hardness to interpret induration properly. Compared to bony indurations, the hardness of the lesions of tuberculosis cutis specified is pretty soft, but compared to that of some other infiltrated processes, it is pretty firm.

erythema infectiosum [ĭn-fĕk′tĭ-, ĭn-fĕk′shĭ-ō-səm] is an exanthematic expression of a systemic infection, of virus cause. Cases occur in epidemics in spring and summer; the course of the disease is relatively mild. The cutaneous expression consists of macules of erythema and papulation principally on the face, arms and legs. The lesions tend to coalesce and then clear in a manner that creates annular and other geometric formations. The condition resolves uneventfully. Alternate titles are *erythema contagiosum* and *fifth disease*. May look like erysipelas. Noted for "slapped face" appearance.

Fifth disease, a childhood exanthem due to B19 (human parvovirus), occurs in young children during the winter and spring months. A single stranded DNA virus capable of autonomous replication.

Incubation period between 4 and 14 days, mild prodrome of headache, pruritus, malaise and chills. Second phase of the illness consists of rash and low grade fever.

Adults tend to have a more serious course, i.e., they have symmetrical arthritis in the hands and knees.

Human parvovirus has been associated with aplastic crisis in children with sickle cell anemia. Parvovirus has been found to cause aplastic crisis in patients with hereditary spherocytosis, hemolytic sickle cell disease, pyruvate kinase deficiency, B-thalassemia intermedia, and acquired hemolytic anemias.

Parvovirus is cytotoxic for erythroid progenitor cells in bone marrow.

Infection with parvovirus during pregnancy can result in death of the fetus. Infection in any of the three trimesters can result in fetal hydrops.

The rash of *erythema infectiosum* (EI) occurs in three phases, beginning with the "slapped cheek" rash, rare in the adult. Then a symmetric rash in a reticular pattern starts on the extensor surfaces of the extremities and on the buttocks and may involve the palms and soles. Then the rash may wax and wane.

Fifth disease can be verified by identification of viral particles or by serologic response. Viral particles can be detected by counterimmunoelectrophoresis (CIE) or by the more sensitive DNA hybridization technique in serum, urine and respiratory secretions during the prodrome.

If an outbreak of EI occurs in a school it is advisable that all pregnant personnel remain at home for 2 to 3 weeks after the last case has been diagnosed.

Serologic testing is recommended for pregnant women in which an EI-like illness develops or who come in contact with a person with the disease. If the results are positive, ultrasound tests to rule out hydrops fetalis should be considered. (Bialecki et al., Journ Am. Acad. Derm., Vol 21, No. 5)

erythema marginatum [măr′jĭ-nā′təm, -nä′təm] describes a redness (*erythema*) that is bordered (*marginatum*). Appearances of this sort are seen in some early cases of rheumatic fever. The condition is probably related to erythema nodosum, erythema annulare centrifugum and erythema multiforme.

erythema migrans [mī′grănz] means a redness (*erythema*) that travels (*migrans*). It is one of several classicized titles for geographic tongue. Sometimes the lesions of erythema marginatum move about and then *erythema migrans* becomes an apt title too.

erythema multiforme (bullosum, exudativum) [mŭl′tĭ-fôr′mē, (bōōl-, bŭl-ō′səm ĕk′sū-də-tī′vəm)] describes a redness (*erythema*) that is of many (*multi-*) shapes (*-forme*) and may be attended by blisters (*bullosum*) and edema (*exudativum*). Most typical instances of the condition are marked by plaques of redness on hands, arms, neck and elsewhere that may develop polychromatically into circles of red to purple colors (iris lesions) or evolve into blisters and edema herpetically (herpes iris). There are many other conditions with erythematous, edematous and bullous lesions resembling what has been described that are clearly traceable to drugs, systemic infections and overt or covert neoplasms and lymphomatoses.

erythema multiforme major (Stevens-Johnson syndrome) shown by blistering lesions involving the mouth, skin and eyes. Very striking extensive lesions heal with a minimum of scarring if properly treated. When the cornea is involved may result in blindness if not treated adequately with systemic steroids. This has many causes, usually due to adverse drug reactions but may occur in the setting of pneumococcal pneumonia, where its presence may help to establish the correct diagnosis.

erythema nodosum [nō-dō′səm] describes a redness (*erythema*) that takes the form of a hard lump (*nodosum*). The condition designated, in typical instances, consists of up to a dozen or so of small-fruit-sized, erythematous nodules on the anterior aspects of legs, sometimes on arms too. Such lesions are known to attend many systemic processes, particularly infections, e.g., streptococcal tonsillitis, rheumatic fever, syphilis, etc. Some drug eruptions take the form of erythema nodosum.

erythema nodosum leprosum [ĕr′ĭ-thē′mə nō-dō′səm lep-rō′-səm] designates a characteristic eruption or erythematous and nodose lesions that sometimes attend lepromatous leprosy. Unlike ordinary erythema nodosum, the lesions of erythema nodosum leprosum are numerous, widespread, persistent, progressive, and attended by constitutional illness (fever, malaise).

erythema nuchae [nōō′-, nū′kē] describes redness (*erythema*) of the back of the neck (*nuchae*). The vascular nevus at the junction of head and neck, so common in children and frequently persistent into adult life, is so designated.

erythema palmare [păl-mā′rē, păl-mä′rē, -mär′ē] describes a redness (*erythema*) of the palm(s) (*palmare*). Conditions ranging from vascular nevi to cardiopathies produce the appearance.

erythema pernio [pûr′nĭ-ō, -nē-ō] describes the redness (*erythema*) of frostbite (*pernio*).

erythema perstans [pĕr′-, pûr′stănz] is a short title for persistent (*perrstans*) erythema of the annular, centrifugal, figurate or gyrate class.

erythema pudoris [p︠o͞o︡-, pū-dō′rĭs, -dôr′ĭs] describes the blush (*erythema*) of shame (*pudoris*).

erythema scarlatiniforme [scär′-, skär′lə-tē′nĭ-fôr′mē] describes a redness (*erythema*) in the character of (*-forme*) scarlet fever (*scarlatini-*). Many febrile, infectious diseases that are not scarlet fever and some drug eruptions are attended by erythemas that may scale in resolution.

erythematodes [ĕr′ə-, ĕr′ĭ-thĕm′ə-tō′dēz, -thē′mə-tō′dēz] is an adjective in classical form meaning like (*-odes*) or having the quality of redness (*erythemat-*).

erythematosus [ĕr′ĭ-thĕm′ə-tō′səs, -thē′mə-tō′səs] is an adjective in classical form that means full of (*-osus*) redness (*erythemat-*).

erythematous [ĕr′ĭ-thĕm′ə-təs, -thē′mə-təs] is an adjective meaning reddened, having the quality of erythema and pertaining or relating to erythema.

erythema toxicum neonatorum [ĕr′ĭ-thē′mə tŏk′sĭ-kəm nē′ō-nə-tō′rəm]. A benign asymptomatic eruption usually starts just after birth. There are macules, papules and large irregular areas of erythema and occasionally pustules. Unknown cause, characteristic histopathology, subcorneal blister, the pustule has a follicular location and is filled with eosinophils. (Lever)

erythemogenic [ĕr′ĭ-thĕm′ō-jĕn′ĭk, ĕr′ĭ-thə-mŏj′ə-nĭk, ĕr′ĭ-thē′mō-jĕn′ĭk] means producing (*-genic*) redness (*erythemo-*). *Rubefacient* would be an equivalent word.

erythralgia [ĕr′ĭ-thrăl′jə, -jē-ə, -jĭ-ə, ē′rĭth-răl′jə, -jē-ə, -jĭ-ə], from its Greek word elements, means a state (*-ia*) of painful (*-alg-*) redness (*erythr-*).

erythrasma [ĕr′ĭ-thrăz′mə] names a superficial infectious process caused by a corynebacterium. As a word *erythrasma* means a reddened (*erythr-*) process (*-asma*).

erythredema [ə-, ē-, ĕ-rĭth′rə-dē′mə] is another title for acrodynia (pink disease, acropolyneuritis). The word says red (*erythr-*) swelling (*-edema*).

erythrism [ə-, ē-, ĕ-rĭth′rĭz′m] literally means a habitus (*-ism*) of redness (*erythr-*). The word is applied, rarely, to that startling ruddiness of some fair-skinned persons.

erythrocyanosis [ə-, ē-, ĕ-rĭth′rō-sī′ə-nō′sĭs], from its Greek elements, means a condition (*-osis*) marked by a red- (*erythro-*) purple (*-cyan-*) color. Unqualified, this word and its adjective (*erythrocyanotic*) can be used descriptively of morphology but cannot be used definitively for diagnosis. *Erythrocyanosis* finds most application with reference to dependent parts, particularly as a sign of peripheral vascular disease.

erythroderma [ə-, ē-, ĕ-rĭth′rō-dûr′mə] is used as a title with modifications for a condition in which the skin (*-derma*) is reddened (*erythro-*). The range of conditions that may be described by this word varies from some of utterly unknown cause to some of somewhat less than utterly unknown cause like psoriasis to a few of better-known cause like generalized allergic eczematous contact dermatitis and atopic dermatitis. In classicized titles *erythroderma* is modified by the neuter singular form of an adjective, since *derma* is a neuter Greek noun, as in the following:

erythroderma desquamativum [dē-squăm′ə-tī′vəm] designates a generalized dermatitis of infants that consists largely of erythema and scaling. It is thought by some to be severe seborrheic dermatitis.

erythroderma exfoliativum [ĕks-fō′lĭ-ə-tī′vəm] denotes a redness of the skin (*erythroderma*) marked by leaf-like scaling (*exfoliativum*). The title is purely descriptive of a condition which may remain of unknown cause, may eventuate in a lymphoma, a leukosis or a reticulosis, or may be discovered at long last to be a drug eruption or a contact dermatitis by sensitization.

erythroderma ichthyosiforme congenitale [ĭk′thĭ-ō′sĭ-fôr-mē kôn-jĕn′ĭ-tā′lē, -ə-tā′lē, -tä′lē, -tăl-ē] designates a dermatosis that begins at or shortly after birth (*congenitale*) and takes the form of fish-like (*ichthyosiforme*) scaling upon a reddened skin (*erythroderma*). Blistering, which is not specified in the title, is a common accompaniment. Better known as congenital ichthyosiform erythroderma (CIE), it may be of either the "wet" or "dry" type, i.e., with or without blisters.

erythrodermia [ə-, ē-, ĕ-rĭth′rō-dûr′mē-ə, -mĭ-ə] is an alternate for *erythroderma*, with exactly the same meaning. In some ways *eryth-*

rodermia is preferable to *erythroderma*, because *-ia*, its terminal element, specifically designates a condition (of red skin), whereas *erythroderma* literally means red skin, since *-ma*, its terminal element, means a result of an action and is part of the formation of the noun *derma* (see under *derma*, *-derma*, *-dermia*, *-ma* and *-oma*). Since *-ia* is a classical Greek and Latin suffix which is feminine singular in form, *erythrodermia*, if used in classicized titles, will take a corresponding form of the adjective, e.g., *erythrodermia desquamativa*.

erythrokeratodermia figurata variabilis [ə-, ē-, ĕ-rĭth′rō-kĕr′ə-tō-dûr′mē-ə, -mĭ-ə fĭg′ū-rā′tə, -rä′tə vâr′ē-, vär′ĭ-ā′bĭ-lĭs, -ä′bĭ-lĭs, -ē-ə-bĭl′ĭs] describes a hereditable condition of the skin (*-dermia*) that is characterized by redness (*erythro-*) around horny (*-kerato-*) plaques that are variable (*variabilis*) in form (*figurata*).

erythroplakia [ə-, ē-, ĕ-rĭth′rō-plā′kē-ə, -kĭ-ə], from its Greek elements, means a red (*erythro-*) flatness (*-plakia*). It amounts to a red plaque, but *plaque* is Dutch, not Greek. In some ways *erythroplakia* is a better word than *erythroplasia* (see next entry) but does not displace it because neither word is anything to get excited about.

erythroplasia [ə-, ē-, ĕ-rĭth′rō-plā′zhē-ə, -zē-ə, -zhə], from its Greek word elements, means a red (*erythro-*) growth or development (*-plasia*). It is used almost exclusively in connection with the eponym *Queyrat*, and the condition is now taken to be that neoplasia on mucous membranes (particularly but not exclusively of the glans penis) that is, on the general expanse of skin, better known by the eponym *Bowen's disease*.

erythroplasia of Queyrat (Bowen's disease of the glans penis) is a striking, rare, insidious skin lesion. It appears as a red, velvety, flat to slightly raised, well circumscribed dermatitis on or over the glans penis. This is a carcinoma in situ but may metastasize if untreated.

erythropo(i)etic protoporphyria [ĕ-rĭth′-rō-pō-ĕt′ĭk; -poi-ĕt′ĭk prō′tō-pôr-fĭr′ē-ə, -ĭ-ə] is a condition based on abnormal metabolism of porphyrins associated with formation (*-poetic*, *-poietic*) of red blood cells (*erythro-*). *Proto-* signifies error in metabolism at the point of synthesis into hemoglobin. Clinical pictures like that of hydroa estivale (which see) are the visible marks of the anomaly.

   Is an inherited disorder of porphyrin metabolism. It is marked by a deficiency of the enzyme ferrochelatase, which results in an accumulation of protoporphyrin in erythrocytes, plasma and liver. On exposure to sunlight, affected children develop a variety of cutaneous manifestations, such as burning, itching, and swelling. The disease can progress to cholelithiasis, portal fibrosis, cirrhosis, and fatal liver failure. Oral beta carotene (Max-Caro, Provatene, Solatene) may decrease photosensitivity; blood transfusions may reduce excess protoporphyrin production; and cholestyramine (Questran) may interfere with its enterohepatic circulation; but nothing has been able to protect against fatal hepatic failure. (Pierini)

érythrose pigmentaire péribuccale [ārētrōz′ pēgmängtâr′ pārēbōōkăl′] is a title in French for a red- (*erythrose*) -brown discoloration (*pigmentaire*) around (*péri-*) the mouth (*buccale*). The phenomenon is probably akin to chloasma in its mysterious mechanism and disagreeable persistence. May be a phototoxic reaction to cosmetics.

eschar [ĕs′kär] derives via Latin and French from the Greek word for fireplace. The word is applied to the necrotic scab or crust caused by a burn, which burn may be from ordinary heat or chemicals.

escharotic [ĕs′kə-rŏt′ĭk] is an adjective meaning pertaining or related to (an) eschar. It is also used as a noun to designate a chemical agent that causes an eschar.

esthiomene [ĕs′thĭ-ŏm′ē-nē, ĕs-thī′ə-mēn] derives from a Greek verb that means to eat and consequently carries the idea of something gnawed, eroded or ulcerated. In clinical application elephantiasic enlargement and ulceration of the genital labia in conditions like syphilis, lymphogranuloma inguinale, and possibly other infections have been designated by the word.

estival [ĕs′tĭ-vəl, ĕs-tī′vəl] and **estivale** [ĕs′tĭ-vā′lē, -vä′lē, -văl′ē] are respectively an English adjective and the neuter singular of a Latin adjective meaning of the summer time. See (*a*)*estival*.

European blastomycosis [blăs′tō-mī-kō′sĭs]. See *cryptococcosis*.

ex, ex- [ĕks; ĕgs, ĕgz] is a Greek and Latin preposition and prefix meaning out of, from, off, away from. See *e-* and *ec-*.

exanthem, exanthema [ĕg′zăn′-, ĕk-săn′thəm; ĕk′săn-thē′mə] from their Greek word elements literally mean a bursting forth (*ex-*) in flowers (*-anthem, -anthema*). In medical sense a bursting forth to the outside is implied. Compare *enanthem, enanthema*. The two forms of measles, chicken pox, smallpox, scarlet fever, etc. have exanthemata as do many other diseases, e.g., syphilis. The word has general uses for any dermatosis that erupts or "flowers" quickly.

exanthema subitum [sōō′bĭ-təm] literally means a sudden (*subitum*) flowering (*exanthema*). What is actually designated is a disease which is attended by extreme drowsiness and high temperature that falls by crisis and is then followed by a morbilliform eruption that clears in a day or two. *Roseola infantum* is an alternate term.

exanthematous [ĕg′zăn-, ĕk′săn-thĕm′ə-təs, -thē′mə-təs] is an adjective meaning pertaining or related to an exanthem(a).

excisional, incisional biopsy [ĕk-sīzh′ən′l, ĭn-sīzh′ən′l bī′ŏp-sē]. The terms *excisional biopsy* and *incisional biopsy* are surgeons' jargon to the understanding of which one has to be admitted. Literally, the one says "cut-out biopsy"; the other, "cut-into biopsy." The average educated person would know what a biopsy is, but that individual or even a physician who is not privy to the arcane ambiguity of the terms would not know that excisional biopsy is intended to mean removal for study of a clinical lesion in entirety (it is hoped) and incisional biopsy is intended to mean removal of only a part of such a lesion. The terms do not say these things clearly; they are not in perfect balance. Excisions are performed by making incisions; incisions by themselves may not result in excisions, but a so-called incisional biopsy is designed to result in an excision. How much more felicitously incisive it would be to speak of biopsy *in toto* (of the whole) and biopsy *in parte* (of a part) instead of the other terms, which do not convey clearly what is done.

exclamation point hairs is a phrase that describes portions of hair shafts as they emerge from the scalp skin in the decalvant phase of alopecia areata. From average girth of hair there is a narrowing of the shaft for a few millimeters to a dot of expansion at the scalp level. The entire appearance is something like, but not quite ! .

excoriate, excoriation [ĕk-skō′- , ĕks-kôr′ē-āt′; -ā′shən] are respectively a verb and a noun derived from Latin *corium*, skin. The verb means to expose corium by mechanical removal of epidermis; the noun means the action and result of such removal. Both words carry connotations of scratching or other physical violence.

excrescence [ĕks-krĕs′əns, -′ns] means a growth (-*crescence*, from Latin *crescere*, to grow, increase) outward (*ex-*). Verrucous lesions are well described by the word.

exfoliate, exfoliation [ĕks-fō′-, ĕk-sfō′lē-āt′; -ā′shən] are respectively a verb and a noun derived from the Latin word *exfoliatus*, stripped of leaves (-*fol-*, from *folium*, leaf); the noun means the action and result of such shedding. Leaf-like scaling is the dermatologic sense of both words.

exfoliativa [ĕks-fō′lĭ-ə-tī′və] and **exfoliativum** [-tī′vəm] are respectively the feminine singular and the neuter singular of a New Latin adjective meaning shedding like leaves. The words appear in titles like *dermatitis exfoliativa* and *erythroderma exfoliativum.*

exfoliative [ĕks-fō′-, ĕk-sfō′lē-ā′tĭv, -ə-tĭv] is the English adjective corresponding to *exfoliativa, -tivum* and means characteristic of or causing exfoliation.

exfoliative dermatitis (erythroderma). The clinical picture may look the same despite the cause, i.e., usually head to toe, virtually universal, firey, red skin. There are many different causes for this syndrome, Red Man (please see) from benign to malignant.

exo- [ĕk′sō] is a combining form from the Greek prefix *ex-* and means outside, out of, outer. Before vowels it appears as *ex-.* See *ec-.*

exocrine [ĕk′sō-, ĕk′sə-krīn, -krēn, -krĭn] literally means separate (*-crine*) to the outside (*exo-*). It is antonymous to *endocrine.* The glands of the skin are, of course, exocrine.

exocytosis [ĕk′sō-sī-tō′sĭs, -sĭt-ō′səs] is used to describe a condition (*-osis*) in which cells (*-cyt-*) are out of (*exo-*) place. The word is applied in dermatohistopathologic descriptions to the appearance of leukocytes in the epidermis as a part of inflammatory process.

extra- [ĕk′stră, ĕks′trə], taken directly from Latin, means outside of, outside the scope of, beyond, above and beyond and in addition to. It is interesting that in Latin *extra* was often used as an adverb and preposition but rarely as a prefix, whereas in English it is used not only as an adjective, adverb and noun but also extensively and extraordinarily as a prefix. Moreover, new words (like *extrasensory*) are constantly being formed by affixing *extra* to the front of existing words.

extracellular cholesterosis [ĕks′trə-sĕl′ū-lĕr, -lər kə-, kō-lĕs′tĕr-ō′sĭs, -səs]. See *cholesterosis, extracellular.*

exudation, exude [ĕg′zū-, -zōō-, ĕk′ū-dā′shən; ĕks-ūd′, ĕg-zūd′, -zōōd′, -sōōd′] are respectively a noun and a verb derived from Latin word elements that mean to sweat out (*ex-*, out, plus *-uda-*, *-ud-* from *sudare*, to sweat, with the *s* dropped out in spelling because of the sound of *s* in *ex-*, as in *expect* from *exspectare*). The noun suggests the action and result of oozing, the verb suggests "to ooze." Both words have application to intensely edematous and vesiculating process.

exudative [ĕks-ū′-, ĕk-sōō′də-tĭv] and **exudativum** [ĕks-ū′-, ĕk-sōō′də-tī′vəm, -vŭm] are respectively an English adjective and the neuter singular of a Latin adjective meaning pertaining or relating to exudation, act or process of oozing out. The English adjective appears in the title *distinctive exudative discoid* and *lichenoid chronic dermatosis*, the Latin adjective, in the title *erythema multiforme exudativum*; in both titles the words suggest succulence or oozing, as from intense edema or blistering.

F

fabism [fā′bĭz′m]. See *favism*.

Fabry's disease is eponymic for angiokeratoma corporis diffusum universale. This is a metabolic disease of glycosphingolipids transmitted in an X-linked recessive pattern. The characteristic skin lesions, angiokeratomas, are an excellent marker for the disease. These may be scattered widely over the body and oral mucosa.

Systemic changes are pain and paresthesias, eye, renal and heart involvement. This is not a "skin" disease; however, electron microscopy findings of skin biopsies in Fabry's disease are diagnostic for this disorder.

Fabry's syndrome [fā′brē]. Angiokeratoma corporis diffusum.

faciale [fā′shē-ā′lē, -ä′lē, -ăl′ē] and **facialis** [-ā′lĭs, -ä′lĭs, -ăl′ĭs] are respectively the neuter singular and the masculine or feminine singular of a New Latin adjective meaning pertaining to the face or visage. They appear in the titles *pyoderma faciale* (neuter) and *pyodermia facialis* (feminine).

faciei [fā′shĭ-ē-ī, -shē-ī], the genitive singular of Latin *facies*, face, means of the face. It appears in a title like *lupus miliaris disseminatus faciei*.

facies [fā′shĭ-ēz, -shēz] is a Latin word for the face. In anatomical nomenclature, a surface or the aspect of a surface is designated by the word. In clinical usage, the word by itself carries a connotation of the expression of the face, physiognomy or visage rather than the face merely as a structure. *Facies* is so used in the following:

facies Hippocratica [hĭp′ə-, hĭp′ō-krăt′ĭ-kə, -ə-kə], also known as the *Hippocratic* [hĭp′ə-, hĭp′ō-krăt′ĭk] *face, countenance, look* or *visage*, is applied to Hippocrates' description (*Prognosis* II) of the mask of impending death.

facies, leonine [lē′ō-, lē′ə-nīn] means lion-like aspect, a fancied appearance of a face distorted by lepromatous nodules or infiltrations of some lymphomatoses.

facies, moon. *Moon facies* designates the rounding of the face caused by administration of adrenocorticosteroids. Emendation:

The condition is usual in Cushing's disease; it develops noticeably during adrenocorticosteroid therapy, when dosage is high.

factitia [făk-tĭsh′ə] and **factitious** [făk-tĭsh′əs] are respectively the feminine singular form of a Latin adjective and an English adjective meaning artificial. The Latin form appears in a title like *urticaria factitia*.

fagopyrism [făg′ō-pī′rĭz′m] means a condition (*-ism*) related to buckwheat (*fagopyr-*). There is a principle in buckwheat which is photosensitizing. Therefore, on occasion, ingestion of buckwheat may result in some form of polymorphous light eruption.

familial benign chronic pemphigus [fə-mĭl′yəl, -ē-əl bē-, bə-nīn′ krŏn′ĭk pĕm′fĭ-gəs, pĕm-fī′gəs] is a blistering dermatosis (*pemphigus*, as a generalized word for a bullous condition) whose nature is told emphatically by the modifying adjectives *familial, benign* and *chronic*. Characteristic in these respects and in histopathology, the condition is, of course, not related to pemphigus of the vulgar, vegetating, erythematous or foliaceous varieties. The title is unpunctuated, as originally formulated. *Hailey-Hailey disease* is the eponymic title.

familial Mediterranean fever is a hereditary metabolic disease of unknown etiology which consists of fever, peritonitis, and occasionally an erythematous, erysipelas-like skin rash, arthritis, and pleuritis. In some cases it may lead to amyloidosis resulting in renal failure and death.

It is found especially in those areas and peoples about the eastern Mediterranean. Sometimes called familial paroxysmal polyserositis—which is very descriptive except that it does not emphasize the usual always-present fever—it manifests as fever and abdominal pain most commonly but also with a wide variety of other symptoms, e.g., pleuritis, arthritis. There are no specific diagnostic tests. The signs and symptoms complex must be put together in a patient of the appropriate racial extraction to make this elusive but not always difficult diagnosis. Response to colchicine has been effective. (Daniel G. Wright)

farcy [fär′sē] derives via French from a Latin word which means to fill, to stuff or (in the vernacular) to constipate. The word is now applied to the chronic form of infection of horses or humans with *Malleomyces mallei*, i.e., the chronic form of glanders. In signs and symptomatology the condition is somewhat like typhoid or other enteric fevers. The dermatologic interest of the condition lies in granulomas and ulcers that may develop on the visible or accessible mucous membranes. See *glanders*.

farmer's and sailor's skin is one of those homely, occupational designations that have a picturesque quality and nonce usefulness.
What this one is intended to convey is a skin affected by the rav-
ages of prolonged exposure to climatic insult (ultraviolet radiation
from sunlight, caloric heat, windburn and cold). Such insults are
more deleterious to fair skins that do not pigment or thicken well.
The marks of the effects are dryness, erythema, freckling, keratoses
(actinic, senile), telangiectasia and a tendency to malignant degeneration. See *sailor's skin*.

fat-replacement atrophy [ăt′rō, ă′trə-fē, -fĭ] is a story phrase that is
intended to convey the idea of diminution of fat tissue and replacement thereof by infiltrating inflammatory cells.

favism [fā′vĭz′m] looks as if it ought to be derived from or to be synonymous with *favus*. It is not, but derives from *faba*, the Latin
word for bean. (Transition from *b* to *v* is philologically common; in
this instance Latin *faba* became French *fève*.) The word *favism*,
therefore, means a condition (-*ism*) relating to the broad, or horse,
bean (*Faba vulgaris* or *Faba faba*). There is a principle in this le-
gume which is hemolytic and, therefore, on occasion, ingestion of
beans of the genus *Faba* may result in hemolytic anemia. The dermatologic marks of the effect could be icterus, pallor and possibly
purpura.

favosa [fə-vō′sə] is the feminine singular of a New Latin adjective
meaning in the nature of (-*osa*) a honeycomb (*fav*-). It appears in
the classicized title *tinea favosa* and describes a superficial fungous
infection whose lesions have equally superficial resemblance to
honeycomb structure. See *favus*.

Favre-Rocouchot skin [fā′vrə; räkōōshō′]. Cutaneous elastosis with
comedones of the face particularly.

favus [fā′vəs] is Latin for a honeycomb. The word is applied to a superficial fungous infection of the scalp, skin or nails caused by
Trichophyton (*Achorion*) *schoenleinii*. The lesions of the condition
are scutular and in aggregation have a vague resemblance to a honeycomb structure.

feigned eruption [fānd ē-rŭp′shən] is an alternate term for *dermatitis
artefacta* or *factitia*.

felis [fē′lĭs], genitive singular of Latin *felis*, cat, means of the (or a)
cat. It appears in *Microsporon felis*.

fell [fĕl] is a rare word from Anglo-Saxon for a hairy covering or a
head of hair, and an obsolete or archaic word for a skin, a hide of
an animal, or an integument of any kind. As a word it is ultimately

related to *pella,* Greek, and *pellis,* Latin, source words of which elements are found in *pellagra* and *erysipelas.*

felon [fĕl′ən] is a word of uncertain, albeit interesting conjectural etymology. It may ultimately derive from classical Latin *fel,* meaning gall or bitterness. It has also been related to Vulgar Latin *fello,* a wrongdoer or cruel person, a meaning transmitted to us from Middle English via Old French. The medical use of the word *felon* in English goes back to the early twelfth century, when it appeared in a description of a disease of scrofulous nature. Today, an abscess of a fingertip, the so-called "closed space" infection, which is indeed a villainous thing, is called a felon. See *whitlow.*

Ferguson Smith's epithelioma [fûr′gū-s'n smĭth]. Keratoacanthoma, multiple.

fester [fĕs′tĕr] derives through Old French *festre,* from Latin *fistula,* a pipe, a kind of ulcer. More commonly encountered in belles-lettres than in medical writing, the word means to turn into pus or to putrefy.

fever blisters, sores, like *cold sores,* are vernacular terms for the lesions of herpes simplex.

fibr-, fibro-. See *fibro-.*

fibril [fī′brĭl], from Latin *fibrilla,* diminutive of *fibra,* a thread, designates a single, fine thread structure.

fibrillar [fī′brĭ-lĕr] means composed or consisting of fine thread structures.

fibr(o)- [fī′brō] is a combining form from Latin *fibra,* a thread. It finds uses in making words for structures that are composed of elongated elements. While a thread in itself suggests delicacy and no great strength, *fibr(o)-* carries connotations of toughness and great strength as from threads in great number woven or twisted.

fibroblast [fī′brō-blăst] names a cell that produces thread (*fibro-*) structures in the form of shoots (*-blast*). The parenchymal cells of the corium which produce the collagen bundles are fibroblasts.

fibroepithelioma [fī′brō-ĕp-ĭ-thē′lē-ō′mə] names a characteristic neoplasia of epithelial and fibrous connective tissue that is potentially malignant, like a basal-cell epithelioma. The lesion commonly occurs on the lower part of the back.

fibroma [fī-brō′mə] literally means the result of (*-ma*) thread (*fibro-*) formation or a tumor (*-oma*) of thread (*fibr-*) structures. The clinical lesion is a hardish papule, nodule or tumor which histologically shows fibroblasts and their product in a dense formation.

fibroma durum [dōō'-, dū'rəm] designates a fibroma that is distinctly hard (*durum*).

fibroma molle [mŏl'ē, -ē] designates a fibroma that is distinctly soft (*molle*).

fibroma pendulum [pĕn'dū-ləm] literally means a hanging (*pendulum*) fibroma. The term is alternate for *acrochordon* or *cutaneous tag*.

fibrosum [fī-, fĭ-brō'səm] and **fibrosus** [-səs] are respectively the neuter singular and the masculine singular of a New Latin adjective meaning fibrous or tough. They appear in titles like *molluscum fibrosum* and *nevus fibrosus*.

fifth disease [fĭfth dĭ-, də-zēz']. In an ordinal designation of the exanthemata, erythema infectiosum is fifth disease.

figurate [fĭg'ū-rāt', -ūr-ət] and **figuratum** [fĭg'ū-rā'təm, -rä'təm] are respectively an English adjective meaning related to or suggestive of a figure and the neuter singular of a Latin perfect passive participle meaning formed or shaped. Both words are descriptive of lesions whose borders suggest the contours of a recognizable form, like a number. The Latin adjective appears in a title like *erythema figuratum*.

filaria [fī-, fĭ-lā'rē-ə, -rĭ-ə, -lä'rĭ-ə, -lär'ē-ə] written with a small letter means a nematode of the genus *Filaria* (written with a capital letter). The word means something in the nature (*-aria*) of a thread (*fil-*, from Latin *filum*, thread). The plural is *filariae* [fī-, fĭ-lā'rĭ-ē, -rē-ē, -lä'rĭ-ī, -lär'ē-ē] or *filarias* [fə-lär'ē-əz].

filarial [fī-lär'ē-əl, -lär'ē-əl] is an adjective meaning pertaining or related to (*-al*) filaria.

filarial elephantiasis [ĕl'ə-fən-, ĕl'ə-făn-tī'ə-sis] designates elephantiasis specifically caused by a filaria. *Wuchereria* (*Filaria*) *bancrofti* is the usual causal metazoon. See *elephantiasis*.

filariasis [fĭl'ə-rī'ə-sĭs, -səs] is a generic word for a condition (*-iasis*) caused by any filaria.

filiform [fĭl'ĭ-, -lə-, fīl'ĭ-fôrm] and **filiformis** [fĭ-lĭ-, fīl'ĭ-fôr'mĭs] are respectively an English adjective and the masculine and feminine of a New Latin adjective meaning in the shape (*-form*, *-formis*) of a thread (*fili-*). The classicized adjective appears in a title like *verruca filiformis*. For the connecting vowel *i* at the end of *fili-*, see under *zosteriform*.

filiform warts [wôrts] is descriptive of warts as they appear on the face and other relatively protected places where they grow or develop thread-like shapes. *Digitate warts* is an alternate descriptive term. See *verruca filiformis*.

first disease [fûrst dĭ-, də-zēz′]. In an ordinal designation of the exanthemata, measles (rubeola) is first disease.

first-degree burn [dē, də-grē′ bûrn] and **first-degree frostbite** [frôst′bīt′] are terms for the mildest degree of the respective injuries, i.e., mainly erythema.

fish skin [fĭsh skĭn] is descriptive in a homely way of the appearance of the skin in ichthyosis vulgaris. The diamond-shaped exfoliation that occurs in the common form of ichthyosis is reminiscent of the scales of a fish.

fissure [fĭsh′ēr] derives through French from Latin *fissura*, a splitting. Thus, any discontinuity in a surface, especially one that persists, is termed a fissure.

fistula [fĭs′tū-lə] is a direct borrowing of the Latin word for a pipe or tube. In medical usage, a sinus or passage that has developed as a congenital anomaly or as the result of a disease process is designated by this word, e.g., *aural fistula, fistula in ano*. See *dental fistula*.

fixed drug eruption [fĭkst drŭg ē-rŭp′shən] is descriptive of that form of drug eruption that appears in a site and, after clearing and upon recurrence, reappears in that very site.

flaccid [flăk′sĭd] means lacking firmness, flabby, lax or soft. The word is frequently mispronounced flăk′ĭd or flă′sĭd; we asseverate that they are mispronounced but Webster's Third enters the second pronunciation marked by a symbol which is explained in "Explanatory Notes" as indicating a variant which occurs "in educated speech but to the acceptability of which many take strong exception. . . ."

It would seem to be a valid rule that *cc* be pronounced hard (like *k*) before the vowels *a, o, u*, as in *occasion, accord, accuse* and before a consonant as in *occlusion*, but like *ks* before *e, i* and *y*, as in *accent, occident, coccyx* and, of course, *flaccid*. We record the two "wrong" pronunciations in our roles as "prescribing descriptionists" but as "describing prescriptionists" we cannot be permissive enough to accept them.

If anyone wishes to kick against this rule, we do not recommend *soccer*, because this seeming exception does not prove (test) or disprove the rule. *Soccer* is derived from association (football), plus *-er* and an additional *c*. We suppose that when *soc* was pulled out of *association*, it was pronounced as *sock*, and a *c* was added because it was feared a single *c* before *e* of *-er* would be pronounced as an *s*. Had we been asked, we surely would have recommended *socker* as better for both the etymological game as well as the sport.

flammeus [flăm′ē-əs] is the masculine singular form of a Latin adjective meaning fiery, flaming. It appears in the title *nevus flammeus*.

fleck [flĕk] is a word of Old Norse origin meaning a flake, particle, speckle or spot.

flesh-color(ed) is generally used thoughtlessly like *skin-color (ed)* (see) as though the world were populated exclusively by "whites." If one really meant the color of flesh as the color of steak, some sensible application of the designation could be made.

floccosum [flŏk-ō′səm] is the neuter singular of a Latin adjective meaning woolly (literally, full of flocks of wool). It appears in the title *Epidermophyton floccosum*.

florid cutaneous papillomatosis (FCP) is a disease consisting of the rapid onset of numerous warty papules indistinguishable clinically from viral warts. These lesions develop on the trunk and extremities. FCP has been described in association with malignant acanthosis nigricans and internal malignancy. (Gheeraert et al. Int J Dermatol 1991 Vol. 30, No. 3)

flush [flŭsh] derives from a Middle English word meaning to fly up (as in *flushing a bird*). Sudden, transient erythema, particularly of the face and occasioned by heat or emotion (e.g., erythema pudoris), and persistent erythema of some fevers, are described by the word. Simple, reversible vascular dilatation is the basis of the acute phenomenon. Persistent erythema or ruddiness as a natural habitus is better described by the word *erythrism*.

flush area [âr′ē-ə] refers to the center of the face and upper portion of the chest where flushing is common or commonly seen because those parts are exposed.

foam cell [fōm sĕl] is descriptive of a histiocyte that has imbibed lipids and has thus come to appear bubbled. Foam cells are seen in many xanthomatous conditions.

focal acral hyperkeratosis. These skin lesions have the same clinical appearance as in acrokeratoelastoidosis, i.e., firm, shiny papules are noted at the periphery of the palms and soles with some extension to the dorsa of the fingers and the sides of the feet.

focal dermal hypoplasia [fō′kəl dûr′məl hī′pō-plā′zhē-ə] **(Goltz syndrome)** mesodermal and ectodermal defects; areas of skin underdevelopment, i.e., the dermis is virtually absent so that subcutaneous fat tissue presses up to the epidermis and the atrophic skin allows herniation of fat. Nodules may be seen on the buttocks, axillae and elsewhere. Serious bone lesions can occur, i.e., syndactyly, scoliosis, etc. The exact genetics is not settled but appears to be X-linked.

fogo selvagem [fō′gō sĕl-vă′jəm] is too difficult for English speakers to pronounce as do the Portuguese [fô′gou sĕl-vă′jĕng]. *Fogo* derives from Latin *focus*, a fireplace, and derivatively means fire; *selvagem*, also from Latin, means wild or savage, from *silvaticus*, belonging to the forest or woods. Thus the term literally means wild fire and is applied to a dermatosis that occurs in South America (Brazil, particularly) and resembles a severe case of pemphigus foliaceus.

foliaceous [fō′lē-, fō′lĭ-ā′shəs] and **foliaceus** [fō′lĭ-ā′-shē-əs, -sē-əs] are respectively an English adjective and the masculine singular form of a Latin adjective meaning leafy, leaflike, with an extended meaning of resembling a leaf in growth.

foliaceous pemphigus. See *pemphigus foliaceus.*

follicle [fōl′ĭ-k'l] derives from *folliculus*, a Latin word that means a little leather bag. The word is thus applied to any tiny, sac-like structure; in dermatology particulary, it names the housing of the hair apparatus.

folliclis [fōl′ĭ-klĭs] was apparently coined from *follicle* to denote tuberculous process around hair follicles. It is rarely heard or seen nowadays. *Papulonecrotic tuberculid* and *micropapular tuberculid* are more current titles. *Acnitis* is a similarly obsolete word for the same thing as it occurs on the face.

follicular [fə-lĭk′ū-lêr, fə-lĭk′yə-lər] and **follicularis** [fŏl-ĭk′-, fə-, fō-lĭk′ū-lā′rĭs, -lä′rĭs, -lăr′ĭs] are respectively an English adjective and the masculine and feminine singular of a New Latin adjective derived from *folliculus*, a little bag, and meaning related to, consisting of or affecting follicles. For **follicular mucinosis,** see **alopecia mucinosa.**

follicular mucinosis (alopecia mucinosa) these are inflammatory skin plaques with alopecia with a characteristic histology, i.e., mucinous edema of the hair follicles. Usually on the face or upper body but may be anywhere. On occasion have been associated with lymphoma.

Follicular occlusion triad consists of hidradenitis suppurativa, dissecting perifolliculitis of the scalp (perifolliculitis capitis abscedens et suffodiens) and acne conglobata.

folliculitis [fŏl-ĭk′-, fə-, fō-lĭk′ū-lī′tĭs, -lē′tĭs] means inflammation (-*itis*) of the follicle, i.e., housing of the hair apparatus, particularly the upper portion of the structure.

folliculitis, Bockhart's [bŏk′härts]. See *Bockhart's impetigo.*

folliculitis decalvans [dē-kăl′vănz] describes an inflammatory condition of hair follicles that results in baldness (Late Latin *decalvans*, making bald, removing the hair).

folliculitis et perifolliculitis abscedens et suffodiens [pĕr′ĭ-fōlĭk′ū-lī′tĭs ăb-sē′dĕnz ĕt sŭ-fō′dĭ-ĕnz] is the formidable title of a formidable condition in which inflammatory process in and about (*peri-*) hair follicles of the scalp results in a flow (Latin *abscedens*, going away) of pus and an undermining (Latin *suffodiens*, digging under) of tissue. *Dissecting cellulitis of the scalp* is a more quickly understood title in English.

folliculitis keloidalis [kē′loi-dā′lĭs, -dä′lĭs, -dăl′ĭs] is alternate for *dermatitis papillaris capillitii.*

folliculitis narium perforans [nā′rĭ-əm, nā′rĭ-əm, năr′ē-əm pĕr′-, pûr′fō-rănz, -fô-rănz] describes inflammation of vibrissal follicles of the nostrils (*narium*) that eventuate in perforation (*perforans*) toward the skin side of the nose.

folliculitis ulerythematosa reticulata [ū-lĕr′ē-, ū-lĕr′ĭ-thĕm′ə-tō′sə rĕ-, rē-tĭk′ū-lā′tə, -lä-tə] describes a characteristic inflammation of follicles that results in scarring (*ul-*) that is full of redness (*-erythematosa*) and is in a netted pattern (*reticulata*). The process is seen on the cheeks of the face.

Fordyce's disease [fôr′dĭs] Ectopic sebaceous glands in the lips and thereabout.

foreign-body granuloma [grăn′ū-lō′mə] or, **reaction** [rē-ăk′shən], describes the tissue response to relatively inert foreign matter. Materials like silica and beryllium, however, provoke sarcoid responses. It used to be thought that such response was inherent from the nature of the material but it may be that the response is allergic or immunologic.

forelock [fôr′lŏk′] derives from Anglo-Saxon and means the tuft of hair (*-lock*) that grows on the front (*fore-*) of the scalp.

forelock, white frontal [whīt frŭn′təl, -t'l] *White frontal forelock* tautologically describes a lock of hair that is depigmented and located on the front of the head hair. *White forelock* is enough.

formication [fôr′mĭ-kā′shən] derives from the Latin words *formica,* an ant, and *formicare,* to creep like an ant. It is a word that is used in the manner of a figure of speech to suggest a sensation as might result from the crawl or scamper of an ant on the skin.

fourth disease [fôrth dĭ-, də-zēz′] is another ordinal designation for an exanthematic disease, of viral cause. Also known eponymically as *Duke's disease,* it is a mild systemic infection whose cutaneous expression is a rapidly evolving (in a matter of hours), bright red, generalized erythema.

Fox-Fordyce [fŏks fôr′dīs] **disease** is eponymic for a papular, intensely pruritic dermatosis of the axillae and pubes and around the nipples that is an inflammatory condition of the apocrine glands of the region.

frambesia [frăm-bē′zhē-ə, -zē-ə, -zhə] is a New Latin formation from the French word for a raspberry (*framboise*). Some common lesions of this treponematosis vaguely resemble raspberries. *Yaws* is a synonymous title for the disease.

freckle [frĕk′'l] derives from a Middle English word that means the same thing, namely, one of the familiar spots of pigmentation so common on faces, shoulders and beyond, especially in the young. *Lentigo* is nearly synonymous. See also *ephelis.*

  freckle of Hutchinson [hŭtch′ĭn-sŭn, -s'n, -sən], **melanotic** [mĕl′ə-nŏt′ĭk], is eponymic for a pigmented and neoplastic process, commonly on the face of women, that resembles a flat, enlarging scborrheic keratosis and tends to development of malignant melanoma of less than the usual fearful quality.

Frei antigen [frī ăn′tĭ-, ăn′tə-jĕn, -jən, -jĭn] is an eponymic designation for a material used to test for present or past infection with the virus of lymphogranuloma venereum. Frei processed the material from bubo pus; modern methods employ cultures of the causative virus on chick embryos or mouse brains.

Frey's syndrome is a complication from diabetic neuropathy resulting in gustatory sweating. (Patterson & Blaylock)

friction blisters occur on the hands and feet from excessive use caused by shearing forces within the epidermis. These are superficial lesions due to necrosis of keratinocytes in the stratum malpighii. (Naylor)

frontalis [frŭn-, frŏn-tā′lĭs, -tä′lĭs, -tăl′ĭs] is the masculine and feminine singular of a New Latin adjective derived from Latin *frons,* *frontis,* forehead or front, and means of a frontal area, usually of the scalp. It appears in the title *alopecia liminaris frontalis.*

frostbite [frôst′bīt′] derives from Anglo-Saxon and Middle English words for freeze and bite. The word describes the sharp, painful sensation both of freezing and thawing of skin and is also used to designate any degree of freezing that results in appreciable skin changes. *Congelation* is a synonym.

fulguration [fōōl′-, fŭl′gū-rā′shən] derives from the Latin word for lightning. It is applied to that procedure of destroying tissue with an instrument that emits heat in the form of sparks. See *electrodesiccation.*

fulvum [fōōl′-, fŭl′vəm] is the neuter singular form of a Latin adjective meaning deep yellow, reddish yellow, golden and tawny. The word is found in the title *Microsporum fulvum.*

fungal [fŭng′gəl] is an adjective meaning pertaining or relating to or caused by a fungus. See *fungous* and *fungus.*

fungicidal [fŭn′jĭ-sīd′əl] is an adjective meaning pertaining or related to a fungicide.

fungicide [fŭn′jĭ-sīd] names an agent that kills (*-cid-*) fungi.

fungistatic [fŭn′jĭ-stăt′ĭk], as an adjective means arresting (*-static*) the growth of fungi and, as a noun an agent that does the arresting.

fungoid [fŭng′goid] means like (*-oid*) a fungus.

fungoides [fŭng-goi′dēz] is a New Latin adjective meaning like (*-oides*) or in the nature of a mushroom (*fung-*). It appears in the titles *granuloma fungoides* and *mycosis fungoides.*

fungous [fŭng′gəs], like *fungal,* with which it is synonymous, means pertaining to or relating to a fungus. Its literal meaning is having the characteristics of or being full of (*-ous* from Latin *-osus,* full of) a fungus. For almost 100 years *fungous* has been used in the sense of infected by or caused by a fungus, and occasional exception has been taken to this usage. However, nothing need be done about it, for such usage is well-established and has ample precedents and parallels.

fungus [fŭng′gəs] is the classical Latin word for a mushroom and derivatively, a growth on the body. Celsus used it in the phrase *fungo simile ulcus,* "a sore like a fungus." Etymologically, it is related to the Greek word *sfongos,* or *spongos,* a sponge. In botany, the word is applied to primitive forms of plant life in a subphylum of *Thallophyta* that are not differentiated into roots, stems and leaves and contain no chlorophyll. The plural is *fungi* [fŭn′jī]; an alternate plural form, *funguses* [fŭng′gəs-ĕz, -əz, -ĭz], entered the dictionaries many years ago and has been creeping up on us, especially from nonmedical quarters.

Also, lay persons use *fungus* itself to denote a disease caused by a fungus as they use *virus* when they say, "I have a virus." Then too, one hears and sees *fungus* used as an adjective, e.g., *fungus disease*. This would not be very objectionable if there were not already two established adjectives, *fungal* and *fungous* from *fungus*. Enough is enough.

furfur [fōōr′fōōr, fûr′fēr] is a classical Latin word that originally meant bran and then scurf and scales on the skin, head, etc. The word appears in *Malassezia furfur*, formerly thought to be the organism of tinea (pityriasis) versicolor. The *furfur* designation must have been derived from the clinical infection rather than from any characteristic of the organism, which does not have a scaly appearance on mount. The causative organism is Pityrosporum orbiculare.

furfuracea [fōōr′fōōr-, fûr′fēr-, fûr′fū-rā′shē-ə, -sē-ə, -shɔ] and **furfuraceous** [fər′fər-, fûr′fū-, fûr′fēr-ā′shəs] are respectively the feminine singular form of a Latin adjective and an English adjective derived from *furfur*, both meaning in the nature of bran or fine scales. The Latin adjective appears in the title *impetigo furfuracea*.

furfuraceous impetigo [ĭm′pĕ-tī′gō, -tē′gō] is a title for a superficial and finely scaling dermatosis, commonly on the face, that is thought by some to be a streptoderma (streptogenous impetigo), by others an aspect of atopic dermatitis (pityriasis alba), and by still others, a chapping from environmental cold.

furrowed tongue [fûr′ōd tŭng]. See *lingua plicata*.

furuncle [fū′rŭng-kəl] derives from *furunculus*, diminutive of *fur*, a Latin word for thief. Thus it means a small-time or petty (*-uncle*) thief (*fur-*). It was used by Pliny and Celsus, much as we use it today, for a boil. One may amuse oneself by reflecting on how often words relating to crime designate body ills and their causes. *Felon* and *latrodectus mactans* (murdering biter-thief, the black-widow spider) come to mind quickly.

furuncular [fū-rŭng′kū-lēr, -lər] is an adjective meaning pertaining or related to a furuncle.

furunculoid [fū-rŭng′kū-loid] means like (*-oid*) a furuncle.

furunculosis [fū-rŭng′kū-lō′sĭs, -səs] means a condition (*-osis*) of boils, i.e., multiple, simultaneous or recurrent boils.

furunculous [fū-rŭng′kū-ləs] is another adjective which, like *furuncular*, means pertaining or related to a furuncle.

fusco-c(a)eruleus [fŭs′kō-sē-r$\overline{oo}$′lē-əs] is a New Latin formation of a masculine singular form of a compound adjective consisting of a combining element, *fusco-*, from *fuscus*, dark, tawny, and *c(a)eruleus*, sea- or sky-blue. It appears in the title *nevus fusco-c(a)eruleus.*

fusiform [fū′zə-, fū′zĭ-, fū′sə-, fū′sĭ-fôrm] is an adjective derived from Latin word elements and meaning spindle-shaped (*fusi-*, combining form from *fusus*, spindle, and *-form*, from *forma*, shape. For discussion of combining forms and the connecting vowel *i* in the word element *fusi-*, see comments under *zosteriform*).

Futcher's lines [f$\overline{oo}$-chĕr] are sharp lines of different grades of pigmentation running longitudinally on the arms of blacks, lighter medially.

G

gallery [găl′ẽr-ē, -ĭ, -ər-ē, -ī] is sometimes used like *burrow, channel, cuniculus* or *passage* to designate the housing in the skin of an infesting metazoal parasite.

gamasoidosis [găm′ə-soi-dō′sĭs, -səs] means a condition (*-osis*) of human infestation with a mite (*Dermanyssus gallinae*) of the family of *Gamasidae*. The word is a New Latin formation, but the origin of *gamas* is uncertain.

gamma [găm′ə], the third letter of the Greek alphabet, like nearly all the other Greek letters, is used in many sciences as an identifier, e.g., *gamma globulin, gamma rays*, etc. It is frequently written in the lower-case Greek form, γ, less often Γ, upper case.

ganglion [găn(g)′glĭ-, găn(g)′glē-ən] derives from Greek and Latin words that mean a swelling or tumor under the skin. Nowadays we apply the word to cystic masses that are related to tendons or joints and to knot-like formations of nerves. The plural is *ganglia* [găn(g)′glē-ə] or *ganglions* [găn(g)′glē-ənz].

gangrene [găn(g)′grēn] derives from a Greek word that was used by Hippocrates and Galen and, taken over into Latin quite early, it was also used by Celsus to mean a consuming, gnawing, or eaten-out ulcer. Nowadays we apply the word to severe necrotizing and sloughing processes. "Dry" and "wet" forms are spoken of, the former, based on circulatory inadequacy, being like a mummification and the latter, based on infection in addition to circulatory inadequacy, being like a putrefaction.

gangrenosa, gangrenosum [găn(g)′grə-, găn(g)′grē-nō′sə; -səm] are respectively the feminine singular and neuter singular of a classicized adjective formed from *gangrene*. Literally, they mean full of (*-osa, -osum*) gangrene. They appear in titles like *pyodermia gangrenosa* and *pyoderma gangrenosum*. See *gangrenous*.

gangrenous [găn(g)′grē-, găn(g)′grə-nəs] is an English adjective meaning pertaining to, related to, like or affected by gangrene.

gangrenous stomatitis [stō′mə-tī′tĭs, -tē′tĭs, -təs]. See *noma*.

Gardner's syndrome [gärd′nērz sĭn′drōm] is a potentially malignant polyposis of intestines associated with cysts and tumors of skin and bone.
    Cutaneous cysts, fibromas, and lipomas; dentiginous cysts; intestinal polyposis with a tendency to malignant degeneration.

gargoylism [gär′goil-ĭz'm] derives through Old French from a Latin word for the gullet. In architecture, gargoyles are grotesque carved faces that are used as waterspouts or adornments on buildings. In medical connotation, then, *gargoylism* means a condition (*-ism*) of extreme facial ugliness, specifically, appearances like those seen in acromegaly and Hurler's syndrome. This does not exhaust all the possibilities.

-gen [jĕn, jən], **-genetic** [jə-nĕt′ĭk], **-genic** [jĕn′ĭk] and **-genous** [jə-nəs] are combining forms from Greek that have to do with conception, gestation and birth, and have senses of producing or arising from. *-Gen* makes nouns; *-genetic, -genic* and *-genous* form adjectives. While there is a tendency to interchangeable use of the adjectival forms, some writers recommend a distinction, particularly between *-genic* and *-genous*, making one active (*-genic*, producing) and the other passive (*-genous*, arising from). On this basis one can get excited about *iatrogenic*, which would mean giving rise to a physician and refer to a physician's biological mother or his alma mater, whereas *iatrogenous* would clearly mean arising from the actions of a physician in his medical functioning.
    There is a related Latin root, *gen*, that also deals with birth and giving birth to, and by extension with a group or class, i.e., those of the same origin. This root appears in the next two entries.

generalisata and **generalisatus** [jĕn′ēr-ăl′ĭ-sā′tə, -sä′tə; -təs, -tŭs, -tōōs] are respectively the feminine and masculine singular of a New Latin adjective (from *genus, generis*, of a class, group or kind) meaning generalized or widespread. The words appear in titles like *alopecia generalisata* (feminine) and *herpes zoster generalisatus* (masculine).

generalized [jĕn′ēr-əl-īzd, -ər-əl-īzd] is said of the lesions of a cutaneous disease when they are widespread and exempt no important region of the skin.

generalized melanosis this is a widespread, very striking, pigmentation of the skin resulting in skin darkening. Can be associated with an occult primary melanoma.

genodermatosis [jĕn′ō-, jē′nō-dûr′mə-tō′sĭs] is generic for a condition of the skin (*-dermatosis*), particularly a significantly abnormal condition, that is dependent on mutation to, or transmission of, abnormal genes (*geno-*).

genotype refers to the genetic make-up of an individual with respect to a single trait or set of traits.

geographic tongue [jē′ō-grăf′ĭk tŭng] is picturesquely descriptive of that process on the tongue which consists of areas of redness that slowly change shape and location over days. *Erythema migrans, exfoliatio areata linguae* and *glossitis areata exfoliativa* are alternate terms.

geotrichosis [jē-ŏt′rĭ-, jē′ō-trĭ-kō′sĭs] means a condition (*-osis*) caused by an organism of the genus *Geotrichum.*

Geotrichum [jē-ŏt-rĭ-, jē′ō-trĭ′kəm] derives from Greek words that mean earth or ground (*ge-*) and hair (*-trich-*). The *o* is a joining insert or link vowel. The word designates a genus of fungi which has characteristics of hair in culture and is largely earthbound, i.e., finds comfortable enough habitat in the ground alone, although it also has feeble pathogenicity for man.

German measles [jûr′mən mē′z′lz] is one of those eponymic and parochial designations that seem ineradicably established. The German designation *röt* (*h*)*eln* and New Latin *rubella* convey the idea of the slight or transient (*-ella*, diminutive, like *-ish* of *reddish*) redness (*rub-*), or reddishness, of the disease in contrast to *rubeola*, or ordinary measles, which is marked by a longer duration of cutaneous erythema. (It is interesting to note that, as a seeming paradox, *-ola* in *rubeola* is also a diminutive ending, but this can be explained by the fact that in earlier medical writing *rubeola* referred, among other things, to small red spots and was also associated with smallpox. Today, the diminutive force of *-ola* in *rubeola* is largely lost and etymologically, the basic meaning of the word is given as reddishness.) In any event, that relatively minor, viral, disease that is characterized by cervical adenopathy, one- to two-day erythema and mild constitutional symptoms is designated by the term *German measles.*

germinativum [jĕr′-, jûr′mĭ-nə-tī′vəm] is the neuter singular of a New Latin adjective meaning relating to birth. It appears in the designation *stratum germinativum.*

gestationis [jĕs-tā′shĭ-ō′nĭs, -shē-ō′nĭs, -shō′nĭs] is the genitive singular of a classical Latin word meaning a carrying; as used in New Latin it means of pregnancy. It appears in the titles *herpes gestationis* and *impetigo gestationis.*

Gianotti-Crosti syndrome [jă-nôt′ē-krôs′tē dĭ-, də-zēz′] is an acute, transient, papular dermatosis of children that is attended by mild fever and malaise being now called papular acrodermatitis of childhood. Due to hepatitis B virus acquired through the skin or a mucous membrane. Also may be due to other viruses such as Coxsachie B, Epstein-Barr virus and cytomegalovirus. (Lever)

giant congenital nevus [jī′ənt kōn-jĕn′ĭ-t'l nē′vəs] designates an extensive hamartoma that consists of a combination of junction, compound and intradermal nevi, hairiness and, frequently, neurofibromas, and has a tendency to malignant melanomatous degeneration. When such a dysplasia covers a large portion of the body like a ragged garment (see *bathing-trunks nevus*) the title is apt; but the designation fails when the lesion is small and has little malignant potential, though it is congenital. In the latter instance, the old term *nevus pigmentosus et pilosus* is simpler and adequately descriptive.

giant eccrine acrospiroma. Eccrine acrospiromas occur typically as small, incidental cutaneous lesions. If allowed to grow for years, some may become gigantic. Malignant transformations may occur. The most important distinguishing features of large benign eccrine acrospiromas are the relative circumscription, the lack of cellular atypia and the absence of stromal, perineural, and angiolymphatic invasion. (Hunt et al. *J. Am. Acad. Dermatol.* 1990; 663-8)

giantism [jī′ənt-ĭz′m] derives from Greek *gigas*, giant, genitive *gigantos*, of a giant, via Latin, French and Middle English. The word is used to denote any condition (*-ism*) of great development as a whole or unusually large size of a part. A superbly functioning seven-foot basketball player and the massive face and hands of an acromegalic are examples of giantism.

giant lichenification [lī′kən-, lī-kĕn′ĭ-fĭ-kā′shən] describes a lesion that is huge in amount of thickening of skin by agmination of papules.

giant urticaria. See *angioneurotic edema*.

Gibert's disease [zhēbĕr′]. Pityriasis rosea.

gigantism [jī-găn′tĭz′m] is synonymous with *giantism*, and was derived more closely from its Greek original.

glabrosa [glă-, glə-brō′sə] and **glabrous** [glā′brəs] are respectively the feminine singular of a New Latin adjective and an English adjective derived from the Latin adjective *glaber*, smooth, and by extension, without hair. The suffixes (*-osa, -ous*) emphasize the smoothness and the absence of hair. The classicized adjective appears in a title like *tinea glabrosa.*

gland [glănd] derives from Latin *glans,* acorn. The size and shape of some glands, particularly the most accessible ones, may have suggested the name of the familiar object for the designation.

glanders [glăn′dĕrz] derives from Old French *glandres,* glands. The clinical appearance of lymph-node enlargement caused by infection with *Malleomyces mallei* must have suggested aptness of *glanders* as a name for the disease.

glans [glănz] is a direct borrowing of Latin *glans,* acorn.

glans penis [pē′nĭs] literally means the acorn (*glans*) of the penis, i.e., the portion which resembles the seed or fruit of the oak.

glomangioma [glō′măn-jĭ-ō′mə] is alternate for glomus tumor. It was probably coined to mean a tumefaction (*-oma*) of the vessels (*-angi-*) of a glomus (*glom-*) body, but the better way to derive the meaning of the word is to consider it formed as a reduplication (*-ma*) of the vessels (*-angio-*) of a glomus (*glom-*) body. When reference is made to so-called multiple glomus tumors, a still better word would be *glomangiomatosis.* This word more accurately fits the histologic facts of glomus tumors in multiplicity because they show more of neoangiogenesis in larger or conglomerate masses and less of myoepithelioid-cell reduplication than does the solitary glomus tumor.

glomera [glō′mĕr-, glŏm′ĕr-ə, -ēr-ə, ər-ə] is the plural of *glomus* (which see).

glomus [glō′məs] derives from a Latin word that means a ball of wool or yarn. In classical Latin it was less used than *globus,* which means the same thing. Both words are in modern medical use, *globus* still more than *glomus.*

  The plural of *glomus* as an original Latin word is *glomera.*

glomus body designates one of those microscopic structures which consist of an arterio-venous shunt. They are abundant on fingertips and some other acral areas.

glomus tumor [tōō′-, tū′mər, -mēr] is a neoplasia of a glomus body. The usual manifestation is a point of pain under a nail or a small, tender swelling on an acral area. The histology is characteristic in the form of reduplication of myo-epithelial cells and vascular structures.

gloss- and **glosso-** [glŏs, glŏs′ō] are combining forms from *glossa,* the Greek word for tongue. The final *o* is a connecting insert; see under *zosteriform.*

glossitides [glŏ′sĭ-tĭ′dēz] is the plural of *glossitis.*

glossitis [glŏ-sī′tĭs] means inflammation (*-itis*) of the tongue (*gloss-*). Since the word is generic, below are placed a few examples of titles that are more distinctive.

glossitis areata exfoliativa [ā′rē-ā′tə, är′ē-ä′tə, ăr′ē-ăt′ə ĕks′fō-lĭ-ə-tī′və] is alternate to *exfoliatio areata linguae* and *geographic tongue.* It means an inflammation of the tongue (*glossitis*) characterized by scaling (*exfoliativa*) in spots (*areata*).

glossitis rhombica mediana [rŏm′bĭ-kə mē′dĭ-ā′nə, -ä′nə, -dē-ăn′ə] describes an inflammatory condition of the tongue (*glossitis*) characterized by a roughly rhomboid (*rhombica*) swelling in the central (*mediana*) portion.

glosso-. See *gloss-.*

glossodynia [glŏs′ō-dĭn′ē-ə, -ĭ-ə, -dī′nē-ə, -nĭ-ə] derives from Greek and means a painful (*-odyn-*) condition (*-ia*) of the tongue (*gloss-*).

glossy tongue [glôs′ē tŭng] is not tautological. In this instance *glossy* derives probably from Scandinavian, certainly not from Greek *glossa,* tongue, and means glowing, shimmering, or lustrous. *Tongue* is Middle English from Anglo-Saxon. The term then ascribes a shiny appearance to the organ, such as one might see in some glossitides, avitaminoses and fevers.

gnathostomiasis [nā′thō-, năth′ō-stō-mī′ə-sĭs] designates the condition (*-iasis*) of infestation with a species of *Gnathostoma,* a genus of nematode worms.

Goeckerman [gĕk′ər-mən, gû′kĕr-män] **treatment** refers to a method of treating psoriasis with ointments of tar followed by irradiation with ultraviolet light. (UVB)

Goltz-Gorlin syndrome [gōltz; gôr′lĭn]. Focal dermal hypoplasia.

gonorrhea [gŏn′ə-rē′ə], from its Greek word elements, literally means a flow (*-rrhea*) from the organ of generation (*gono-*). Of course, the flow of neither urine nor semen is meant, but the purulent discharge of infection with the gonococcus.

goose flesh is a picturesque description of the perifollicular papulation of the skin caused by cold or strong emotion. The allusion to the appearance of the skin of plucked geese may not be evocative to many by now. *Cutis anserina* is a Latinization. Horripilation is a related phenomenon.

Gorlin-Goltz syndrome [gôr′lĭn; gōltz]. Basal-cell nevus syndrome (see *nevus, basal-cell*).

Gottron's sign. Violaceous flat topped papules seen over the knuckles in dermatomyositis suggested as pathognomonic of the disorder.

Gougerot-Blum syndrome [go͞ozhərō′; blŭm]. Pigmented purpuric lichenoid dermatitis.

Gougerot-Carteaud syndrome [go͞ozhərō′; kärtō′]. Confluent and reticulated papillomatosis.

gout [gout] derives from Latin *gutta*, a drop, via French. In Medieval Latin *gutta* was applied to diseases that were attributed to a "defluxion of humors." Theories change; names persist longer. In any event, the dermatologic marks of the condition which are due to elevated serum uric acid levels are tophi, particularly on the ears, and painful swelling and acrocyanosis, particularly of the great toes. Treatment with allopurinol corrects the disease. One of the truly great achievements of modern day therapeutics.

graft versus host disease is classically associated with bone marrow transplantation (graft) and/or blood transfusions with immunocompetent cells which are introduced into a host that is unable to reject the graft as he or she is not immunocompetent. There are two distinct clinical entities, acute and chronic types, and two forms of the disease, iatrogenic and congenital.

Patients have widespread often severe skin lesions starting as a minor macule-papular rash which may eventuate in exfoliation.

grain itch [grān ĭch] is another of those folk designations, this time for infestation with *Pyemotes* (*Pediculoides*) *ventricosus*.

granular [grăn′ū-lẽr, -lər] is an adjective from *granule*. The word, then, describes materials that are finely particulate or appearances that are marked by graininess. A word of this sort, of course, refers to no absolute scale of size but has clarity in a context of macroscopic or microscopic viewing.

granular-cell myoblastoma [mī′ō-blăs-tō′mə] is a neoplasm or tumor (*-oma*) of cellular elements of the muscle-making variety (*myoblast-*) whose cytoplasm has finely particulate (*granular*) structure.

granular cell tumor (granular cell myoblastoma) usually solitary; multiple in 10% of cases; most common site tongue (40%). Characteristic faint granules PAS-positive and diastase resistant. Suddan Black positive on occasion. Do not mistake hyperplastic epidermis for squamous cell carcinoma. Once the granular cells are visualized, it establishes the diagnosis of granular cell tumor. (Lever)

granular degeneration [də-, dē-jĕn'ĕr-ā'shən] describes degradation of material from some original structure into a new appearance of fine graininess.

granule [grăn'ūl] derives from Late Latin *granulum*, diminutive of *granum*, grain, and means a little (*-ule*) grain (*gran-*).

granuloma [grăn'ū-lō'mə] literally means the result of (*-ma*), or the development of a mass of (*-oma*), granulation. This common word is used in gross clinical and histologic descriptions of processes that consist of packed cellular elements of the reticulo-endothelial system in grain-like conglomerations, especially such as are common in tuberculosis, syphilis, leprosy, the deep mycoses, etc. It is also used in titles as follows:

granuloma annulare [ăn'ū-lā'rē, -lä'rĕ, -lăr'ē] names that condition in which hard papules appear and arrange themselves in a ring (*annulare*) around a center of more or less normal-looking skin.

granuloma, beryllium [bē, bə-rĭl'ĭ-əm, -ē-əm]. *Beryllium granuloma* designates the clinical tumor and histologic formation of a granuloma following entry of beryllium salts into the skin.

granuloma, eosinophilic. See *eosinophilic granuloma*.

granuloma, foreign-body. See *foreign-body granuloma*.

granuloma inguinale [ĭng'gwĭ-nā'lē, -nä'lĕ, -năl'ē] names a characteristic infection caused by the organism, *Donovania granulomatis*. Commonly on and around the genitalia, the lesions are ulcero-vegetating plaques of red granulation.

granuloma, monilial [mō-nĭl'ĭ-əl, -ē-əl]. *Monilial granuloma* describes tumid process resembling similar lesions of tuberculosis, syphilis and other diseases of that class, but here clearly caused by *Candida albicans*. The phenomenon probably stems from immunologic developments like those that obtain in the deep mycoses.

granuloma pyogenicum [pī'ō-jĕn'ĭ-kəm] names a characteristic nodule of pea-size or thereabouts that is red, thinly epithelized, frequently crusted and composed of vascular elements resulting from endothelial proliferation. Such a lesion commonly follows upon a minor trauma and presumably secondary infection with banal pyogens.

granuloma telangiectaticum [tĕl-ăn'jē, tĕl-ăn'jĭ-ĕk-tā'tĭ-kəm] is preferred by some to *granuloma pyogenicum*. It emphasizes the neo-angiomatous development of end (capillary) blood vessels (*telangiectaticum*).

granuloma, zirconium [zər-, zĭr, zēr-kōʹnĭ-əm, -nē-əm]. *Zirconium granuloma* designates the clinical papulation and histologic formation of granulomas following entry of zirconium salts into the skin as has been known to occur particularly in the axillae from the use of antiperspirants containing the agent.

granulomatosa [grănʹū-lōʹmə-tōʹsə] and **granulomatous** [-təs] are respectively the feminine singular of a New Latin adjective and an English adjective derived from it, both meaning in the nature of, like or having qualities of granuloma. The classicized adjective appears in a title like *cheilitis granulomatosa.*

granulomatosis [grănʹū-lōʹmə-tōʹsĭs] means a condition (*-osis*) of development of granulomatous process.

granulomatosis, Wegener's [vāʹgə-nûrz] is eponymic for a complex, usually fatal, process of unknown cause that manifests itself clinically on the skin and in other organs as tumefactions and ulcerations. Histologically, angiitis, necrosis and cellular infiltrates of granulomatous nature are present.

granulomatous. See *granulomatosa.*

granulosis rubra nasi [grănʹū-lōʹsĭs rōōʹbrə nāʹsī] names a condition (*-osis*) in which small masses (*granul-*) that are red (*rubra*) form on the nose (*nasi*). The condition results from occlusion and cystic dilatation of the epidermal portion of sweat ducts.

granulosum [grănʹū-lōʹsəm] is the neuter singular of a Late Latin adjective meaning granular. It appears in the designation *stratum granulosum.*

gravidarum [grāʹvə-, gräʹvĭ-, grāʹvĭ-, grāʹvĭ-dāʹrəm, -däʹrəm] is the genitive plural of a classical Latin adjective used as a noun and means of pregnant women. It appears in the title *chloasma gravidarum.*

grenz [grĕnts] is a German word meaning border. There may be a proper name *Grenz,* but that is not the source of the designation *grenz rays.* Therefore, *grenz* should not be capitalized when it appears in a sentence internally. The sense of *grenz* in *grenz rays* is one of size of wave length, namely, electromagnetic energy of the order of 2Å in wave length, compared to 0.1 to 0.5Å for conventional X rays and lesser sizes for cosmic rays. The implication of *grenz* then is that the power of rays of this quality is on the border or limit of the sort of biological effect one may expect of electromagnetic energy of small wave lengths.

grocer's itch [grō′sĕrz ĭch]. *Grocer's itch* is another of those titles with an occupational attribution which is not exact. An acariasis caused by a *Tyroglyphus* is meant. *Copra itch* and *vanillism* are alternate, equally inadequate, titles.

ground itch [ground ĭch]. *Ground itch* is again an inadequate vernacular title for an infestation from a metazoal parasite acquired by contact with soil that harbors it. The title does not suggest signs of the papular, urticarial or vesiculo-pustular lesions that appear at the cutaneous portal of entry of the larvae of *Ancylostoma* and *Strongyloides*.

Grover's disease (transient acantholytic dermatosis). A benign skin disease occurring mainly on sun-exposed areas (chest, back, thighs) of patients over 40 years of age. Clinically, there are scattered discrete papules or papulovesicles and microscopically variable acantholysis, dyskeratosis, spongiosis and suprabasal clefting. Benign papular acantholytic dermatosis has been proposed to name the disease as some cases have persisted for more than two years. (Fitzpatrick)

gumma [gŭm′ə] is a New Latin word that derives from Egyptian via classical Greek and Latin, Old French and Middle English. It means something in the nature of gum. That characteristic lesion of tertiary syphilis that clinically is a rubbery lump and histologically an indifferent mass of scar is given this word.

gummatous [gŭm′ə-təs] is an adjective meaning pertaining or relating to a gumma.

guttata [gŭ-tā′tə] and **guttate** [gŭt′āt′] are respectively the feminine singular of a Latin adjective and an English adjective derived from it, both meaning having spots that resemble drops. The Latin adjective appears in the title *parapsoriasis guttata;* the English adjective appears in the two following titles.

guttate parapsoriasis [păr′ə-sə-rī′ə-sĭs] names a more or less characteristic picture of finely scaling, drop-like macules that are reminiscent of psoriasis.

guttate psoriasis designates ordinary psoriasis in which the lesions are small and discrete like drops of process upon the skin.

gynecomastia [gī′nē-, jī′nē-, jĭn′ē-kō-măs′tē-ə, -tĭ-ə] is the condition (*-ia*) in males wherein the breasts (*-mast-*) take on womanish (*gyne-*) proportions.

gypseum [jĭp′sē-əm] is a Late Latin word meaning chalky in senses of both color and consistency. It is found in *Microsporon gypseum*.

gyrata [jī-, jĭ-rā′tə, -rä′tə] and **gyratum** [jī-, jĭ-rā′təm, -rä′təm] are the feminine singular and neuter singular respectively of a Late Latin adjective meaning made in circular form, rounded—hence, winding or coiled in round or spiral fashion. These forms appear in the titles *cutis verticis gyrata* and *erythema gyratum*.

gyrate [jī′rāt′], meaning coiled or winding round, is the English derivative and equivalent of *gyrata* and *gyratum*.

H

haem- [hēm]. See *hem-*. In American printing the ligatures æ and œ, which technically are not diphthongs but digraphs because they are pronounced in English as single sounds, are written as a single character by omission of the first element of the combination. Thus *hæm-* becomes *hem-*; *ædema* becomes *edema*; etc. The British practice is still to print them as ligatures or seeming diphthongs (i.e., æ, œ).

Hailey-Hailey disease [hā′lē dĭ, də-zēz′]. Familial benign chronic pemphigus.

hair [hâr] derives from Middle English through Anglo-Saxon and cognates in Old High German, Danish and Swedish. The single structure, as a thread of keratin, is too well known to define. One may remark, however, that the word used as a collective immediately suggests scalp hair to most persons, especially women.

    hair follicle nevus, often present at birth, is a rare tumor consisting of a small nodule on the face. Histologically these are hair follicles and perhaps sebaceous glands. (Pippione et al)

Hallopeau's disease [ălōpō′]. Several: lichen sclerosus et atrophicus, acrodermatitis continua, dermatitis vegetans.

haloderm(i)a [hăl′ō-dûr′mə, -mē-ə, -mĭ-ə] is a generic word for skin changes (*-derma, -dermia*), usually a drug eruption, caused by a halide (*halo-*), usually a bromide or an iodide. Conceivably, skin changes caused by chlorides and fluorides and by elemental bromine, chlorine, fluorine and iodine would be designated by this word but it is not done. Allergic contact dermatitis and primary irritation (chemical burns) from this class of agents are not ordinarily called haloderm(i)as.

halo nevus [hā′lō nē′vəs] is an alternate title for *leukoderma acquisitum centrifugum*. *Halo* refers to a circle of light and the title is picturesquely descriptive, but not really good because it suggests that the acquired depigmentation and the enclosed pigmented nevus are one process.

    An important entity as it may be confused with malignant melanoma. In this lesion, the host makes antibodies against a nevus cell nevus resulting in a regression or disappearance of the nevus. Clinically usually presents as a pigmented nevus with a depigmented area or halo surrounding it.

hamartoma [hăm′ər-tō′mə] is New Latin coinage from Greek *hamartia*, a fault, plus -*oma* in the sense of tumor. In the specialized language of theology the root of the word appears in *hamartiology*, the doctrine of sin. Merely for skin, however, Albrecht defined *hamartoma* as a tumor formation from misplaced embryonal cells. The application of the word then depends on what one considers embryonal cells and what one considers misplaced about them. In Albrecht's view identical twins and supernumerary units (digits, nipples) are hamartomata. But what of reduplication or overdevelopment of tissue that belongs in situ, like angiomata? It is doubtful if *hamartoma* is a useful word unless one makes it synonymous with *nevoid anomaly* or generic for any defective development stemming from faulty embryogenesis.

hand-foot-mouth disease [hănd fŏŏt mouth dĭ-zēz′] is febrile, exanthematous, maculopapular, and eventually vesicular. The lesions appear first in the mouth and then on the hands and feet. The cause is a virus (Coxsackie or echo-virus). This down-to-earth English title tolls the knell of Latinization loudly. A century or so ago, *manus*, *pes*, and *os* would have gotten into the act. It would have been something like *morbus manus, pedis, et oris*.

Hand-Schüller-Christian disease [hănd′-, hând′shŏŏ′lər-krĭs′chən dĭ-, də-zēz′]. Histiocytosis X.

hangnail [hăng′nāl′] is a corruption of Anglo-Saxon *agnail*, which derives from *ang-*, painful, and *naegl*, nail. The sense of *ang-* is further seen in common modern words like *anger* and *anguish*. *Hangnail* refers to those ragged, "hanging" tags of eponychium that are so commonly formed by accident or promoted by a compulsive habit of picking on the cuticles, a form of onychotillomania.

Hansen's disease [hän′sən]. Leprosy.

hapalonychia [hăp′ə-lō-nĭk′ē-ə, -ĭ-ə], derived from Greek word elements for soft (*hapal-*) and nail (-*onych-*), means a condition (-*ia*) of soft nail plates. Such a condition may be natural and relative (as fine, soft hair might be) or acquired as an aspect of malnutrition and debility.

hapten(e) [hăp′tən, -tēn] derives from the Greek verb *haptein* meaning to grasp, clutch or make contact. The word is applied to a substance (-*en*, -*ene*) that becomes antigenic when it complexes (*hapt-*) with proteins.

"hardening" [här′də-nĭng, -d′nĭng] refers to the phenomenon of more or less clearing of allergic eczematous contact dermatitis, in spite of continued exposure to a causative eczematogenic allergen. It is an event more hoped for than expected. If it occurs at all, it is more likely a result of reactive thickening of the stratum corneum, which holds off absorption of allergen from the skin surface, rather than the result of a new immunologic development.

harelip [hâr′lĭp] is descriptive of the congenital defect in children that resembles the cleft lip of the hare. The human anomaly is usually of the upper lip, lateral or central when single, and off-center when bilateral or double. The condition is frequently associated with additional incomplete development of the palate as a result of failure of fusion of branchial clefts.

harlequin fetus [här′lə-kwĭn, -kĭn fē′təs] is a picturesque description of a severe grade of ichthyosis in which hyperkeratosis and diamond-shaped exfoliation is so marked as to suggest the design, color and patchy condition of the traditional costume of a clown (*harlequin*). The condition is so severe that the afflicted infant is either stillborn or not viable for long. *Ichthyosis lethalis* is an alternate term.

The most severe form of congenital ichthyosis. The infant is totally deformed by being encased in thick, contracted skin resulting in enfacement of the ears, lips, nose and digits. Most such infants die within weeks of birth.

Harter's syndrome is familial rosacealike dermatitis with warty keratotic plaques on trunk and limbs.

Hartnup's disease [härt′nŭp]. Pellagroid dermatitis, photosensitivity, tryptophan dysmetabolism.

harvest mite [här′vəst mīt] is a parochial designation for *Trombicula irritans*. See *chigger*.

head louse [hĕd lous] is a lay designation for *Pediculus humanus capitis*.

heavy chain disease is a lymphoma like disease with excessive production of heavy-chain proteins. Skin manifestations may include urticaria. Serum protein electrophoresis will show a marked decrease in albumin, near absence of gamma globulin, and a narrow band or abnormal protein in the region of beta or gamma globulin that is similar in the serum or urine.

Hebra's disease [hĕb′rä]. Prurigo agria or ferox, and prurigo mitis.

helicis [hĕl′ĭ-, hē′lĭ-sĭs], genitive singular of Latin *helix*, means of something spiral. In the title *chondrodermatitis nodularis chronica helicis* the spiral indicated is the outer rim of the pinna.

helminthiasis [hĕl′mĭn-thī′ə-sĭs] means a condition (*-iasis*) caused by a worm (*helminth-*). There are a few worms that infest the skin but direct invasions of the skin by helminths, e.g., *Dracunculus medinensis* and larvae of *Strongyloides* and *Ancylostoma*, are not referred to as helminthiases although they well might be. The word seems to be reserved for infestations of the gut, solid viscera and muscles by worms. There may be cutaneous marks of such remote helminthiases in the form of urticaria and erythema-multiforme-like eruptions.

heloma [hē-lō′mə] and **helosis** hē-lō′sĭs] derive from the Greek word *helos*, nail (of carpentry, not anatomy) or nail-head. Thus, the words mean respectively a tumefaction (*-oma*) in the shape of a nail or nail-head (*hel-*) or a condition (*-osis*) of resemblance to a nail-head or nail and are uncommon synonyms for *callosity, callus, clavus* or *corn*. In ancient Greek *helos* itself designates a wart or callus. See *ephelis* for a related etymological subtlety.

hem- [hĕm], **hema-** [hē′mə], **hemat(o)-** [hē′mə-tō, hĕm′ə-tō], **hemo-** [hē′mō, hĕm′ō] are combining forms from the Greek word for blood. See *haem-*.

hemangioma [hē-măn′jē-ō′mə, -jĭ-ō′mə] is New Latin from Greek words meaning massing, overdevelopment or tumefaction (*-oma*) of blood (*hem-*) vessels (*-angi-*). Common varieties are further described by words like *cavernous* (large and deep sinuses), *superficial* (small and shallow blood-vessel elements) and *strawberry* (appearing like the common fruit).

hemangiomatosis [hē-măn′jĭ-, hē-măn′jē-ō′mə-tō′sĭs] is a condition (*-osis*) in which there is massing overdevelopment or tumor formation of blood vessels (*hemangiomat-*). More extensive and complicated processes than single and simple hemangiomata are described by the word, i.e., conditions that are known eponymically by names like Osler, Parkes-Weber, etc.

hemangiopericytoma [hē-măn′jē-ō-pĕr′ĭ-sī-tō′mə] designates a highly malignant neoplasm (*-oma*) of certain cells (*-cyt-*) that are normally present in and around (*-peri-*) the walls of blood vessels (*hemangio-*).

   A tumor of capillaries which can arise wherever these are found. Skin lesions appear as hardened nodules or plaques and have been known to be extensive in size. The deep-seated tumors as opposed to those on the skin with a more ominous-appearing pathology are apt to metastasize. Perhaps it will help to remember this tumor by thinking of it as good, bad and indeterminate, i.e., benign type does not metastasize, malignant types do in 3/4 of the cases, and the indeterminate type would be the borderline malignant type with infrequent metastasis approximately 1/3 of the time.

hemat(h)idrosis [hē′măt-, hĕm′ăt-(h)ĭ-drō′sĭs] and **hematohidrosis** [hē′mə-, hĕm′ə-tō-hĭ-drō′sĭs] are New Latin words from Greek that mean a condition (-*osis*) of bloody or blood-stained (*hemat-*, *hemato-*) sweat (-*hidr-*, -*idr-*).

hematoma [hē′mə-, hĕm′ə-tō′mə] is New Latin from Greek meaning the result of (-*ma*), or a mass (-*oma*) resulting from, bleeding (*hemato-*, *hemat-*). An extravasation of blood within a tissue in the form of a sizable swelling is designated by the word.

hematoxylin [hē′mə-, hĕm′ə-tŏk′sə-lĭn] is the common dye used in combination with eosin in histologic processing. The word means a material (-*in*) derived from wood (-*xyl-*, in this instance, logwood) and of brownish color (*hemato-*, like blood). As a chemical complex it reacts with alkalies to yield a violet to blue color.

hemi- [hĕm′ĭ, -ē] is a prefix from Greek meaning one half. *Semi-* and *demi-* are Latin equivalents.

hemi(-)atrophy [hĕm′ē-ăt′rə-fē, -fĭ] means failure of complete development (-*atrophy*) of half (*hemi-*) a part or region.

hemochromatosis [hĕm-ō-, hē′mō-krō′mə-tō′sĭs] literally means a condition (-*osis*) in which the skin is colored (-*chromat-*) from the blood (*hemo-*). The actual color has been likened to bronze. The phenomenon occurs in connection with atrophic and cirrhotic processes of the liver and pancreas. Diabetes and marks of hepatic insufficiency are associated phenomena. Hemosiderin is the basis of the cutaneous hyperpigmentation.

Emendation: The hyperpigmentation is actually from increased melanin in the epidermis. The iron of hemosiderrin in itself is not brown in vivo as though it were in the form of rust.

hemophilia [hĕm′ō-, hē′mō-fĭl′ē-ə, -ĭ-ə], from its Greek word elements, literally means a blood- (*hemo-*) -loving (-*phil-*) condition (-*ia*). Continuous hemorrhage from a failure of coagulation of blood is designated by the word. The condition is inherited and exhibited only by males but transmitted only by females.

hemorrhage [hĕm′ə-rĭj], from its Greek word elements, means a bursting forth (-*rrhage*) of blood (*hemo-*). The common phenomenon is too well-known to require extensive description beyond saying that a considerable letting of blood externally is usually meant.

Extravasations of blood into tissue are also hemorrhages but usually other descriptive words like *ecchymosis, hematoma, peliosis, petechia, purpura, suggillation* and *vibex* are used to denote contained hemorrhages, especially when they have special characteristics.

hemosiderin [hĕm′ō-, hē′mō-sĭd′ĕr-ĭn, -ə-rĭn] is the material (*-in*) derived from the iron (*-sider-*) fraction of blood (*hemo-*).

hemosiderosis [hĕm-ō-, hē′mō-sĭd′ĕr-ō′sĭs, -ə-rō′sĭs] is New Latin from Greek word elements that mean a condition (*-osis*) related to the iron (*-sider-*) fraction of blood (*hemo-*). The word is used synonymously with *hemochromatosis*, but can also be used to designate deposition of iron from any hemorrhage in any tissue. In the skin a rust-colored pigmentation results which may be transient or long-enduring.

Henoch-Schoenlein purpura. [hĕn′ŏk; shôn′lĭn] Allergic nonthrombocytopenic purpura.

herald patch [hĕr′əld pătch] is the initial lesion of pityriasis rosea that is a presage (*herald*) of more to come.

hereditary hemorrhagic telangiectasia (Osler-Weber-Rendu disease). A bleeding disorder resulting from a vascular developmental abnormality. Autosomal dominant.

The telangiectases result from dilation and convolutions of vesicles and capillaries in the skin and mucous membranes.

The most common hereditary vascular disorder associated with a hemorrhagic diathesis. (A.J. Marcus, *Cecil Textbook of Medicine*, 18th Edition, Wyngaarden and Smith, editors, Saunders)

Hermansky-Pudlak syndrome is an unusual type of albinism; hair bulbs are tyrosinase positive. Platelet suppression with bleeding tendency, low platelet count usually present.

herpangina [hûr′păn-jī′nə] is derived from Greek word elements via Latin and literally means a creeping (*herp-*) strangulation (*-angina*). The word names an infection of the throat by the Coxsackie virus that is marked by intense swelling of the area.

herpes [hûr′pēz] is a Latin word taken over from Greek and meaning a creeping. The Greek root means to creep; etymologically related to this root are the English words *reptile* and *serpent* (derived from Latin). *Herpetology* is literally the study of creeping things. Greek writers used the word *herpes* to designate shingles; Pliny, the Roman writer on natural history, used it to designate "a cutaneous eruption that creeps and spreads." Today the word is applied to vesicular processes in which there is a tendency for the blisters to form rather quickly, to cluster and to seem to creep along. The "creep" idea is more one of succession of blister formation in a linear fashion rather than one of movement.

herpes genitalis is caused mainly by herpes simplex virus type II, resulting in vulvovaginitis and herpes of the penis. Serious common problems. Diagnosis must be established by viral cultures and typing. Present treatment is with systemic and local acyclovir.

herpes gestationis [jĕs-tā′shĭ-ō′nĭs, -shē-ō′nĭs, -shō′nĭs] is a title for an uncommon eruption that resembles dermatitis herpetiformis, occurs in pregnancy (*gestationis*) and tends to remit following delivery and to re-occur in subsequent pregnancies. It is characteristic in the grouped and creeping (*herpes*) morphology of its papulo-vesicular, pruritic lesions and intractable chronicity during pregnancy. May be difficult to separate from bullous pemphigoid.

An extremely rare interesting blistering disease associated with pregnancy and or the puerperium. Clinically similar to bullous pemphigoid but immunologically a distinct entity. Immunoelectronmicroscopy shows deposits of IgG in skin of lesions.

The lesions may vary from pruritic papules to bullae and can be widespread. Systemic steroids may be necessary to control. Not truly associated with infant mortality or morbidity.

herpes iris [ī′rĭs] describes an arc arrangement (*iris*, rainbow) of creeping (*herpes*) vesicular process. The phenomenon is seen in erythema multiforme.

herpes labialis [lā′bē-, lā′bĭ-ā′lĭs, -ä′lĭs, -ăl′ĭs] specifies the location of herpes simplex on the oral lips (*labialis*). Usually due to herpes virus type 1.

herpes progenitalis [prō-jĕn′ĭ-tā′lĭs, -tä′lĭs, -tăl′ĭs] specifies the location of herpes simplex on or of the genitalia (*progenitalis*). Invariably due to herpes virus type II. This is oncogenic when it occurs on the uterine cervix.

herpes simplex [sĭm′plĕks] is the title for that common viral infection in which a rapidly evolving cluster of vesicles (*herpes*) occurs. The condition is common on the oral lips but possible almost anywhere else on the skin, on accessible mucous membranes and on the cornea. Due to herpes simplex virus types I and II.

herpes simplex recurrens [rē-kŭr′ĕnz] describes repeated (*recurrens*) episodes of herpes simplex in a fixed site.

herpes zoster [zōs′-, zŏs′tĕr, -tər] is another well-known viral infection due to the varicella-zoster (VZ) virus, which usually causes varicella in children and zoster in adults, in which creeping vesiculation (*herpes*) tends to assume a belt or girdle (*zoster*) arrangement on the trunk. In reality, the allusion to *girdling* on the trunk is inaccurate because even where it could be reasonably pictorial, as on the waist, it does not fit the incomplete, unilateral fact. On the face and limbs there is, of course, no girdling at all, but an arrangement that is determined by the distribution of the peripheral sensory nerves in those regions. Nevertheless, there are those who are more exercised by the *herpes* part of the title than by the *zoster*. They would have the title merely as *zoster*. They do have it as one word, in synonymy at that, in *zona* and *shingles*. Both *zoster* and *zona* are words of Greek origin meaning belt or girdle, which were taken over into Latin. Both the Greeks and the Romans applied these unmodified words to herpes zoster so that those moderns who favor *zoster* alone as a title for the disease make a commendable bow to antiquity. Trouble arises, however, with a phrase like *post-herpetic neuralgia*. *Shingles* derives from Latin *cingulum*, a belt, a word which was not applied by the Romans to *herpes zoster*.

HZ also **zona, shingles,** is a dermatomal cutaneous infection caused by reactivation of the varicella-zoster virus that normally lies latent in sensory ganglia following an early attack of varicella. A creeping vesiculation (herpes) tends to assume a belt or girdle (zoster) arrangement on the trunk. On the face and limbs there is no girdling at all, but an arrangement that is determined by the distribution of the peripheral sensory nerves in those regions. In addition to its cutaneous manifestations, zoster is accompanied by neuritic symptoms and may be complicated by an array of neurologic sequelae. (R.W. Price, *Cecil Textbook of Medicine* 18th Edition, Saunders Co., Wyngaarden & Smith, editors)

herpes zoster generalisatus [jĕn'ĕr-ăl'ĭ-sā'təs, -sä'tŭs, -tōōs] describes the widespread dissemination (*generralisatus*) of varicelliform lesions and it amounts to the supervention of chicken pox (*varicella*) following herpes zoster. Occurs in the immune deficient host.

herpetic, herpeticum [hər-, hûr-pĕt'ĭk; -ĭ-kəm, -ə-kəm] are respectively an English adjective and the neuter singular form of a New Latin adjective meaning pertaining or relating to herpes, a creeping.

herpetiform, herpetiformis [hər, hûr-pĕt'ĭ-fôrm, -ə-fôrm; -fôr'mĭs] are respectively an English adjective and the masculine and feminine singular of a New Latin adjectival formation from Greek and Latin elements meaning like, or in the shape of (*-form, -formis*) a creeping (*herpeti-*) lesion.

herpetoid [hûr'pē-, hər'pə-, hûr'pə-toid] means in the nature of or like (*-oid*) herpes.

Herxheimer reaction [hûrks′hī-mər rē-ăk′shən] designates an augmentation of clinical response of reactions of allergic nature when antigen is suddenly released by the action of a therapeutic agent.

Exacerbation of disease process by sudden release of antigens from the action of a therapeutic agent, e.g., aggravation of a syphilitic chancre upon inception of penicillin therapy.

heter(o)- [hĕt′ər-, hĕt′ēr-ō] is a combining form taken from Greek and meaning other, other of two, other than usual, different, opposite of *hom* (*o*)-, same, *is* (*o*)-, equal, and *orth* (*o*)-, straight, correct—all from Greek.

heterochromia [hĕt′ər-, hĕt′ēr-ō-krō′mē-ə] is New Latin from Greek elements meaning a condition (-*ia*) of other than usual (*hetero-*) color (-*chrom-*). As a matter of description, a condition of two or more colors simultaneously, one of which may be normal is described by the word. Eyes of different color are so designated, but piebaldism, vitiligo and tinctorial developments in histology could also be described by the word.

hibernoma [hī′bər-, hī′bēr-, hī′bēr-nō′mə] literally means a mass or tumor (-*oma*) related to the wintertime (*hibern-*, from Latin *hibernus*, wintry). Recalling the deposits of fat laid down by hibernating animals in preparation for sleeping out winter rigors, certain masses of brown (embryonal) fat found in certain tumors have been termed *hibernomas*. Perhaps the effect is a phylogenetic atavism.

hickey [hĭk′ē, -ĭ] is one of those words of unknown origin that invite humorous or playful applications. From original application to devices used in electrical trades (certain switches, conduit-pipe benders) it was quickly embellished to *do-hickey*, meaning a gadget or tool used to manage some simple operation. Of further interest is the use of the word *hickey* to denote a device, gadget or tool whose name one cannot remember or does not know. Of still further interest is the variety of picturesque expressions for the same concept and idea, like *do* (*o*)*dad*, *rigamajig*, *thingum* (*a*)*bob* and *what-do-you-call-it*, corrupted to *whatchamacallit*. Of dermatologic interest is application of the word to a pimple (papulo-pustule) and to the erythematous and later ecchymotic mark (*passion purpura*) of a playful bite or pinch, usually on the cheeks (of the face or buttocks), the neck or breasts, inflicted or incurred in hanky-panky.

hidebound disease [hīd′bound′ dĭ-, də-zēz′] is a descriptive reference to the condition of the skin in diffuse scleroderma. The immobilized tightness of the face, chest and extremities, as though wrapped in contracted leather, is told by the term.

hidradenitis [hĭ-drăd′′n, hĭ-drăd′ə-nī′tĭs, -nē′tĭs, -təs], a New Latin formation from Greek word elements, literally means inflammation (*-itis*) of sweat (*hidr-*) glands (*-aden-*). However, not the ordinary sweat or eccrine glands are meant, but specifically apocrine glands.

hidradenitis suppurativa [sŭp′ū-rə-tī′və] describes inflammation of apocrine glands (*hidradenitis*) that is going to, or has gone to, purulence (*suppurativa*). The common process is located in the axillae, where apocrine glands are abundant. The umbilical, genito-perineal and areolar areas may be affected since apocrine glands are present in these places, albeit sparsely.

hidradenoma [hĭ-drăd′′n-, hĭ-drăd′ə-nō′mə], a New Latin formation from Greek word elements, means a neoplasia or tumor (*-oma*) of a sweat (*hidr-*) gland (*-aden-*). Reduplication of the deep portion and massing of the cells thereof are the histologic marks of the process.

hidr(o)- [hī′drō, hĭd′rō] is a combining form from Greek *hidros*, sweat. It is not to be confused with *hydr* (*o*)-, which is a combining form from *hydor*, the Greek word for water. It is true that sweat is largely water but the iota (*ι*) of difference displaces the transliterated upsilon (*υ*).

hidrocystoma [hī′drō-, hĭd′rō-sĭs-tō′mə], a New Latin formation from Greek elements, means cystic deformation (*-cystoma*) of sweat (*hidro-*) glands.

hidromeiosis a disease of sweating resulting from poral occlusion by hyperhydration of the stratum corneum.

hidrosis [hĭ-drō′sĭs, -səs] is a learned word for ordinary sweating or perspiration. However, the term may also be applied to excessive sweating or a skin disease affecting the sweat glands.

In addition *hidrosis* is used in word composition as an alternate for *idrosis*, a state of sweating. The *h* represents the aspirate present in the Greek word for sweating, and perhaps the *idrosis* form is an unnecessary way of transcribing the original, but it's too late and we have to sweat it out now.

hiemalis [hē′ə-, hē′ĕ-, hī′ē-mā′lĭs, -mä′lĭs, -măl′ĭs] is a Latin adjective meaning belonging to, pertaining to or relating to (*-alis*) winter (*hiem-*). It appears in the titles *prurigo hiemalis* and *pruritus hiemalis*.

Hippocratic facies, or **face.** See *facies Hippocratica*.

Hippocratic facies, fingers, nails [hĭp′ō-krăt′ĭk]. "The mask of impending death," clubbed fingers and convex nails.

Hippocratic fingers [fĭng′gẽrz] designates bulbous enlargement of the terminal phalanges of fingers seen in certain conditions of pulmonary insufficiency. See *clubbed fingers.*

Hippocratic nails [hĭp′ə-, hĭp′ō-krăt′ĭk nālz] is a term applied to the broad, convex nails of clubbed, or Hippocratic, fingers.

hirsute [hĭr′-, hər′-, hûr′sūt′, -sōōt′] is an adjective derived from Latin *hirsutus* meaning hairy, bristly or rough with hair.

hirsuties [hĭr-, hər-, hûr-sū′shĭ-ēz, -sōō′shē-ēz, -shēz] is a New Latin noun meaning hairiness. The word probably should not be used merely for ordinary hairiness that is still normal for a person but quite especially for unusual, coarse hairiness that is abnormal development. *Hypertrichosis* is nearly synonymous but simply implies acquired, excessive (*hyper-*) hairiness (*-trichosis*) of any quality. *Hirsutism* is an alternate word, simpler to say than *hirsuties.*

hirsutism means excessive growth of body hair in women. May or may not be associated with pathology. This is growth of terminal hairs where it would not normally be found in females.

hirudiniasis [hĭr′ū-, hə-, hĭ-rōō′dĭ-nī′ə-sĭs] means a condition (*-iasis*) of infestation with leeches (*hirudin-*, from Latin *hirudo*, genitive *hirudinis*, a leech).

histi- and **histio-** [hĭs-tĭ, -tē; hĭs′tĭ-ō, -tē-ō] derive from Greek *histion*, web, and are often used for *hist* (*o*)- in the sense of tissue. See *hist-(o)-.*

histiocyte [hĭs′tē-ə-, hĭs′tĭ-ō-sīt′] derives from Greek elements that mean a tissue (*histio-*) cell (*-cyte*). The cell designated is not just any tissue cell but a particular one that derives from the reticuloendothelial system and is then found visiting and acting special roles in many tissues. The structural and tinctorial properties of histiocytes are difficult to specify because they appear in many guises, even disguises, depending upon functions the cells assume in health and disease.

histiocytic cytophagic panniculitis, a frequently fatal systemic disease, is characterized by recurrent widely distributed, painful subcutaneous nodules associated with malaise and fever. A low-grade form of malignant histiocytosis is at first confined to the skin but then strikes vital organs. Patients usually die of sudden hemorrhage. (Lever)

Rare disease but causes severe skin lesions. May cause acute destruction of fatty tissue and more rarely of the visceral organs involved.

Patients have cutaneous nodules and plaques that sometimes are ecchymotic and ulcerated and are characterized by infiltration of the subcutaneous tissue by large benign histiocytes with cytophagic features. Deaths may be due to hemorrhagic complications. May respond to aggressive polychemotherapy. (Alegre & Winkleman)

histiocytoma [hĭs′tē-ə-, hĭs′tĭ-ō-sī-tō′mə] designates a tumor (-*oma*) consisting of histiocytes. *Nodulus cutaneus, cutaneous nodule* and *subepidermal nodular fibrosis* are alternate terms.

histiocytosis X [hĭs′tē-ə-, hĭs′tĭ-ō-sī-tō′sĭs ĕks] comprises three distinct clinical entities due to proliferation of histiocytes: Letterer-Siwe disease, Hand-Schüller-Christian disease, and eosinophilic granuloma. The most striking skin findings are seen in Letterer-Siwe disease which usually develops in the first year of life. It very often appears like severe seborrheic dermatitis which may be the first manifestation of the disease. If the visceral involvement is extensive, prognosis is poor. Anemia, thrombocytopenia, lymphadenopathy, enlargement of the liver and spleen, and pulmonary infiltrates may be part of the clinical presentation. (Lever)

hist(o)- [hĭs′tō-, -tə] is a combining form from the Greek word *histos*, web, warp. It is used with meanings of web, net and tissue.

histology [hĭs-tŏl′ə-jē, -jĭ] is the study (-*logy*) of tissues (*histo-*). Study at microscopic levels, i.e., fine structure, is implied.

Histoplasma [hĭs′tō-plăz′mə] is the name of a genus of fungi whose cell cytoplasm has a webbed or retiform (*histo-*) appearance.

Histoplasma capsulatum [kăp′sōō-, kăp′sū-lā′təm, -lä′təm] is the name of a species in the genus *Histoplasma* which has pathogenicity for humans and whose cells are marked by a distinctive capsule which is an artifact of preparation.

histoplasmin [hĭs′tō-plăz′mĭn] is an "antigen" crudely processed from species of *Histoplasma* in the manner of actinomycin from *Actinomyces* and tuberculin from the tubercle bacillus. Its manner of use and interpretation of test results parallel those of the similar materials.

histoplasmosis [hĭs′tō-plăz-mō′sĭs] is a coinage designed to name a condition (-*osis*) caused by a fungus that bears the name *Histoplasma capsulatum*.

This is usually a deep funguus infection. There is a primary cutaneous disease caused by *Histoplasma capsulatum* usually the disease starts with inhalation of air borne spores. Endemic in the eastern and central United States. Cutaneous histoplasmosis results from skin dissemination in less than 10% of cases especially in those who are immunosuppressed. No organisms are found in these lesions. Treatment is with amphotericin B. Primary skin lesions are self-limited in the normal host. (Tomecki et al)

HIV, human immunodeficiency virus, is the viral causative organism of AIDS.

hive, hives [hīv; hīvz] are words of uncertain origin. Originally there was but *hives* as a word meaning an eruption of wheals. Nowadays, *hive*, as a back formation, is used as a singular meaning a wheal or urtica.

Hodgkin's disease [hŏdj′kĭnz dĭ-, də-zēz′] is eponymic for that lymphomatous process or reticulo-endotheliosis that is marked clinically by intense pruritus, excoriations, specific and nonspecific cutaneous lesions and lymphadenopathy. Histologically, it is notable for a characteristic giant cell (Dorothy Reed-Sternberg cell) within lymph nodes and other sites of cellular infiltration.

holocrine [hōl′-, hŏl′ō-krīn, -krēn, hŏl′ə-krən] literally means separating (-*crine*) in entirety (Greek, *holo-*, whole). The word is sometimes applied to describe the sebaceous gland whose product is a sort of complete shedding cellular substance altered to fats.

holocrine gland is alternate for *sebaceous gland*.

hominis [hŏm′ĭ-, hō′mĭ-nĭs] is the genitive singular of the Latin noun *homo*, human being, and therefore means of, belonging to or pertaining to a human being. It is found in titles like *Actinomyces hominis* and *Sarcoptes hominis*.

homme rouge [ôm, ŭm rōōzh] is a French term that means red (*rouge*) man (*homme*). It is applied descriptively to individuals who are affected by an erythroderma when the redness of the process is startling. See *l'homme rouge*.

Hopf, acrokeratosis verruciformis of [hŭpf]. Wartiness of hands and feet.

hordeolum [hôr-dē′ō-ləm, -dē′ə-ləm] is New Latin from *hordeolus*, diminutive of *hordeum*, barley. *Hordeolus* was used in Late Latin to mean a sty(e) in the eye. One may assume that the word suggested itself for the common lesion because at its most bothersome stage it looks like a grain of barley.

Hormodendron, -um [hôr′mə-, hôr′mō-dĕn′drŏn, -drən; -drəm] derives from Greek elements that mean chain (*hormo-*) and tree (*-dendron, -dendrum*). The -*on* ending is Greek; -*um* is a corresponding Latin ending. The words name a genus of fungi with cultural characteristics that are suggestive of chains and trees from the arrangement of hyphae and spores. Two species of the genus (*compactum, pedrosoi*) cause chromoblastomycosis.

horn [hôrn] is Anglo-Saxon with cognates in Danish, German and Gothic and probable relationship to Latin *cornu*, horn, and Greek *krangon*, a small crustacean. Ultimate derivation may be Sanskrit *kar*, hard. In any event hard keratin of all mammalian kinds is now designated by the word.

horny [hôr′nē, -nǐ] is an adjective meaning pertaining to, relating to, in the nature of horn, and hard or tough.

human herpes virus 6 (HH6, HBLV) roseola infantum (exanthem subitum, sixth disease), always considered a very aptly named disease now known to be due to human herpes virus 6. These patients age 6 months to about 3 years develop sudden high fever, then on approximately the fourth day the fever breaks suddenly and a widespread morbilliform rash develops not involving mucous membranes. HH6 has been implicated in making the HIV virus more virulent.

humectant [hū-mĕk′tənt] is an adjective and noun derived from *humectans*, present participle of the Latin verb *humectare*, to moisten, to wet, and literally it means wetting, moistening. Related to it are the unusual words *humect* and *humectate*, to wet or become wet, and *humectation*, a wetting or moistening, as well as the simpler words *humid* and *humor*. The first three are marked "rare" in Webster's Second, "archaic" in the Third but *humectant*, meaning, when used as a noun, a substance that helps to retain moisture, is very much alive among the hucksters of Madison Avenue as a gimmick word to advertise real or fancied "moisturizing" properties of some cosmetics.

Hunterian chancre [hŭn-tēr′ǐ-ən]. The well-developed, "classical" chancre of syphilis: a painless, crateriform ulcer with an indurated border on the penis.

Hurler's disease [hûr′lērz, -lûrz dǐ-, də-zēz′], **syndrome (MPS I-H)** [sǐn′drōm], is a mucopolysaccharidoses characterized by gargoylism, ocular hypertelorism and shagreen skin among other signs and by urinary excretion of chondroitin sulfate B and heparitin sulfate.

Hutchinson-Gilford syndrome [hŭtch′ǐn-sən; gǐl′fôrd]. True progeria.

Hutchinson's freckle. See *melanotic freckle of Hutchinson*.

Hutchinson's freckle, teeth [hŭtch′ǐn-sən]. Lentigo maligna; notched incisors in congenital syphilis.

Hutchinson's sign. Periungual spread of pigmentation into the proximal and lateral nail folds; a most important indicator of subungual melanoma.

hyalin(e) [hī′ə-lĭn, -lən, -līn, -lēn], derived from a Greek word for glass, means glassy.

hyaline degeneration [də-, dē-jən′ēr-ā′shən, -ə-rā′shən] describes degradation from a more definite structure to something like glassy character.

hyalinosis cutis et mucosae [hī′ə-lĭ-nō′sĭs kū′tĭs ĕt mūkō′sē] is alternate for *lipoid proteinosis*. By this title the condition is described in its histologic aspect as a glassy (*hyalin-*) condition (*-osis*) of the skin (*cutis*) and mucous membranes (*mucosae*).

hydr(o)- [hī′drō], a combining form indicating water, is derived from Greek and Latin *hydr* (*o*)-, which ultimately goes back to the Greek word *hydor*, water. The *Hydra*, which refers to the famous water snake killed by Hercules, *hydraulic*, operated by water, and *hydrogen*, literally, generating water, are some simple words containing this combining form. It is not to be confused in spelling or pronunciation with *hidr* (*o*)-, which derives from Greek *hidros*, sweat. See *hidr* (*o*)-, and *hidrosis*.

hydroa [hī-drō′ə] is a bothersome word both because of the problem associated with its derivation and also because of confusion about its gender. One theory about its etymology is that it is composed of the Greek word element *hydr-*, water, and *-oä*, the plural form of the Greek noun *oön*, which is of neuter gender and means egg. Thus, *hydroa* would mean literally water-, or watery, eggs, and would adequately describe the eggs (like caviar and roe) of an aquatic animal. The relationship between such eggs and an eruption of blisters would then have to rest upon some fancied or fanciful resemblance.

Another and more plausible theory is that *hydroa* is an alteration of the Greek neuter plural noun *hidroa* used by Galen and others to designate heat spots or pustules. In this case *hydr-* would be construed as a case of confusion with *hidr-*.

In any event, *hydroa* and its modifiers bespeak an eruption of delicate blisters on exposed skin (arms, face, legs) that appears in some patients during the summertime. Such blisters heal with scars faintly reminiscent of cowpox (*vacciniform-*, resembling vaccinia).

hydroa vacciniforme are tense umbilicated vesicles resembling smallpox that appear on the face, backs of hands, and chest. These will break, crust, and may scar. Usually clears after puberty. Rx:

avoid sun. Sunscreens, group 5 topical steroids, wet compresses, and antimalarials can control these diseases.

hygroma [hī-grō′mə] is New Latin from Greek word elements meaning a moist (*hygr-*) tumor (*-oma*). Certain lymphangiomas of the face and thereabouts, especially those with cavernous or cystic structure, are called hygromas. The word is also used for distended bursae and fluid-filled cysts or sacs of other character in other locations.

hyper- [hī′pēr, hī′pər] is a direct borrowing of the Greek prefix meaning more, over, above, excessive, high, above normal, etc. It is equivalent to the Latin *super-*. In the following words beginning with *hyper-* only the first pronunciation is given, the other is possible.

hypergammaglobulinemia of Waldenström is characterized by hypergammaglobulinemia, recurring purpura, an elevated erythrocyte sedimentation rate, and the presence of rheumatoid factor indicative of circulating immune complexes. There is a significant association with auto-immune diseases, especially Sjögren's syndrome and lupus erythematosis. This is a chronic relapsing purpura and usually benign. (K.A. Finder et al. *J. Am. Acad. Dermatol.* 1990; 23: 669-76)

hyper(h)idrosis [hī′pēr-(h)ĭ-drō′sĭs] means excessive (*hyper-*) sweating (*-hidrosis, -idrosis*).

hyperimmunoglobulinemia E syndrome is a primary immunodeficiency characterized by recurrent staphylococcal abscesses and markedly elevated serum IgE concentrations. There is often a lifelong history of severe recurrent staphylococcal abscesses involving the skin, lungs, joints and other sites. The pruritic dermatitis that occurs is not typical atopic eczema and does not always persist. (Rebecca H. Buckley, *Cecil Textbook of Medicine*, Wyngaarden & Smith, editors, 18th Edition, W. B. Saunders, 1988).

hyperkeratosis [hī′pēr-kĕr′ə-tō′sĭs] means excessive (*hyper-*) cornification (*-keratosis*).

hyperkeratosis follicularis et parafollicularis in cutem penetrans [fō-lĭk′ū-lā′rĭs, -lä′rĭs, -lär′ĭs ĕt păr′ə-, ĭn kū′tĕm, -təm pĕn′ə-, pĕn′ē-tränz] describes a condition (*-osis*) in which excessive (*hyper-*) horn (*-kerat-*) forms in and about hair follicles (*follicularis et parafollicularis*) and tends to penetrate (*penetrans*) the living structure of the skin (*in cutem*, into the skin).

hyperpigmentation [hī′pēr-pĭg′mĕn-tā′shən, -mən-tā′shən] means excessive (*hyper-*) coloration (*-pigmentation*).

hyperplasia [hī'pĕr-plā'zhē-ə, -zē-ə, -zhə] means over or excessive growth or development (-*plasia*).

hyperprebetalipoproteinemia. Individuals with this lipid abnormality may develop eruptive xanthomata.

hypersensitivity reactions, four types:

1. Immediate or anaphylactic reaction, IgE-mediated, comes from an antigen reacting with specifically sensitized IgE that is fixed to mast cells and basophils resulting in degranulation of these cells and the release of mediators which cause vasodilation.

2. Cytotoxic reaction (does not occur in skin)

3. Immune complex reaction, in which an antigen reacts with specific circulating antibodies produced by plasma cells. The resulting antigen-antibody complexes fix complement resulting in Arthus phenomenon, etc. This attracts neutrophils or eosinophils which participate in the inflammatory response, e.g., allergic vasculitis, bullous pemphigoid.

4. Delayed hypersensitivity or cell-mediated reaction, mediated by specifically sensitized T lymphocytes. Lymphokines are released from sensitized lymphocytes at the site of the antigen and produce tissue damage, e.g., allergic contact dermatitis, including garden variety poison ivy.

hypertrichosis [hī'pĕr-trī-kō'sĭs] means excessive (*hyper-*) hairiness (-*trichosis*).

hypertrichosis lanuginosa is a rare hereditary syndrome in which lanugo hair is retained throughout life (congenital type). The acquired type may be associated with an underlying malignancy. In that instance it is given the most apt name of malignant down.

hypertrophic scar [hī'pĕr-trŏf'ĭk, -trō'fĭk skär] describes a complication of the healing of wounds that results in exuberant cicatrization that resembles keloid formation. Some aver that the condition is a keloidosis; others maintain that hypertrophic scars, unlike keloids, do not extend beyond the limits of the wound and eventually flatten of themselves.

hypertrophicus [hī'pĕr-trŏf'ĭ-kəs, -trō'fĭ-kəs] is the masculine singular of a New Latin adjective from Greek elements and means over- (*hyper-*) -grown (-*troph-*, literally nourishing, plus -*icus*, adjective ending). It appears in the titles *lichen corneus hypertrophicus* and *lupus erythematosus hypertrophicus.*

hypertrophy [hī-pĕr'trə-fē, -fī] means over (*hyper-*) -development (-*trophy*, literally, nourishment).

hypha [hī′fə] is New Latin from a Greek word for a web. The word now designates a single thread-like element of fungal mycelium.

hyphen, use of. There is a tendency in modern technical writing to string along adjectives, adjectival and adverbial phrases, and nouns—all without intervening punctuation—to modify nouns. Also letters and parts of words are slapped together thoughtlessly to make unpronounceable and un-understandable acronyms and non-sensical neologisms. Such formations are ambiguous, to say nothing of being unreadable or inelegant.

For example, would it not be better to write and say *pico-RNA-viruses* [pē′kō-är′ĕn′ā′-vī′rə-səs] instead of *picornaviruses* [pə-kôr′nə-vī′rə-səs] and *per-iodic* [pûr′ī-ŏd′ĭk] acid rather than *periodic* [pēr′ĭ-ŏd′ĭk] acid? The hyphens make the meanings clearer. Notice what happens if the hyphen is omitted in a formation like *un-ion-ized.* The cure of much ambiguity and the promotion of clarity in modern technical writing lies in liberal use of the hyphen and other simple, nonverbal marks. Omission of such marks is convenient for a writer who knows what he or she has in mind and is a minor saving in printing, but may incommode or confuse readers for all time. There is more to be gained than lost by using a hyphen even when omission of it is already a recognized custom. To give one more example and recommendation about it, a hyphen should be used when there has to be a pause in pronunciation of elements in newly formed words, especially when omission of it creates an "un-natural" diphthong and suggests there need be no pause, e.g., *kerato-acanthoma* and *micro-organism.*

hyp(o)- [hī′pō] is a Greek prefix that means less, under, beneath, diminished, down, below normal, etc. It is equivalent to Latin *sub-*.

hypoderm [hī′pō-dûrm] designates the region immediately subjacent (*hypo-*) to the true skin (*-derm*). It is that region where there is an intermingling of panniculus adiposus and corium at the level of the lowest hair bulbs and sweat glands.

hypomelanosis of Ito An important rare neurocutaneous disorder, onset at birth, infancy or childhood. Skin shows hypomelanosis over Blaschko's lines. More than seventy-five percent have seizures, mental retardation and an abnormal EEG may ensue. Hearing and visual exams are important.

hyponychium [hī′pō-nĭk′ĭ-əm, -ē-əm] names the barely discernible but still viable remnant of embryonal periderm that persists under (*hyp-*) the free edge of the nail (*-onychium*). Compare *eponychium.*

hyposensitivity [hī′pō-sĕn′sə-tĭv′ə-tē, -tĭ] means a condition of less (*hypo-*) sensitivity than average.

hystrix [hĭs′trĭks], the transliteration of the Greek word for a porcupine, relates particularly to the sharp character of its spines or quills. The word is used in the title *ichthyosis hystrix* to describe, not so sharply, the verrucous character of this form of ichthyosis. The stem of the word is found in *hystriciasis*.

I

-ia [ē′ə, ĭ′ə, yə] is a common abstract noun ending used in New Latin formations. In French and German it is found as *-ie*; in English it can appear as *-y*. For example, *dermatologia* is New Latin; *dermatologie* is French and German; *dermatology* is English. In many medical words, *-ia* comes to signify a pathologic condition (e.g., *onychia*).

-iasis [ī′ə-sĭs, -səs] is a compound combining form (*-ia-* plus *-sis*) from Greek meaning, in our special contexts, a pathologic condition of sorts, e.g., *psoriasis*, or a pathologic condition caused by something, e.g., *acariasis*. The plural is *-iases* [ī′ə-sēs]. See comments on this suffix under *zosteriform*.

-ic, -ical [ĭk; ĭ′k'l, ə-kəl] are adjectival endings from Greek *-ikos*, Latin *-icus* and Late Latin *-icalis* with the force of relating or pertaining to. The choice of which to use is sometimes clear and simple, sometimes fuzzy and complicated. For example, there is little uncertainty about *economic* and *economical* or *politic* and *political*, but should it be *dermatologic* or *dermatological*? In these instances where *-ic* and *-ical* do not confer a distinctly different meaning, as they do in the first examples, the choice seems to matter little except in that *-ical* is longer by one syllable. The older habit favored *-ical*; the modern tendency is to favor *-ic*. It has been suggested that *-ic* be used to denote close or intimate relationship and *-ical* to denote more remote or loose relationship. There are some instances in which *-ic* is not likely to displace *-ical*, e.g., *chemical, medical*, etc. In our specialty *dermatologic* would seem more often appropriate than *dermatological* in most connotations.

ichthyosis [ĭk′thē-ō′sĭs], from its Greek word elements, literally means a fishy (*ichthy-*) condition (*-osis*). The genodermatoses commonly designated by the word are marked by desquamation in roughly polygonal or spinous fragments of stratum corneum that vaguely resemble the scales or other surface characteristic of fish.

There are four major types, three minor forms and numerous syndromes with ichthyosis as part of the findings.

Ichthyosis vulgaris, the most common type, develops a few months after birth. There are scales on the extensor surfaces of the extremities, the distribution is opposite to atopic dermatitis in that the antecubital and popliteal fossae are spared. Smaller scales are present over the body. Pathology shows hyperkeratosis with a thin or abstract granular layer. May be an acquired condition in underlying cancers and sarcoidosis. (Lever)

Other major forms are X-linked ichthyosis, epidermolytic hyperkeratosis and autosomal recessive ichthyosis which in former times was divided into congenital ichthyosiform erythroderma and the very severe lamellar ichthyosis.

The three minor forms are harlequin ichthyosis, erythrokeratoderma variabilis and ichthyosis linearis circumflexa. (Lever)

icterus [ĭk′tər-, ĭk′tĕr-əs] is New Latin from the Greek word for jaundice that is found in Hippocrates. Pliny cites a legend to the effect that when a jaundiced person perceived a certain yellow-green bird called *icterus,* the patient recovered but the bird died. It's a flight of ornithological and medical fancy that is sad for the birds.

-id(e), id [ĭd, ed; ĭd]. *-Id (e)* is a suffix from Greek and Latin. French and British practice favors the spelling *-ide;* American hurry and efficiency tend to shorten the suffix to *-id,* although *-ide* persists in some American terminologies, especially in chemistry. In the main we may dispose of *-id* from the Latin source by saying that it derives from *-idus,* an adjectival ending, and gives us the ending of modern adjectives and nouns like *acid, stupid,* etc. *-Id (e)* from the Greek source is more complicated. It derives from *-ides,* which is patronymic, i.e., means son or daughter (descendant) of. There are words where it is difficult to decide whether the suffix *-ide* derives from the Greek or Latin source, but wherever it appears in a noun it carries the sense of formal or figurative family relationship.

idiopathic guttate hypomelanosis is a common acquired-type of leukoderma characterized by multiple discrete angular or circular macules, usually 2 to 8 mm in diameter. The macules are off-white or porcelain in color without scale or atrophy and are located predominantly on the exposed areas of the upper and lower extremities. Seen in patients over 30 years of age. Cause unknown. (Polysangam et al. *J. Am. Acad. of Dermatol.* 1990, v. 23, p. 681.)

idr(o)- [ĭd′rō]. See *hidr (o)-.*

ignis, sacer. See *sacer ignis.*

il- [ĭl] is an assimilated form of the Latin prefix *in-* found before word elements beginning with the letter *l,* as in *illegal* and *illusion.* See *in-.*

im- [ĭm] is an assimilated or changed form of the Latin prefix *in-* found before word elements beginning with the letters *b*, *m* and *p*, as in *imbrication, immunization* and *implantation*. See *in-*.

immediate hypersensitivity consists of all the allergic responses that begin within minutes of antigen-antibody interaction and may be divided into cytotoxic or anaphylactic on the basis of the mediation of the clinical response.

immediate hypersensitivity reaction, e.g., anaphylaxsis, occurs following stimulation of tissue mast cells and circulating basophils. These reactions are frequently mediated by the interaction of multivalent allergens with specific, cell-surface IgE antibodies. It is now recognized that mast cells and basophils also are stimulated by a number of other non-IgE associated mechanisms. (M.D. Tharp, *Dermatology Clinics*, W. B. Saunders; October 1990)

immersion foot [ĭ-mûr′zhən fo͞ot] refers to conditions that are consequences of prolonged wetness of the feet, such as are incurred in wars and in some industrial and agricultural operations. Those consequences are maceration and intertrigo primarily and inevitably, and bacterial or fungal infections secondarily and usually.

immitis [ĭ-mī′lĭs, -mētĭs, ĭ-mĭt′ĭs, ĭm′ĭ-tĭs] is the masculine and feminine singular form of a Latin adjective meaning not (*im-* = *in-*) mild, gentle or benign (*-mitis*), that is to say, harsh, merciless or cruel. It appears in the title *Coccidioides immitis*.

immune [ĭ-mūn′] is an adjective derived from Latin and literally meaning without (*im-* = *in-*) obligation (*munus*, duty). The original Latin meaning of the word was exemption or protection from things disagreeable. In some present-day connotations, however, an opposite sense appears, especially in a term like *auto-immune*. Not self-protection but self-harm is the sense and the fact. In the older literature of allergy, particularly the French, *immune* was used to denote an artifically induced state of sensitization, and so it is still used among laboratory workers in the field of immunology.

In addition to the sense of being protected or not being susceptible to something, *immune* has an extended meaning of being unresponsive or impervious to, as in "immune to all pleas for mercy." Extending this meaning still further lay persons are heard to say, "I have become immune to the medicine." Failure to benefit is thus implied by *immune*.

immune complex diseases. These are caused by the deposition or formation of antigen-antibody complexes in tissues. Inflammation results and leads to acute or chronic disease of the organ system in which the immune complexes have been deposited.

Examples are the autoimmune diseases, rheumatoid arthritis, systemic lupus erythematosus, cutaneous vasculitis, Sjögren's syndrome, mixed connective tissue disease, polyarteritis nodosa and systemic sclerosis. Infectious diseases: bacterial, viral and parasitic diseases. Neoplastic diseases and many other conditions, e.g., atopic disease, sickle cell anemia, thrombotic thrombocytopenic purpura, kidney and bone marrow transplantation, xanthomatosis, oral ulceration, Behçet's syndrome, pemphigus, bullous pemphigoid, IgA deficiency and ankylosing spondylitis. (Adapted from Charles G. Cochron. *Cecil Textbook of Medicine*, 18th Edition. Saunders, 1988, Wyngaarden and Smith, Editors.)

immunity [ĭ-mū′nə-tē, -tĭ] means a state or condition (*-ty*) of protection (*immuni-*) against something disagreeable. Unlike *immune* (which see), *immunity* can hardly be applied in an opposite sense, although if one were going to be consistent, a state of auto-immunity should be considered as, and is indeed, a sort of waiver of immunity.

immunization, immunize [ĭm′ū-nĭ-zā′shən, ĭ-mūn′ĭ-zā′shən, -ĭ-zā′shən; ĭm′ū-nīz, ĭ-mūn′īz] refer to the state of, and the process of achieving, protection against something disagreeable. Again, from the modern ambiguity of *immune*, induction and establishment of a sensitized state that can be harmful or fatal can also be designated by the words in clarified context.

immunodeficiency diseases. More than three dozen different primary immunodeficiency syndromes have been reported. These may involve all components of the immune system, including lymphocytes, phagocytic cells, and the complement proteins. These diseases often have striking cutaneous manifestations, i.e., widespread uncontrolled infection. Please see acquired immunodeficiency syndrome (AIDS). (Rebecca H. Buckley, *Cecil Textbook of Medicine*, Wyngaarden & Smith, editors, 18th Edition, W. B. Saunders, 1988).

immunofluorescence. Primarily of two types, direct and indirect, which are of crucial importance in diagnosing the bullous diseases, connective tissue diseases, especially lupus erythematosus and allergic vasculitis. Direct immunofluorescence is performed on fresh or frozen tissue in a special fixative to show if identifying antibodies are present. Indirect immunofluorescence in dermatology is usually performed on serum to see if culprit antibodies are present, and if so, in what titer, thereby at times indicating severity.

immunology [ĭm′ū-nŏl′ō-jē, -ə-jē, -jĭ] encompasses the study (*-logy*) of humoral changes of diverse sorts, protective or adverse, and especially those that seem to depend upon antigen-antibody interactions. Not only specific, acquired alterations in reactivity (allergic transformations) but native and inherent phenomena like blood types, heterophile antibodies, properdin, etc. are subjects of immunologic investigation.

impetiginization, impetiginize [ĭm′pĕ-tĭj′ə-nĭ-zā′shən, -nĭ-zā′shən; ĭm′pĕ-tĭj′ə-nīz] refer to the condition of super-imposed pyogenic superficial infection and process of becoming superficially infected as a secondary event upon something original. See *impetigo.*

impetigo [ĭm′pə-, ĭm′pĕ-tī′gō, -tē′gō], from its Latin word elements, means an attack (*im-*, for *in-*, against *-peti-*, for *pete*, stem of *petere*, to seek: *-go*, noun ending; the preceding *i* is a modified form of the thematic vowel of the verb used as a connecting vowel. (For comments on stems, thematic vowels, connecting vowels see under *zosteriform* and compare *intertrigo*). The word was used in classical Latin for a scabby eruption. In modern times, we apply *impetigo* to the well-known superficiality of inflammation and friable, "stuck-on" crusts. The plural of the word in classical consistency is *impetigines* [ĭm′pə-, ĭm′pĕ-tĭj′ĭ-nēz, -tĭ′jĭ-nēz]. Varieties of impetigines follow.

impetigo contagiosa [kŏn-tā′jĭ-ō′sə, -jē-ō′sə] as a title emphasizes easy transmissibility, which, however, is a relative quality. Impetigo, except in the immunologically immature (the very young) housed in crowded nurseries, does not rank in contagiosity with the viral exanthemata, typhoid, cholera, yellow fever, bubonic plague, etc. *Impetigo vulgaris* is an alternate title.

impetigo herpetiformis [hər-, hûr-pĕt′ĭ-fôr′mĭs]. Generalized pustular psoriasis of von Zumbusch, acrodermatitis continua of Hallopeau and impetigo herpetiformis represent the same disease process. There is considerable resemblance and overlapping in the clinical picture of these three diseases, and they have the same histologic appearance. They differ mainly in mode of onset and in distribution of the lesions.

impetigo neonatorum [nē′ō-nə-tō′rəm, -nä-tôr′əm, -nă-tôr′əm] is the title for a severe bullous form of superficial pyoderma that is seen in the immunologically immature (the very young). The condition is not different from impetigo contagiosa, or vulgaris, in cause. The course may be stormy because the subjects are immunologically undeveloped, and the clinical lesions persist longer as bullae rather than evolve quickly into crusts.

impetigo vulgaris [vŭl-gā′rĭs, -gä′rĭs, -gär′ĭs] names the common (*vulgaris*) variety of impetigo. See *impetigo contagiosa.*

implantation cyst [ĭm′plăn-tā′shən sĭst] is a title for a cystic process that results from traumatic or other artificial implantation of one tissue into another.

in, in- [ĭn], **-in(e)** [ĭn; īn, ēn] are respectively a preposition, prefix and suffix. The first is Anglo-Saxon and is akin to Latin *in* and Greek *en*; the second is both Anglo-Saxon and Latin and is also akin to Greek *en-*; the third is derived from Greek *-inos* and Latin *-inus*, often via French *-in* (*e*). All three word elements have both common and uncommon contextual meanings.

In Latin phrases, *in* as a preposition meaning into, to, toward (expressing motion) takes the accusative case (e.g., *in cutem*) and meaning in or within (expressing position) takes the ablative case (e.g., *in utero*). As a prefix, *in-*, in addition to meaning in, into, within and toward, means not or without (equivalent to Anglo-Saxon *un-*). *In-* also seems to intensify meaning (e.g., *flammable* means able to burn; *inflammable* means able to be set on fire easily or able to burn fiercely). Before words of Latin origin beginning with *b* and *p*, *in-* is changed to *im-* (e.g., *imbibe, impalpable*) and before *l*, *m* and *r*, it is assimilated (e.g., *illegitimate, immune, irradiate*). *In-* in both its senses of in-ness and negation may appear as *em-* or *en-* especially in words of Latin origin coming into English via French (e.g., *employ, enclose, enemy*); *em-* and *en-* also mean to make (e.g., *embitter, endear*). There are also Greek *em-* and *en-* of the *in* meaning (e.g., *empathy, endemic*). *-In* (*e*) is a suffix which, as a noun ending, means a material (e.g., *gelatin, chlorine*) and, as an adjectival ending, means having the nature of (e.g., *opaline, crystalline*). The suffix *-ine* (from Latin *-ina* via French *-ine*) is also used to form feminine nouns and names (e.g., *chorine, Josephine, Geraldine, Maxine*, etc.).

incarnatus, incarnati [ĭn′kär-nā′təs, -nä′təs, -tŭs; -nā′tī, -nä′tī, -tē] are classical Latin adjectives (masculine singular and plural respectively) that literally mean converted into flesh (from *incarnare*). (Compare *The Incarnation*.) In the titles *unguis incarnatus* and *pili incarnati* the sense is changed to enclosed by or inserted into flesh, a meaning which the Oxford English Dictionary lists as obsolete and rare! See *ingrowing*, or *ingrown hair*, or *nail*.

incisional biopsy [ĭn-sĭzh′ən′l bī′ŏp-sē]. The terms *excisional biopsy* and *incisional biopsy* are surgeons' jargon to the understanding of which one has to be admitted. Literally, the one says "cut-out biopsy"; the other, "cut-into biopsy." The average educated person would know what a biopsy is, but that individual or even a physician who is not privy to the arcane ambiguity of the terms would not know that excisional biopsy is intended to mean removal for study of a clinical lesion in entirety (it is hoped) and incisional biopsy is intended to mean removal of only a part of such a lesion. The terms do not say these things clearly; they are not in perfect balance. Excisions are performed by making incisions; incisions by themselves may not result in excisions, but a so-called incisional biopsy is designed to result in an excision. How much more felicitously incisive it would be to speak of biopsy *in toto* (of the whole) and biopsy *in parte* (of a part) instead of the other terms, which do not convey clearly what is done.

inclusion body [ĭn-klōō′zhən bŏ′dē, -dĭ] is a term used in histopathology to describe appearances in cells (virus colonies, other artifacts) that are caused by parasites or pathogens that obligatorily require intracellular conditions.

inclusion cyst [ĭn-klōō′zhən sĭst] has about the same meaning as *implantation cyst.*

incontinentia pigmenti [ĭn-kŏn′tĭ-nĕn′shĭ-ə, -shē-ə, -shə, -tē-ə, -tĭ-ə pĭg-mĕn′tī] is the title of a potentially widespread dysplastic process whose most common and obvious effect results from an inability to hold (*incontinentia*) pigment where it normally belongs. Instead of rising in the epidermis in the usual manner, melanin seems to descend into the cutis where it is picked up by phagocytes. The clinical result is bizarre pigmentation, commonly in the form of zebra-like stripes. The range of dysplasia is, however, wider than mere pigmentary anomaly and is not encompassed by the title. In infancy, bullae may precede the pigmentation; later, neoplasias in the eyes, nervous system and other organs and failure of good dentition may occur. The pigmentary oddity alone has a strong tendency to correct itself around and after puberty; the other dysplasias persist.

incubation period [ĭn′kū-bā′shən pĭr′-, pēr′ĭ-əd, -ē-əd] is generally taken to mean the time that elapses from the moment of infection to the first clinically recognizable symptoms or signs of an infectious disease. This definition is suitable for infectious diseases like botulism, diphtheria and tetanus whose first clinically recognizable symptoms or signs depend on the actions of toxins, in which case incubation period depends on how soon an adequate amount of toxin becomes operative. Such incubation periods are generally short, a matter of days. In the case of infectious diseases like leprosy, tuberculosis and syphilis whose signs and symptoms depend on the development of immunologic transformations, incubation period must be redefined as the period from the moment of infection to the development of the first immunologic transformation. Such first immunologic transformation may be evinced by a clinically recognizable sign like a chancre (if the skin is the portal of entry of the causative micro-organisms) or it may be an event detectable only by a laboratory procedure like a serologic or skin test. In general, such incubation periods are those of delayed hypersensitivity, i.e., a matter of one to three weeks. Clinical events may never be obvious in some such circumstances (e.g., in tuberculosis) or only at long last (e.g., in leprosy). It is therefore not proper to speak of an incubation period of ten to twenty years, as is sometimes done for leprosy, when first immunologic changes must have occurred in the usual way and in the usual time.

indeterminate leprosy [ĭn′dē-tûr′mə-nāt, -de-tər′mə-nət lĕp′rə-sē, -rō-sē, -sĭ] describes a type or stage of the disease in which it cannot be told clinically and especially not histologically whether progression and differentiation will be toward lepromatous or tuberculoid forms of the disease.

India-rubber skin [ĭn′dĭ-ə, -dē-yə rŭb′ēr, -ər skĭn] is descriptive, in terms of a familiar object, of elasticity of skin and softness of tissue as may be appreciated in the Ehlers-Danlos syndrome.

indolent [ĭn′də-, ĭn′dō-lənt, -lĕnt], from its Latin word elements, literally means not (*in-*) suffering (*-dolent*). Its modern everyday meaning is lazy or idle. In a medical phrase, then, like *indolent ulcer* the implication is chronic, slow to heal or long enduring without significant pain or discomfort.

indurata [ĭn′dū-rā′tə]. See *indurativa*.

indurated, induration [ĭn′dū-rāt′ĕd, -ĭd, -əd; ĭn′dū-rā′shən] are respectively a participial adjective and a noun that relate to events or a state (*-tion*) in which things have gotten very (*in-*, intensive sense) physically hard (*-dura-*).

induratio plastica penis [ĭn′dū-rā′shĭ-ō, -shē-ō, -shō, -rä′tĭ-ō, -tē-ō plăs′tĭ-kə pē′nĭs] is the title for a considerably (*in-*, intensive sense) hardened condition (*-duratio*) of the penis, which hardness is still of some flexibility (*plastica*). The condition is a fibrosis following upon inflammatory changes that may result from trauma or infections, particularly gonorrheal infection. Better known as Peyronie's disease.

indurativa, indurativum, induratum [ĭn′dū-rə-tī′və; -vəm; ĭn′dū-rā′ təm, -rä′təm] are respectively (the first two) the feminine and neuter singular of a New Latin adjective and (the third) the neuter singular of a classical Latin adjective meaning very (*in-*, intensive sense) hard or hardened (*-durat-*). The words appear in classicized titles, e.g., *tuberculosis cutis indurativa, erythema indurativum*, or *induratum. Indurata*, the feminine singular of the classical adjective, appears in the titles *acne indurata* and *tuberculosis cutis indurata.*

-ine. See under *in.*

infantile acropustulosis. A pruritic vesiculopustular eruption of the hands and feet seen from infancy to age 3, then usually clears. Some feel this may be due to prior scabies. (James)

infantile eczema. See *eczema, infantile.*

infect, infection [ĭn-fekt′; ĭn-fĕk′shən] derive from Latin *inficere*, first meaning to dip, then to dye or stain and finally to taint, spoil or corrupt. Thus *infect* and *infection* come to mean to us to corrupt and the result of corruption by microbial pathogens.

infectiosum [ĭn-fĕk′shĭ-ō′səm, -shē-ō′səm, -tĭ-ō′səm, -tē-ō′səm] is the neuter singular form of a New Latin adjective meaning infectious. It appears in the title *erythema infectiosum.*

infectious [ĭn-fĕk′shəs] means caused by microbial agents and contagious, communicable or "catching." In epidemiology *contagious* is more often used than *infectious* to express easy communicability of disease.

infectious eczematiod dermatitis [ĕg-zĕm′ə-toid dûr′mə-tī′tĭs, -tē′tĭs] is the title for a characteristic superficial inflammatory dermatosis that results from the run of pus on the skin from some remote focus, e.g., within the meatus and on the pinnae of ears from purulent otitis media, on the upper lip from intra-nasal pyogenic infections, around sinuses from apical dental abscesses, around colostomies, etc. Some persons apply the title to any impetiginization, especially secondary infection upon primary irritant dermatitis of the hands, nummular eczema, etc. It is not wise.

infest, infestation [ĭn-fĕst′; ĭn′fĕs-tā′shən] have dubious or complicated etymologies. The short of it is that the words seem to derive from elements that came to mean at first not able to be defended and then, by a transfer of agency, made unsafe, troublesome, hostile, dangerous, etc. To us now the words mean respectively to harbor metazoal ("animal") parasites on or in the body and the act, process or result of such harboring.

infiltrate, infiltration [ĭn′fĭl-trāt; ĭn′fĭl-trā′shən]. *Infiltrate* literally means to put into or through (*in-*) packed wool or felt (*-filt-*); *infiltration* is the result thereof. Medically the words describe seepage into tissue of matter that is not ordinarily present and invasion by cells that are not normal to the location.

inflame, inflammation, inflammatory [ĭn-flăm′; ĭn′flə-mā′shən; ĭn-flăm′ə-tôr′ē, -tō′rē, -rĭ] derive from Latin via French and carry senses of burning or blazing (-*flam* [*m*]-) fiercely (*in*-, intensive sense). Medically, the signs and symptoms of the phenomenon have long been described mnemonically by the Latin words *calor* (fever or increased local temperature), *rubor* (redness or erythema), *tumor* (swelling or edema), *dolor* (pain or itching in the case of skin) and *laesa functio* (failure or fault of function).

infundibulum [ĭn′fŭn-dĭb′ū-ləm] is a word applied to that part of a hair follicle that extends from the pilosebaceous ostium to the opening of the sebaceous gland into the follicular structure. *Infundibulum* means a funnel in Latin, and is applied at large to anatomic structures that are more or less funnel-shaped, as is the structure in point.

ingrowing, or **ingrown, hair**, or **nail** [ĭn′grō′ĭng, ĭn′grōn′ hâr, nāl], are simple statements about hairs that continue to grow but have failed to emerge from the pilosebaceous ostium, and of nails that grow pushed or dug into flesh at the edges. *Pili incarnati* and *unguis incarnatus* are classicized titles for the conditions.

inguinal [ĭng′gwĭ-nəl], **inguinale** [ĭng′gwĭ-nā′lē, -nä′lĕ, -năl′ē] and **inguinalis** [ĭng′gwĭ-nā′lĭs, -nä′lĭs, -năl′ĭs] are respectively an English adjective, the neuter singular and the masculine or feminine singular of a Latin adjective meaning belonging, pertaining or relating to the groin. The neuter form appears in the titles *Epidermophyton floccosum* (*inguinale*) and *lymphogranuloma inguinale* and the feminine, in *tinea inguinalis*.

integument [ĭn-tĕg′ū-mənt] and **integumentum** [ĭn-tĕg′ū-mĕn′təm], its Latin original, are derived from the Latin verb *tegere*, to cover. There exist also the English word *tegument* and the Latin word *tegumentum* meaning the same things as *integument* and *integumentum*, and both are used in medical writing today. The prefix adds a descriptive detail, which is supplied in the English expression *a covering upon*, i.e., it rounds out the word. Or else, one may look upon it as an intensive adding stress to the word, giving *integument* a special sense of a complete or thorough cover, such as the skin surely is.

inter and **inter-** [ĭn′tûr, -tĕr, -tĕr, -tər] are respectively a preposition and a prefix taken from Latin and meaning between, among.

interdigital [ĭn′tər-, ĭn′tĕr-dĭj′ĭ-təl, -ə-təl] and **interdigitalis** [ĭn-tĕr-, ĭn-tûr-dĭj′ĭ-tā′lĭs, -tä′lĭs, -tăl′ĭs] are respectively an English adjective and the masculine or feminine singular of a New Latin adjective meaning between (*inter-*) the anatomical digits, i.e., fingers or toes. The Latin adjective appears in the title *erosio interdigitalis blastomycetica* (feminine).

intermediate leprosy [ĭn-tẽr-mē′dē-ət, -dī-ət lĕp′rə-sē, -rō-sē, -sī] describes a type or stage of leprosy in which lesions are not yet differentiated into the more common lepromatous and tuberculoid forms. *Borderline, dimorphous* and *indeterminate* are words alternate for *intermediate.*

intertriginous [ĭn′tər-, ĭn′tẽr-trĭj′ĭ-nəs] is an adjective meaning relating or pertaining to intertrigo.

intertrigo [ĭn′tər-, ĭn′tẽr-, ĭn′tẽr-trī′gō] is Latin, meaning a rubbing (-*tri*-, from *terere*, to rub, plus -*go*, noun ending; for the *i* see *impetigo*) between (*inter*-). The dermatosis so named is a superficial inflammatory process that occurs in places where skin is in apposition (i.e., intertriginous) and thus is subject to the friction of movement, increased local heat, maceration from retained moisture and irritation from accumulation of debris. Given enough of these effects, dissolution of stratum corneum, exudation of intercellular serum and secondary infection arc inevitable. The Romans used the word to denote chafing of the skin from riding or walking. We get the effect from sitting too much.

intra and **intra-** [ĭn′trə] are respectively a Latin preposition and prefix meaning within or on the inside.

intracutaneous [ĭn′trə-kū-tā′nē-əs] means relating or pertaining to (-*aneus*) the inside (*intra*-) of the cutis.

intradermal [ĭn′trə-dûr′məl] is a hybrid adjective from Latin and Greek with the same meaning as *intracutaneous*, which purists prefer. *Endodermal* would satisfy them only in part because -*al* is still of Latin origin while the rest is of Greek origin.

intra-epidermal and **intra-epithelial** [ĭn′trə-ĕp′ĭ-dûr′məl; -ĕp′ē-, -ĕp′ĭ-thē′lĭ-əl, -lē-əl, -thēl′yəl] are other hybrid adjectives composed of Latin and Greek elements and designating things within (*intra*-) the epidermis or any epithelial structure. Purists not only excoriate themselves when they see these formations but must be all the more irritated when the hyphen is omitted. *Endo-epidermal* and *endo-epithelial* would keep them only slightly more sedate.

inunct, inunction [ĭn-ŭngkt′; ĭn-ŭngk′shən] derive from Latin *ung-(u)ere* and respectively mean to rub or smear and result of rubbing or smearing an oil or salve into the skin. The noun also means an ointment or unguent.

inverted follicular keratosis [ĭn-vûr′tĭd fə-lĭk′ū-lẽr kẽr′ə-tō′sĭs] has been coined to designate a small keratotic process which tends to develop into the skin instead of on top. Such lesions are common on the nose as warty papules. Histopathologists argue among themselves about whether lesions so designated are not special forms of seborrheic keratoses or keratoacanthomas.

ioderma, iododerma [ī′ə-, ī′ō-dûr′mə; ī-ō′-, ī′ō-dō-dûr′mə] designate any pathologic condition of the skin (-*derma*) caused by iodine and compounds thereof. A wide range of morphologic possibilities, acneform, vesiculo-bullous, furunculoid, carbunculoid and granulomatous, is encompassed by the words.

ir- [ĭr] is an assimilated form of the Latin prefix *in-* that appears before word elements beginning with *r*, e.g., *irrational, irremediable, irrevocable.* See *in-*.

irradiate, irradiation [ĭr-rā′dē-āt′, -dĭ-āt′; ĭr-rā′dē-ā′shən] refer to the action and result of applying electromagnetic energy (-*radi-*) in considerable amounts or duration (*ir-* = *in-*, intensive sense). Application of electromagnetic energy of 0.1 to 2 Å in wave length (X rays) is usually implied; application of ultraviolet ranges, but not those of the visible spectrum (illumination), is also described by the words.

irritate, irritation [ĭr′ə-, ĭr′ĭ-tāt; ĭr′ĭ-tā′shən] derive from a Latin word meaning inciting or provoking (*irritare*, to incite, provoke, etc.). In medical contexts the words are used to denote both signs and symptoms, i.e., both objective and subjective phenomena, of inflammation and disordered feeling.

ischemia [ə-skē′-, ĭs-kē′mē-ə, -mĭ-ə] is New Latin from Greek word elements meaning a condition (-*ia*) in which there has been an impediment (*isch-*) to flow of blood (-*em-*). Not banal first-aid measures for minor hemorrhages but severe interference with circulation from thromboses and other forms of arterial occlusions are designated by the word.

ischidrosis [ĭs′kə-, ĭs′kĭ-drō′sĭs] is a rare word from Greek word elements that mean a condition (-*osis*) of stoppage (*isch-*) of sweat or sweating (-*idr-*). Probably a pathologic diminution or insufficiency of sweating as might occur in congenital ectodermal defect or thermal anhidrosis, rather than the result of applying antiperspirants, deserves so fancy a word.

-ism [ĭz′m, ĭz′əm] is a suffix coming down all the way from Greek *-ismos* through Latin, various periods of French and Middle English and denoting a condition (e.g., *polymorphism*), a characteristic (e.g., *colloquialism*), an act (e.g., *baptism*), an abnormal condition (e.g., *alcoholism*), a doctrine (*monotheism*)—and many more! In its last meaning, *-ism* appears also as an independent word (as in "the battle of the isms").

iso- [ī'sō, ī'sə, ī'zō, ī'zə] is a combining form from Greek, meaning alike, equal, same or uniform (e.g., *isosceles, isotherm*). In a few words it appears as *is-* (e.g., *isanthous*, having equally regular flowers). Among special meanings of *iso-* there are two as follows: from different individuals of the same species (e.g., *iso-antibody*); having a branched chain of carbon atoms (e.g., *isohydrocarbons*).

isomorphic effect [ī'sō-môr'fĭk ĕ-, ə-fĕkt'; see *iso-* for other pronunciations of *iso-*] describes the phenomenon of induction by physical trauma, or by other influence, of lesions of the very same (*iso-*) form (*-morphic*) that is characteristic of a disease. The event is commonly seen in lichen planus and psoriasis. *Koebner phenomenon* is an eponymic designation for the clinical effect and is a distinguishing feature of psoriasis.

isthmus [īs'mŭs] is a literal borrowing from the Greek word for a narrow passage, particularly a strip of land between two bodies of water. Of dermatologic interest is the designation by the word of the region of a hair follicle between the upper part which is called the *infundibulum* and the part immediately subjacent. It is also the part into which the sebaceous gland extrudes its product. As was said for infundibulum, there are other structures in the body that have isthmuses. In fact, wherever there is an infundibular formation, the stem of the funnel becomes an isthmus.

itch [ĭch] is of Anglo-Saxon origin. It is a noun and a verb (mainly intransitive) concerning the well-known uncomfortable sensation. The use of *itch* as a transitive verb meaning to cause an itch is obsolete or poetic; many suffering patients, however, say *itch* for *scratch* in a phrase like "I itched it." Let's excuse the solecism because of the distress.

itch mite [mīt] is a vernacular designation for *Sarcoptes scabiei var. hominis* (which see).

-ite [īt] as a noun ending derives via Latin and French from Greek *-ites* (see next entry). The suffix relates things to a class or group, e.g., *Brooklynite, dendrite, Laborite, nitrite*, etc.

-itis [ī'tĭs, ē'tĭs] is a Greek adjectival ending, feminine in form, that relates thing to a specified something. In Greek medicine it appeared in terms like *arthritis nosos* (disease of joints). Even in Greek the word for disease was dropped in some such instances (e.g., *pleurities*); the adjective was then treated as a noun and was transmitted to us via Latin. See *dermatitis*. In New Latin and modern medical terminology an exclusive meaning of inflammation (which is, of course, not inherent in the suffix) has been added to the exclusion of all else, and the element has become an English noun ending. In nonmedical, metaphorical writing one sees -*itis* in nonce formations that are intended to be mildly humorous in implying something like a disease, e.g., it might be said of a politician that he has *Presidentitis*.

Ito's nevus [ē′tō]. Nevus fuscoceruleus acromiodeltoideus.

ixodiasis [ĭk′sō-dī′ə-sĭs] names a condition (-*iasis*) caused by ticks, particularly those of the family Ixodidae (hard-bodied ticks). *Ixod-* (from Greek) refers to birdlime, a viscid substance derived from certain trees and used to entrap small birds by smearing it on twigs. The Ixodidae have a surface tackiness on their hard bodies. Species (e.g., *andersonii, variabilis, occidentalis*) of the genus *Dermacentor* infest, bite and transmit the agent (*Rickettsia rickettsii, Pasteurella tularensis*) of Rocky Mountain spotted fever and tularemia. They also cause syndromes known as *tick pyrexia* and *tick paralysis* by either a toxin or an allergic mechanism.

J

Jacquet's erythema [zhäkā']. Intertrigo with ulceration.

Jadassohn, anetoderma of [yä'dä-sōn]. Atrophy following upon crops of inflammatory papules of unknown cause.

Jadassohn's epithelioma [yä'dä-sōn]. See Borst-Jadassohn epithelioma.

Jadassohn-Lewandowski syndrome [yä'dä-sōn; lēv'ăn-dov'skē]. Pachyonychia congenita.

Jadassohn-Tièche nevus [yä'dä-sōn; tē-ēsh']. Blue nevus.

jaundice [jôn'-, jän'dĭs] derives from Latin *galbus*, yellow, via French *jaune*. There is no *d* in the original words but in English *d* appears as a phonetic accretion, a common philologic phenomenon also seen, for example, in the English word *sound* from Latin *sonare* and French *sonner*. In any event, *jaundice* describes the distinctly yellow color imparted to the skin, sclerae and mucous membranes by excesses of bile pigments resulting from some hepatic, choledochal and hemolytic diseases. Lay persons speak of yellow jaundice, which is obviously tautologic, but then physicians speak of black jaundice, which is rather paradoxical. Let all be forgiven.

Jessner-Kanof disease [yĕs'nēr, kăn'ôf]. Lymphocytic infiltration of the skin.

jigger [jĭg'ēr, -ə(r)] is a corruption of the word *chigo* (e), which designates the sand flea, *Tunga penetrans*. In the interest of scientific accuracy and clarity, *jigger* should not be confused with *chigger*, which designates the harvest mite, *Trombicula irritans*. However, as a glance through unabridged dictionaries quickly reveals, the words *chigger*, *chigo* (e) and *jigger* have long been equated and confused, especially in the United States, for they look and sound so much alike. All that one can advise is that the tiny creatures be kept apart if the names can't be. See *chigger* and *chigo* (e).

Job's syndrome. These patients often with atopic dermatitis and impaired neutrophil chemotaxis develop repeated severe pyodermatous skin lesions—cold abscesses apparently much in similarity to those of the biblical Job.

jock (strap) itch [jŏk (străp) ĭch] is a racy and lay designation for pruritus (usually with inflammatory changes) in the groins and thereabouts, attributable to friction and enhanced intertriginous conditions occasioned by the wearing of a jock strap. Some among the laity use the term for intertrigo, superficial fungous or pyodermatous infection, seborrheic dermatitis, etc. in the groin even if a jock strap has never been worn, merely because of the location. The *jock* of *jock strap* may derive from *jockey, jack* or *jock,* a male; *strap* derives from Greek and Latin words (*strophos, stroppus*) for a band or cord.

junction(al) nevus [jŭnk′shən-(-əl, -′l) nē′vəs] designates a pigmented macule or a flattish papule that, upon microscopic examination, can be seen to result from collections of pigment-producing cells gathered into thèques and situated at the dermo-epidermal junction. There is little to choose between *junction* and *junctional;* one can argue cogently for the noun used as an adjective or for the adjective itself, but never to any firm conclusion, and what one decides upon is vaguely personal.

jungle rot [jŭng′g′l rŏt] is another of those parochial designations for intertrigines and superficial fungous and pyodermatous infections, especially in intertriginous places, that are common in the heat and humidity of tropical areas. If anyone wishes to know, *jungle* derives from Sanskrit via Hindi from a word for forest or desert, and *rot* is from an Anglo-Saxon word connoting decay, decomposition or putrefaction.

juvenile melanoma [jōō′və-n′l, -nĭl, -nīl mĕl′ə-nō′mə] names a lesion occurring mainly in the prepubertal young that to gross inspection is a reddish or red-brown, solitary papule (not necessarily so deep brown or black as *melanoma* would suggest). Histologically, it consists of pigment-producing cells that appear malignant in mitotic rate and other characteristics. The condition however, is benign, not malignant.

juvenilis, juveniles [jōō′və-nī′lĭs, -nĭl′ĭs; -lēz] are respectively the masculine and feminine singular and the plural of a Latin adjective meaning pertaining to, or of, the young. The singular is found in the title *verruca plana juvenilis,* the plural, in *verrucae planae juveniles* (both feminine).

juxta-articular node(s) [jŭk′stə-, jŭks′tə-är-tĭk′ū-lĕr nōd(z)] refers to swellings (*nodes*) nearby or to the side of (*juxta-*) a joint (*-articular*) that sometimes appear in rheumatic fever and late syphilis. Other swellings in the region of joints, e.g., the furuncular, lymphadenomatous or xanthomatous, are not so called.

K

kala azar [kä′lä ä-zär′] names a leishmaniasis caused by *Leishmania donovani.* The words are Hindi for black (*kala*) disease (*azar*). The clinical condition is notable cutaneously for a grayness of the skin which was originally and exaggeratedly called black. Otherwise, the disease is visceral and gives rise to fever, anemia, leukopenia, emaciation and enlargements of organs (particularly hepato- and splenomegaly) as a result of parasitization of the reticulo-endothelial system. The skin eventually also shows the parasitic invasions when examined in microscopic sections.

Kaposi's disease [kă-pō′sē, shē]. Several: disseminated herpes simplex and vaccinia in atopic dermatitis, xeroderma pigmentosum, lichen ruber moniliformis, pityriasis rubra pilaris, multiple idiopathic hemorrhagic sarcoma (see corresponding entries in the Dictionary). Also prevalent in AIDS but the incidence is diminishing.

Kaposi's sarcoma [kô′pŏ-shĭz, kə-pō′sĭz, -sēz, -shēz sär-kō′mə]. See *multiple idiopathic hemorrhagic sarcoma. Kaposi* is a Hungarian name, which should be pronounced kô′pŏ-shĭ; the variations listed show attempts to anglicize it and are not recommended, but they are heard.

Kaposi's varicelliform eruption [văr′ĭ-sĕl′ĭ-fôrm, -ə-sĕl′ə-fôrm ē-rŭp′shən]. See *eczema herpeticum.*

Kasabach-Merritt syndrome [kăs′ə-bäk; mĕr′ĭt]. Thrombocytopenic hemangiomatosis.

Kawasaki's disease. Mucocutaneous lymph node syndrome. This is an acute febrile illness with a erythematous macular and papular dermatitis. It is of unknown etiology and occurs most often in infants, children and occasionally in young adults. There is a distinctive red dermatitis involving the palms and soles with marked edema.

Fever develops for a few days, then a measles- or scarlet-fever like rash more pronounced on the trunk than on the face and a strawberry tongue with cervical lymphadenopathy in most patients ensues.

Scarlet fever must be ruled out by appropriate antistreptolysin O (ASO) titers. The condition does not respond to antibiotics.

Fatalities have been rarely reported due to coronary thrombosis, coronary arteritis and or aneurysms.

keloid [kēloid]. The etymologic problem for *keloid* is complicated. If the English is from Greek via French *chéloïde*, it would derive from the Greek word for a claw of if via French *kéloïde*, then from the word for tumor or hernia plus the suffix *-oid*, meaning like. In any event, the modern word has come to stand for a type of over-cicatrization, especially of accidental and surgical wounds, that spreads beyond the limits of such wounds and is unpredictable as to when and in whom it will occur and to what sizes it will develop. Blacks are more susceptible to the effect than whites. The condition tends to persist indefinitely.

keloid acne. See *acne, keloid.*

keloidalis [kē′loi-dā′lĭs, -dä′lĭs, -dāl′ĭs] is the masculine and feminine singular of a New Latin adjective meaning of the character or in the nature of (*-alis*) a keloid. It is found in the title *acne keloidalis.*

keloidosis [kē′loi-dō′sĭs] means a condition (*-osis*) of keloid development. The word would probably be applied to extensive process rather than a solitary, small keloid.

kerat- and **kerat(o)-** [kĕr′ət, kĕr′ə-tō] are combining forms from Greek *keras*, genitive *keratos*, the Greek word for horn.

keratin [kĕr′ə-tĭn] designates the protein material (*-in*) that makes up horny (*kerat-*) tissue.

keratinization [kĕr′ə-tĭn′ĭ-zā′shən, -ī-zā′shən, -tən-ə-zā′shən] means the process of formation (*-ization*) of keratin.

keratinous [kĕ-răt′ə-nəs] is an adjective meaning consisting of, pertaining or relating to keratin.

keratitis [kĕr′ə-tī′tĭs, -tē′tĭs, -təs] refers to inflammation (*-itis*) of the cornea (*kerat-*) of the eye, not horny tissue in general.

kerato-. See *kerat-.*

kerato(-)acanthoma [kĕr′ə-tō-ăk′ăn-thō′mə] is a New Latin formation from Greek elements that bespeak a mass or overdevelopment (*-ma, -oma*) of the prickle-cell layer (*-acantho-, -acanth-*) and horny (*kerato-*) layers of the epidermis. In the writing of this word we recommend the use of a hyphen because in speaking there is a pause between *kerato* and *acanthoma* and both the word and its component elements are more clearly understood if a hyphen separates the *o* and the *a* so that these two vowels do not seem to make a diphthong. The lesion now designated by the word *kerato-acanthoma* is a benign nodule that is characterized grossly by a central plug of horn surrounded by reddish or flesh-colored borders, and histologically by that central plug of horn surrounded by epitheliomatous hyperplasia. The lesion resembles squamous-cell carcinoma, sometimes indistinguishably by gross and even microscopic viewing. The condition is, however, benign, self-healing and of unknown cause. Two types exit, solitary and multiple (uncommon).

keratoderm(i)a [kĕr′ə-tō-dûr′mə, -mē-ə, -mĭ-ə], from its Greek elements, literally means a pathologic condition of the skin (*-derma*, *-dermia*) characterized by excessive formation of horn (*kerato-*). In classicized titles modifying adjectives must be in neuter singular form for *keratoderma* and in feminine singular form for *keratodermia*, as for all other *-derma*, *-dermia* words (see *-derma* and *-dermia*). In our listing of such words below and elsewhere, the neuter form of the adjective is put first and the ending of the feminine is put in parentheses to correspond with *-m (i)a*, in which the *i* in parentheses is part of the feminine singular ending. For example, in the next entry *keratoderm (i)a* is a short way of writing both *keratoderma* and *keratodermia*. Since here the neuter form of the noun comes first alphabetically, the neuter form of the modifying adjective is put first and in full, *blennorhagicum*. The final syllable, *-cum*, of the neuter form is replaced by *-ca* in the feminine form, and this is indicated by (-ca). Hence, read in full, the two terms are *keratoderma blennorrhagicum* (neuter) and *keratodermia blennorrhagica* (feminine). *Hyperkeratosis* and *tylosis* are near synonyms of *keratoderm (i)a*; callosities, calluses, clavi and corns are keratoderm(i)as. There are several conditions with *keratoderm (i)a* in their titles, as follows:

keratoderm(i)a blennorrhagicum (-ca) [blĕn′ō-rā-jĭ-kəm (-kə)] is a rupial and psoriasiform hyperkeratosis that is sometimes seen in association with, and presumably as a consequence of gonorrheal (*blennorrhag-*) infection. See *Reiter's disease.*

keratoderm(i)a climactericum (-ca) [klī′măk-tĕr′ĭ-kəm (-kə)] names circumscribed tylosis, usually on palms and/or soles that occurs around the time of, and is thought to be related to, the menopause (*climactericum*, the climacteric).

keratoderm(i)a eccentricum (-ca) [ĕk-sĕn′trĭ-kəm (-kə)] is alternate for *porokeratosis*.

keratoderm(i)a palmare (-ris) et plantare (-ris) [păl′ mä′rē, -mä′rē, -mär′ē (-rĭs) ĕt plăn-tä′rē, -tä′rē, -tär′ē (-rĭs)] designates hyperkeratosis of the palms (*palm-*) and soles (*plant-*). That form of the condition that is common on Meleda, an Adriatic island, has been parochially named *mal de Meleda*.

keratoderm(i)a punctatum (-ta) [pŭnk-tā′təm, -tä′tŭm, -təm (-tə)] describes hyperkeratosis as points (*punctat-*) of process, i.e., dots or scattered small spots of cornification.

keratohyaline granules [kĕr′ə-tō-hī′ə-lĭn, -lēn grăn′ŭlz] are specks seen within the cells of the stratum granulosum that appear glassy (*-hyaline*) and of the character of horn (*kerato-*) in conventional histologic staining. They are correction precursor substances in the formation of finished keratin.

keratolysis [kĕr′ə-tŏl′ə-sīs], from its Greek word elements, literally means solution, dissolution or separation (*-lysis*) of the horny (*kerato-*) layer of the epidermis.

keratolysis exfoliativa [ĕks′fō-lĭ-ə-tī′və] describes a common form of separation of stratum corneum (*keratolysis*) on palms and soles in leaf-like flakes (*exfoliativa*). Sometimes the classicized words *areata manuum* (in circumscribed areas of the hands) are added to the title. The process starts in what has been described as "empty" blisters. No exudation attends the phenomenon, which is of unknown cause.

keratolytic [kĕr′ə-tō-lĭt′ĭk] as an adjective pertains or relates to keratolysis and as a noun designates a material that separates or dissolves horn substance.

keratoma [kĕr′ə-tō′mə], from its Greek elements, means a massing or overdevelopment (*-ma, -oma*) of horn (*kerato-, kerat-*) substance. The word is nearly synonymous with *callosity, callus, clavus* and *corn*.

keratoma hereditare mutilans [hə-, hĕ-, hē-rĕd′ĭ-tā′rē, -tä′rĕ, -tĕr′ē mū′tĭ-lănz] is the title of a hyperkeratotic condition (*keratoma*) that is based on heredity (*hereditare*) and its mutilating (*mutilans*).

keratoplastic [kĕr′ə-tō-plăs′tĭk] as an adjective relates to what builds up (*-plast-*) horn (*kerato-*) substance, and as a noun designates a material that can do that job.

keratosis [kĕr′ə-tō′sĭs], from its Greek elements, means a condition (*-osis*) of excessive development of horny (*kerat-*) tissue. *Keratoma* and *keratoderm* (*i*)*a* are nearly synonymous. *Keratosis* is frequently seen used interchangeably with *keratoderm* (*i*)*a*. Following are some titles in which *keratosis* is traditional:

keratosis, actinic. See *actinic keratosis.*

keratosis blennorrhagica. See *keratoderm* (*i*)*a blennorrhagica* (*-cum*).

keratosis follicularis [fō-lĭk′ŭ-lā′rĭs, -lä′rĭs, -lăr′ĭs] is one classicized title for the condition that is also known by the eponym *Darier's disease.* The flaw of this title is that the hyperkeratotic and
dyskeratotic process is not particularly or exclusively follicular in
position. However, the typical clinical feature of the process in the
form of agminated verrucous papules is well known, as is its pre-
ponderant location on the chest and back. Histology is also stereotypic in the *corps ronds*, grains and other marks of dyskeratization.

keratosis palmaris et plantaris. Three major dominant forms: keratosis palmaris et plantaris of Unna-Thost (either diffuse or localized, occasionally linear); epidermolytic keratosis palmaris et plantaris (clinically indistinguishable from Unna-Thost type,
histologically show hyperkeratosis); keratosis palmo-plantaris
punctata, or papulosa (many keratotic plugs). Two recessive forms:
mal de Meleda, or keratosis palmaris et plantaris of the Meleda
type (diffuse involvement of the palms and soles and marked tendency toward progression to the dorsal hands and feet, ankles and
wrists, elbows and knees); Papillon-Lefêvre syndrome (clinical
characteristics of the meleda type in association with periodontosis
resulting in loss of the deciduous teeth. Keratosis palmaris et plantaris occurs in three syndromes: pachyonychia congenita, hidrotic
ectodermal dysplasia, and Richner-Hanhart syndrome associated
with tyrosinemia (Lever).

keratosis pilaris [pĭ-lā′rĭs, -lä′rĭs, -lăr′ĭs] means hyperkeratosis
around the ostia of hair (*pilaris*) follicles. This common genodermatosis is most frequently situated on the outer aspects of the limbs.

keratosis, seborrheic [sĕb′ə-rē′ĭk]. *Seborrheic keratosis* designates a
highly characteristic papule that clinically is tan to brown (even to
black) in color, slightly to markedly raised, of great variety in size
and distribution, and obviously hyperkeratotic in a greasy (*seborrheic*) sort of way. Histologically too, epithelial hyperplasia and
hyperkeratosis are highly characteristic.

keratosis, senilis [sē-nĭ′lĭs], or **senile** [sē′nĭl, -nĭl] **keratosis,** designates another highly characteristic condition of hyperkeratosis that
is clinically scaly in character and that histologically shows hyperplasia of a sort that begins to suggest squamous-cell carcinoma.
Actinic, senile, and solar keratosis are all the same.

keratosis, solar [sō′lĕr]. *Solar keratosis* is alternate for *actinic keratosis.* Actinic, senile, and solar keratosis are all the same.

keratotic [kĕr′ə-tŏt′ĭk] is an adjective meaning pertaining or relating
to keratosis.

kerion [kē′rĭ-, kē′rē-ŏn, kĭr′ē-ŏn] is a direct transliteration of the Greek word for a honeycomb, beeswax and honey. The original word was used in Greek medicine by Hippocrates *et alii* for tumors that have resemblances to a honeycomb. Nowadays we apply the word to inflammatory tumors developing upon ordinarily superficial fungous infections. On the scalp particularly, such a development may show many points or purulence because of the follicular pattern of inflammation and thus vaguely simulate the honeycomb appearance.

kerionic [kē′rĭ-, kē′rē-ŏn′ĭk, kĭr′ē-ŏn′ĭk] is an adjective meaning pertaining or relating to kerion.

Kettle's syndrome [kĕt′l]. Malignant degeneration in lymphedema of the lower extremities

kinky hair [kĭngk′ē hâr]. The word *kinky* derives from Danish or Swedish *kink*, twist into a rope. Hence, kinky hair is hair twisted in tight bends. It is a characteristic of some ethnic groups.

Klein-Waardenburg syndrome. Congenital deafness, piebaldism (congenital circumscribed hypomelanosis). There is also lateral displacement of the inner canthi of the eyes and heterochromia of the irides.

Klippel-Trenaunay syndrome [klĭpĕl′; trĕnōnā′]. Unilateral hemangiomatosis with hypertrophy of bones and soft tissues

knotted hair [nŏt′ĕd hâr] describes an acquired condition in which hairs turn on themselves and make simple grannies. The phenomenon is artificial and dependent on neglect of elementary hygiene, although certain kinds of fine hair with a natural tendency to curl may be unusually susceptible to the effect.

knuckle pads [nŭk′l pădz] are thickenings over knuckles of fingers (possibly toes) that are simple hypertrophies of full thickness of skin. The condition may be a congenital (and hereditary) anomaly or an occupational artifact. See *heloma*. Treatment is to know what they are and keep hands off!

Koch's phenomenon, postulates [kôkh]. The phenomenon is reinvocation of tuberculous process within a reaction time of a day or two by reinoculation of tubercle bacilli in a subject already infected or sensitized by previous infection; the postulates are proof of infection by a specific microbe by (1) recovery of that microbe from an infected subject, (2) production of the same infection by it in a new, previously uninfected subject, and (3) recovery of the same microbe from the latter

Koebner phenomenon [kûb′nẽr, -nər fə-nŏm′ə-nŏn]. See *isomorphic effect*. Isomorphic response to scratch or other trauma in certain diseases like psoriasis and lichen planus.

Koebner reaction or **isomeric response** is a distinguishing feature of psoriasis. The phenomenon consists of the appearance of lesions at sites of trauma.

Kogoj's pustule [kô′goy]. Neutrophilic microabscess amid edematous epidermal cells in pustular psoriasis

koilonychia (koi′lō-nĭk′ē-ə, -ĭ-ə] derives from Greek and Latin elements meaning a condition (*-ia*) of hollow (*koil-*) nails (*-onych-*). *Spoon nail* is synonymous and describes the concavity of nail plates in terms of a nearly universally familiar object.

Koplik's spots [kōp′lĭk]. Pale, round spots on the mucous membranes of the buccal mucosa, particularly in measles.

kraurosis [krô-rō′sĭs] is New Latin from Greek elements meaning a condition (*-osis*) that is dry or brittle (*kraur-*). The word is applied to dry conditions of mucous membranes, particularly of the female genitalia, and may serve usefully and tentatively until more definite diagnostic resolution can be made.

Kveim "antigen" [kvām ăn′tə-jĕn] and **test.** When tissue (lymph node, spleen, skin) that is infiltrated with epithelioid cells in the manner of "naked" tubercles and characteristic of sarcoidosis is processed by crude grinding and diluted 1:10 with normal saline, an "antigen" is produced which, when injected into a subject who has sarcoidosis, will generally cause a nodule to appear in four to six weeks. Upon histologic examination the lesion produced by the test will show sarcoid structures. The type of sarcoid tissue from which the "antigen" can be made and the type of sarcoidosis to which the test is applicable are of that process of disputed cause, and not those types that are caused by materials like beryllium and silica.

Kveim test [kvām]. Reaction to intracutaneous deposition of a crude extract of tissue affected by sarcoidosis

kwashiorkor [kwăsh′ē-ôr′kôr, -kər] is said by some to mean red boy in a South African dialect, by others to be a native name in Ghana. The word names a disease of malnutrition that is characterized by faded redness of hair, erythema and superficial scaling of the skin and variable systemic signs of protein and vitamin deficiencies (hepato- and splenomegaly, anasacra, etc.). Some say the word *kwashiorkor* is from a Ga dialect of Ghana and means "the sickness of the weaning."

Kyrle's disease [kûrlz dĭ-, də-zēz′]. See *hyperkeratosis follicularis et parafollicularis in cutem penetrans*.

L

labial, labialis [lā′bĭ-əl; lā′bĭ-ā′lĭs, -ä′lĭs, lā′bē-āl-ĭs] are respectively an English adjective and the masculine and feminine singular of a Medieval Latin adjective meaning pertaining or relating to a lip (*labium*). The words may apply to either the oral or vulvar lips. The Latin word appears in a title like *herpes labialis*.

labium [lā′bĭ-əm, -bē-əm] is a direct borrowing of the Latin word for lip. The word is most commonly applied to the oral and vulvar lips. In reference to the vulvar lips there may be further specification of *major* and *minor* by modifying *labium*, a neuter noun, with the corresponding Latin adjectives in neuter form, respectively *maius* [mä′-, mā′yəs], *minus* [mĭ′-, mĭ′-nəs]. The plural of *labium* is *labia* [lā′bē-ə, -bĭ-ə] and the corresponding Latin adjectives in neuter form are respectively *maiora* [mä-, mə-yō′rə, -yôr′ə] and *minora* [mī-, mĭ-nō′rə, -nôr′ə].

lacerate, laceration [lăs′ĕr-āt′; lăs′ĕr-ā-shən] derive from *laceratus*, perfect passive participle of the Latin verb *lacerare*, to tear to pieces, and mean respectively to mangle, rend or cut crudely and the result of such action.

lacuna [lă-kū′nə, lə-kōō′nə] is a direct borrowing of the Latin word for a discontinuity like a ditch, pit, hole, gap, hollow, cavity, etc. In medicine, the word is used for natural, pathological and artificially created discontinuities of gross or microscopic size in organs or surfaces.

lame foliacée [lăm fəlyăsā′] is a French phrase that means a thin blade, plate or sheet (*lame*) that is laminated in composition as though by layered leaves (*foliacée*). It is applied to the histologic appearance of neuro-ectodermal structures in the skin that appear as thin, stratified formations.

lamella [lə-mĕl′ə] is a direct borrowing of a Latin word which is a diminutive of *lamina* (whence *laminate*), a thin slice of metal or wood, a layer, leaf or plate. We use the word in connection with scales and scaling.

lamellar [lə-mĕl′ĕr] is an adjective from *lamella* and means pertaining or relating to things that are thin slices or formed of delicate sheets.

lamellar dyshidrosis (keratolysis exfoliativa) very fine scaling seen typically on the palms. This has zero significance but should be differentiated from tinea manum by KOH exam of skin scrapings. "Responds" to anything which is put on it. A not infrequent minor skin finding.

lamellar exfoliation of the newborn is the title of a congential condition in which the emerging infant is covered by a membrane of epitrichium (periderm) which eventually exfoliates in keratinous sheets post partum. A form of ichthyosis supervenes later in childhood. See *collodion baby.*

Langerhans' cell [läng′ĕr-häns, lăng′ĕr-hănz sĕl] is eponymic for a dendritic cell found among the cells of the stratum mucosum of the epidermis in positions higher than the stratum germinativum. Such cells are thought to be descendants of melanocytes that are present among basal cells. The dendritic cell found high in the stratum mucosum.

Langer's lines [läng′ērz, lăng′ērz līnz]. See *lines of cleavage.*

Langhans' cell [läng′häns, lăng′hănz sĕl] is eponymic for a foreign body type of giant cell.

lanosum [lă-, lə-nō′səm] is a Latin neuter singular adjective literally meaning full of (-*osum*) wool (*lan-*). It appears in *Microsporum lanosum* and probably describes the woolly character of the aerial growth of this fungus in culture.

lanugo [lə-nū′gō, lă-nōō′gō] is a direct borrowing of a Latin word for a woolly substance or the down of plants, cheeks, etc.

lanugo hair designates the fine hairs that are present on the body everywhere except on the truly hairless areas. In some animals the sum of lanugo hair constitutes a vellus or fleece that is distinct from the rest of hair or fur. In the human animal the vellus or fleece coat is vestigial.

large cell lymphoma (histiocytic lymphoma). usually of B-cell origin but may be due to histiocytes. Nodules occur on the skin which may get quite large and may ulcerate. Prognosis depends on cell of origin; large cell histiocytic lymphomas have a worse prognosis. Hard to distinguish from mycosis fungoides; usually requires special studies. (Lever)

larva [lär′və] is a direct borrowing of the Latin word for a ghost, specter or mask. Its technical use for an insect in the grub state dates from Linnaeus.

larva migrans [mī′grănz] is the title of an infestation, commonly by one or more larvae of *Ancyclostoma braziliense,* in which the grubs move erratically (*migrans*) in superficial channels which the creatures form within the stratum corneum as they travel. *Creeping eruption* is an alternate title.

lata [lā′tə, lä′tə] and **latum** [lā′təm, lä′to͞om] are Latin adjectives meaning flat or broad. The first appears as a neuter plural in a title like *condylomata lata* and the second as a neuter singular in *condyloma latum.*

latent [lā′t′nt] derives from Latin and means lying hidden, concealed or lurking.

latent infection [ĭn-fĕk′shən] in some contexts carries the idea of hidden, concealed or luking infection that is doing its dirty work without clear, outward signs, and in other contexts the idea that what is latent will eventually become patent. The concepts are best understood in the next entry.

latent syphilis [sĭf′ĭ-lĭs, -ə-lĭs] is said of those stages of the disease in which there are no clinical signs of disease process. There is further specification of *early latent* and *late latent syphilis* and implication that more disease will eventually supervene.

lateralis [lā′tĕr-ā′lĭs, lä′tə-rä′lĭs, lăt′ĕr-āl′ĭs] is a Latin adjective meaning belonging or pertaining to a side, hence, *lateral.* It is commonly misused for *lateris* (which see) in the title *nevus unius lateris,* literally meaning "nevus of one side," not "lateral nevus."

lateris [lā′tĕr-ĭs, lä′tə-rĭs, lăt′ə-rĭs] is the genitive singular of the Latin noun *latus,* side, and means of a (the) side. It appears in the title *nevus unius lateris.*

Latrodectus mactans [lăt′rō-dĕk′təs măk′tănz] is the technical designation for the black-widow spider. The term is New Latin, composed as a hybrid of one Greek and two Latin elements, and means a killing (L., *mactans*), bandit- (L., *latro-*) -biter (G., *dectus*). The poor creature is maligned; she merely devours her mate after the orgy of copulation, bites in fear or self-defense and otherwise engages in the joys and sorrows of natural zoologic struggle. Its bite results in arachnidism (see).

lattice fibers [lăt′ĭs fī′bĕrz] is an alternate for *reticulum fibers,* those newly formed proteins that appear in healing processes of the cutis and go to make up mature collagen. The *lattice* or *reticulum* designation is descriptive of a lacy, webbed or netted characteristic of the material as seen in conventional and other histologic processing.

lazarine leprosy [lā′zēr-, lăz′ə-rĭn, -rēn, -rĭn lĕp′rə-sē] is a type of leprous process marked by severe ulceration, mutilation and scarring. *Lazarine* derives from *lazar*, a leper or beggar, and ultimately from *Lazarus*, the name of the biblical beggar who was considered to have had leprosy because he is described as "full of sores" (Luke 16:20).

LE, or **L.E.** [ĕl ē] is an almost unavoidable acronym for *lupus erythematosus.* See comments under *acronym.*

LE cell, factor, phenomenon [sĕl, făk′tēr, fə-nŏm′ə-nŏn]. These are designations for some of the findings with respect to laboratory aspects of lupus erythematosus. In patients afflicted with lupus erythematosus (and some other diseases) the LE cell is that characteristic leukocyte that appears on slide preparations of blood with engulfed, foreign nuclear material in its cytoplasm (or in variant poses like rosettes); the LE factor requires antibodies reactive with DNA-histone and complement. The LE cell is found in about 80% of patients with lupus.

Leiner's disease [lī′nēr]. Erythodermia desquamativa in infants.

leiomyoma [lī′ō-mī-ō′mə] is New Latin from Greek elements that mean an overdevelopment (*-ma*) or tumor (*-oma*) of smooth (*leio-*) muscle (*myo-, my-*) cells. The clinical lesion is a papule of no visible distinction, but palpably tender. It is benign.

leiomyosarcoma [lī′ō-mī′ō-sär-kō′mə] is a malignant development in which smooth (*leio-*) muscle (*-myo-*) cells proliferate into a fleshy (*sarc-*) mass (*-oma*).

Leishmania [lēsh-mā′nē-ə, -măn′ē-ə] is the name for a genus of protozoal micro-organisms. Species of the genus (*donovani, orientalis, tropica*) are pathogenic for humans. The word is, of course, eponymic (after General William Bing Leishman, surgeon, British Army, born in 1865) and, as a designation for a genus, takes a capital initial letter.

leishmaniasis (-osis) [lēsh′mə-nī′ə-sĭs; -mā′nē-ō′sĭs] are general terms for any condition (*-iasis, -osis*) caused by any pathogenic species of the genus *Leishmania.* Used as a common noun the word takes a small initial letter.

leishmanid [lēsh′mə-nĭd] designates any lesion within the possibility of infection with a species of the genus *Leishmania.* See *-id.*

lens [lĕnz] is a direct borrowing of the Latin word for a lentil. Owing to the shape of this fabaceous seed, the word is applied to objects, particularly transparent ones, that are doubly convex.

lenticular [lĕn-tĭk′ū-lêr] means in the shape or form of a lentil.

"lentigine" [lĕn′tĭ-jĭn, -jĕn, -jĭn] is back formation of an erroneous singular from *lentigines*, plural of *lentigo*. See comparable instances under "*comedone*" and "*ephilide*."

lentigines [lĕn-tĭj′ĭ-nēz] is the proper plural of *lentigo*, according to its declension in Latin.

lentiginosis [lĕn-tĭj′ĭ-nō′sĭs] designates a condition (-*osis*) marked by profusion of lentigines.

lentiginosis profusa [lĕn-tĭj′ĭ-nō′sīs prō-fū′sə] designates a genetic syndrome whose major signs and symptoms are gathered in a strained mnemonic term, namely, the "leopard" syndrome, in which the *1* stands for *lentigines*; the *e* for *electrocardiac abnormalities*; the *o* for *ocular hypertelorism*; the *p* for *pulmonary stenosis*; the *a* for *abnormalities of the genitalia*; the *r* for *retardation of growth*; the *d* for *deafness*.

lentiginous [lĕn-tĭj′ĭ-nəs] means full of (-*ous*) lentigines: i.e., marked by many lesions of the type, and, by extension, pertaining or relating to a lentigo.

lentigo [lĕn-tī′gō] is a direct borrowing of the Latin word for a lentil-shaped spot like a freckle.

lentigo maligna [lĕn-tī′gō mə-lĭg′nə] is new coinage for what has long been called Hutchinson's freckle and circumscribed precancerous melanosis of Dubreuilh. The term is too final. The condition so named more often stays clinically benign in course for years (or forever), then progresses eventually to true malignancy.

lentigo maligna melanoma [lĕn-tī′gō mə-lĭg′nə mĕl′ə-nō′mə] is intended to mean supervention of malignant melanoma upon lentigo maligna. If *lentigo maligna* is a regrettable term, *lentigo maligna melanoma* is even more regrettable. It is awkward to parse. One must figure out that *lentigo maligna* is made adjectival to *melanoma* and that *melanoma* means *malignant melanoma*.

lentil [lĕn′tĭl, -t′l] derives via French *lentille* from Latin *lenticula*, diminutive of *lens*, lentil. It designates the common fabaceous plant and the seed thereof.

leonine [lē′ō-nīn, lē′ə-nīn, -nən], deriving from Latin *leoninus*, means pertaining to, appearing like, or having the aspect of a lion.

leonine facies [fā′shĭ-ēz, -shē-ēz, -shēz] is descriptive of infiltration of the face, particularly on and about the brow, that imparts a resemblance to the face of a lion. The appearance is common in lepromatous leprosy and occasional in some other conditions (e.g., some lymphomatoses).

leontiasis [lē′ŏn-tī′ə-sĭs] means a lion-like (*leont-*) condition (*-iasis*). It is alternate for *leonine facies.*

"leopard" syndrome. See *lentiginosis profusa.*

leper [lĕp′ēr] designates an individual afflicted with leprosy.

lepothrix [lĕp′ō-thrĭks], deriving from Greek word elements, means scaly (*lepo-*) hair (*-thrix*). The word is applied to a fungous infection of the hair shafts of the axillae caused by a species of *Nocardia.* The clinical appearance is that of tan or reddish, hard concretions attached to the hair shafts. *Trichomycosis axillaris* is an alternate title.

lepr- and **lepro-** [lĕpr, lĕp′rō] are combining forms from Greek and Latin *lepra*, leprosy.

lepra [lĕp′rə]. The original Greek and Latin word for modern leprosy.

lepra bacillus [bə-sĭl′əs] is an ordinary designation for *Mycobacterium leprae.*

leprid(e) [lĕp′rĭd, -rīd, -rēd] designates any lesion or type of process within the possibilities of infection with *Mycobacterium leprae.*

lepro-. See *lepr-.*

leprologist, leprology [lĕp-rŏl′ō-jĭst, -ə-jĭst; lĕp-rŏl′ō-jē, -ə-jē, -jī] are words applied to a student of, and the study of, leprosy. The disease is so ancient, still so common and so complex that it has merited and still merits specialized students and study.

leproma [lĕp-rō′mə] designates a tumorous (*-oma*) process of leprosy.

lepromatous [lĕp-rŏm′ə-təs] is an adjective meaning pertaining or relating to a leproma or characterized by formation of lepromas.

lepromatous leprosy is that form of the disease that is marked clinically by lepromas and histologically by abundant lepra bacilli within hydropic epithelioid cells.

lepromin [lĕp′rō-mĭn] is an "antigen" made from lepromatous tissue. Materials designated as lepromins are crudely processed from lepromatous tissue that is heavily laden with lepra bacilli. What is obtained is an unstandardized soup of bacillary fragments and other indefinable substances derived from diseased tissue.

lepromin test and **reaction.** Injection of lepromin in a patient with tuberculoid leprosy generally produces an enduring infiltration several weeks later and sometimes a 48-hour tuberculin-like reaction;

in lepromatous leprosy the reaction is generally negative. The name of Mitsuda is associated with the long-postponed positive reaction, and that of Fernandez with the 48-hour reaction.

leprosarium [lĕp′rō-să′rē-əm, -să′rē-əm] is a place (*-arium*) for the care or confinement of lepers.

leprosy [lĕp′rō-, lĕp′rə-sē], the modern name of the disease, derives from Late Latin *leprosus*, which means full of (*-osus*) the disease (*lepr-*).

leprosy, anesthetic, borderline, dimorphous, indeterminate, intermediate, lazarine, lepromatous, Lucio, macular, maculo-anesthetic, mixed, neural, neuro-, nodular, tuberculoid. So protean are the clinical, histologic and other aspects of leprosy that a large number of more or less specifying adjectives have been attached to *leprosy* to make distinctions. Those listed are still in current use. There are many more that are obsolescent, obsolete or rare. *Anesthetic, macular, maculo-anesthetic, neural, neuro-* and *tuberculoid* have synonymy and specify the sign of localized anesthesia, the morphe of lesions (macules), involvement of nerves (neural, neuro-) or histology (tuberculoid). *Lepromatous* and *nodular* specify the clinical characteristic of that form which is tumorous. *Dimorphous* and *mixed* designate leprous process which has characteristics of both major forms (lepromatous and tuberculoid). *Borderline, indeterminate* and *intermediate* imply leprous process that is not yet sufficiently differentiated to be classified *lepromatous* or *tuberculoid*. *Lazarine* and *Lucio* have been applied to severe ulcerating and mutilating leprous process.

leprous [lĕp′rəs], deriving from Late Latin *leprosus*, literally means full of leprosy and, by extension, pertaining or relating to leprosy.

Lesch-Nyhan syndrome [lĕsh; nī′ən]. Mental retardation and self-multilation by biting; deficiency of hypoxanthine guanine phosphoribosyl transferase

lesion [lē′zhən] derives from Latin *laesio*, a hurt or injury, and in modern medical parlance means any detectable deviation from normal structure.

lesion, primary, special, secondary. Primary lesions may be defined as appearances that are the first grossly recognizable, or the most characteristic, structural changes of skin diseases. Special lesions are also primary in the sense given above but carry the connotation of "special" because they are of exceptionally peculiar structure or odd mechanism in production or limited to a few dermatoses. Secondary lesions are those that evolve or develop as natural progressions from primary lesions or from adventitious events like scratching, irritation and secondary infection of primary lesions.

lethal [lē′thəl], **let(h)alis** [lē-t(h)ā′lĭs, -tä′lĭs, -tăl′ĭs] are respectively an English and a Latin adjective derived from *letum*, death, and mean relating to death, deadly, fatal. The word *letum* sometimes appears as *lethum* in classical Latin because of a fancied relationship with *Lethe*, the river of forgetfulness in Hades (the Lower World, Hell). The English adjective appears in the title *midline lethal granuloma* and the Latin adjective, in *ichthyosis let (h)alis.*

Letterer-Siwe disease [lĕt′ēr-ēr-, -ər sē′vĕ, -sī′wē dĭ-, də-zēz′]. See *histiocytosis X.*

leuc(o)- and **leuk(o)-** [loo̅′ko̅] are alternate spellings of a combining form from the Greek word *leucos*, or *leukos*, meaning white. Which spelling is used depends on whether one transliterates the kappa (κ) in the Greek word with a *c* or a *k*. Some prefer the *c* because of practice long established by the Latin method of transliteration, others, the *k*, because it is closer to the original Greek letter. There is a growing tendency by translators of Greek classics to stick closer to the Greek spelling. Moreover, when the word element to which this combining form is attached begins with an *e*, the hard sound of the transliterated kappa is more easily kept by the letter *k*, as in *leukemia*. Hence, all entries for words beginning with *leuc (o)-, leuk (o)-*, will begin with the latter form, e.g., *leukoderm- (i)a* will be listed instead of *leucoderm (i)a*, etc.

leukemia [loo̅-kē′mē-ə, -mĭ-ə] does not, of course, mean white blood but a condition (*-ia*) in which the blood (*-em-*) contains an abnormally large number of white (*leuk-*) cells as a constant feature. Compare *leukocytosis.*

leukemia cutis [kū′tĭs] has to be understood as a condition (*-ia*) in which there has been an invasion of the skin (*cutis*) by the white (*leuk-*) cell elements of the blood (*-em-*) in the course of the disease leukemia.

leukemid [loo̅′kə-mĭd], a coinage by analogy with other *-id* words, can be used to designate any cutaneous expression of leukemia. Both specific infilitrates and nonspecific lesions are encompassed. Implication of allergy should not be read into this word. See *-id.*

leuk(o)-. See *leuc (o)-.*

leukocytosis [loo̅′ko̅-sī-to̅′sĭs] means a condition (*-osis*) of increased number of white (*leuko-*) blood cells (*-cyt-*) as a transient phenomenon, usually associated with transient infection.

leukoderm(i)a [loo′ko-dûr′mə, -dûr′mē-ə, -mĭ-ə] literally means a condition of the skin (-*derma,* -*dermia*) in which it is abnormally white (*leuko-*). The whiteness, of course, is always predicated upon failure of production of melanin. One hardly ever comes across *leucoderma* or *leukodermia*; *leukoderma* is the word and appears in the two titles that follow.

leukoderma acquisitum centrifugum [ăk′wĭ-sī′təm, -sē′təm, ə-kwĭ z′ĭ-təm sĕn-trĭf′ū-gəm, -ə-gəm] is the title of a depigmenting process that begins around pigmented nevi. The thrust of the title is that the depigmentation is acquired (*acquisitum*) and does not come on as a part of the genetic nature of the nevus, and that the depigmentation progresses away from the center (*centrifugum*) toward an expanding periphery. One knows now that depigmentation progresses toward the center too, and thus *et* (We realize now that *centripetum* is bad Latin and that the better word would be *centripitens.*) could very well be added to the title. *Halo nevus* is a poor alternate title.

leukokeratosis [loo′ko-kĕr-ə-tō′sĭs] designates a condition (-*osis*) of hyperkeratinization (-*kerat-*) which is distinctly white (*leuko-*). Such whiteness is the appearance of hyperkeratinization on mucous membranes.

leukokeratosis oris [ō′rĭs, ôr′ĭs] describes hyperkeratinization in its white character about or in the mouth (*oris*).

leukonychia [loo′ko-nĭk′ē-ə, -ĭ-ə] is a New Latin formation from Greek word elements that mean any condition (-*ia*) in which the nails (-*onych-*) are unduly white (*leuk-*). A whiteness of the entire nail plate is termed *leukonychia totalis*; horizontal streaks of whiteness, *leukonychia striata*; and shots of whiteness, simply *leukonychia* or *gift spots.*

leukoplakia [loo′ko-plā′kē-ə, -kĭ-ə] is a New Latin formation from Greek word elements that mean a white (*leuko-*) flatness (-*plakia*). Those well-known patches of hyperkeratinization on mucous membranes (particularly in the mouth and on the genitalia) that are bluish white or stark white and have a tendency to become squamouscell carcinoma are designated by the word.

leukoplasia [loo′ko-plā′zhē-ə, -zē-ə, -zhə] is a New Latin formation from Greek word elements that mean a white (*leuko-*) development (-*plasia*). It is not a commonly used word, but in many ways it is as good as or better than *leukoplakia*, just as *erythroplasia* is better than *erythroplakia*. The betterness lies in the idea of continuous development rather than finished quality. Both sets of words can be discriminatingly used, depending on what stage of process one wishes to describe.

leukotrichia [lo͞o'ko-trīk'ē-ə, -ĭ-ə] is a New Latin formation from Greek word elements that mean a white (*leuko-*) condition (*-ia*) of the hair (*-trich-*). *Canities* and *poliosis* are alternate words.

Lewandowsky, rosacea-like tuberculid of [lĕv'ăn-dŏv'skē]. Papulosis of the face resembling rosacea.

Lewandowsky-Lutz, epidermodysplasia verruciformis of [lĕv'ăn-dŏv'skē; lo͞ ots]. Verrucous dyscrasia of the epidermis with a tendency to malignant degeneration.

l'homme rouge [lôm, lŭm ro͞ozh] is alternate for *homme rouge* (which see), with the addition of a form of the French definite article (*l'* for *le*).

lichen [lī'kən, -kĭn] is given in dictionaries as probably deriving from a Greek verb meaning to lick. No explanation is given or conjecture advanced as to why from a word of this original meaning a noun was adapted both in Greek and Latin for those symbiotic forms of plant life (a fungus and an alga) that are now designated lichens, and also for those dermatoses that vaguely resemble the botanical formations because they present to the eye a surface pattern of more or less closely agminated papules. One may suggest that the slow growth of lichens on rocks and seasonal covering and uncovering of them may have suggested licking in the same sense as a gentle wave is poetically said to lap or lick a shore in its ebb and flow. With such a fancy in mind, the topologic morphe of botanical lichens may then have suggested the word *lichen* as appropriate for the surface characteristics of some dermatoses. Following are many titles, still more or less current, which we note largely for the etymology of their modifying adjectives. There is much about the conditions that is unknown and, of course, cannot be told by the titles, which are mainly and but partially descriptive of morphology.

lichen amyloidosus [ăm'ə-loi-dō'səs] designates a papular dermatosis (*lichen*) that is full of (*-osus*) amyloid, i.e., amorphous material that looks like (*-oid*) starch (*amyl-*) in certain histologic processing. Many textbooks and articles carry this title erroneously as "*lichen amyloidosis.*"

lichen chronicus simplex [krŏn'ĭ-kəs sĭm'plĕks] describes a papular eruption (*lichen*) that endures long (*chronicus*) and is uncomplicated (*simplex*). One may wonder what is simple about that intractable, inscrutable and pruritic condition commonly about ankles, elbows, and the nape and postero-lateral aspects of the neck. The alternate title *circumscribed neurodermatitis* (which see) is even worse.

lichen corneus hypertrophicus [kôr′nē-əs hī′pĕr-trŏf′ĭ-kəs] describes a papular eruption (*lichen*) whose lesions are palpably horny (*corneus*) and usually overgrown (*hypertrophicus*).

lichen myxedematosus [mĭk′sə-dĕm′ə-tō′səs, -dē′mə- tō′səs] describes a papular eruption (*lichen*) whose lesions are full of (-*osus*) swollen (-*edemat-*) mucin (*myx-*). The modifying word refers, of course, to the histologic appearance of the papular content.

lichen nitidus [nĭt′ĭ′dəs] describes a papular eruption (*lichen*) whose lesions are visibly shiny (*nitidus*). The condition has been interpreted as a form of lichen planus.

lichen obtusus corneus [ŏb-tū′-, ŏb-tōō′səs kôr′nē-əs] is a title for a rare papular dermatosis (*lichen*) in which the lesions are described as blunt (*obtusus*) in surface characteristic and otherwise horny (*corneus*).

lichen pilaris seu (or sive) spinulosus [pĭ-lā′rĭs, -lä′rĭs, -lär′ĭs sēōō, sū (sī′vē) spī′nū-, spī′nōō-, spĭn′ū-lō′səs] describes a papular eruption (*lichen*) whose lesions are situated about hairs (*pilaris*) and/or (*seu, sive*) are pointed (*spinulosus*). *Seu* is an alternate form of *sive*, meaning originally "if you please," then "or if" and finally "or."

lichen planopilaris [plā′nō-pĭ-lā′rĭs, -lä′rĭs, -lär′ĭs] describes a papular eruption (*lichen*) whose lesions are flat (*plano-*) and situated around the hairs (-*pilaris*). The condition is a form of lichen planus.

lichen planus [plā′nəs, plä′nōōs] describes a characteristic papular dermatosis (*lichen*) whose lesions are flat (*planus*). The anterior aspects of the arms, the anteromedial aspects of the thighs, the small of the back and the penis are common sites of the process.

lichen planus pemphigoides. Coexisting lichen planus and bullous pemphigoides.

lichen ruber [rōō′bĕr, -bər] describes a papular dermatosis (*lichen*) whose lesions are red (*ruber*). The title is alternate to *lichen planus* and both titles are sometimes combined as *lichen ruber planus*. If *pruriens* (itching) were added to the title even more about the condition would be told.

lichen ruber acuminatus [ə-kū′mĭ-nā′təs, -nä′təs, -tōōs] is a title for a papular dermatosis in which the individual lesions are red (*ruber*) and pointed (*acuminatus*).

lichen ruber moniliformis [mō-nĭl′ĭ-fôr′mĭs] describes a papular eruption (*lichen*) whose lesions are arranged in the form of (*-formis*) a necklace (*monili-*).

lichen sclerosus et atrophicans (atrophicus) [sklĕ-, sklə-, sklē-rō′səs ĕt ə-trŏf′ĭ-kănz (ə-trŏf′ĭ-kəs)] describes a papular eruption (*lichen*) whose lesions both clinically and histologically appear hardened (*sclerosus*) and atrophying (*atrophicans*) or atrophied (*atrophicus*). The chest, upper back and genitalia are common sites of the process. Individual lesions are noted for porcelaneous color and follicular patulousness.

lichen scrofulosorum [skrŏf′ū-lō-sō′rəm, -sôr′əm] describes a papular eruption (*lichen*) that occurs in the tuberculous (*scrofulosorum*, of the tubercular). It is a self-resolving condition that is not so serious as it sounds. *Tuberculosis cutis lichenoides* is an alternate title.

lichen spinulosus. See *lichen pilaris seu* (or *sive*) *spinulosus*.

lichen striatus [strī-, strĭ-ā′təs, -ä′to͞os] describes a papular eruption (*lichen*) whose lesions are arranged in a stripe (*striatus*).

lichen trichophyticus [trĭk′ō-fīt′ĭ-kəs] describes a papular eruption (*lichen*) that may occur in some fungous infections caused by *Trichophyton* as a special immunologic event. Irritation or exacerbation of a focus of fungous infection is sometimes attended by a sudden exanthem of papules that are sterile but clearly related to the pre-existing condition.

lichen urticatus [ûr′tĭ-kā′təs, -kä′təs] describes a papular eruption (*lichen*) whose lesions have a wheal-like (*urticatus*) quality.

lichenification, lichenified [lī′kən-, lĭ-kĕn′ə-fĭ-kā′shən; lī′kən-, lĭ-kĕn′ĭ-fīd, -ə-fīd] are respectively a noun and an adjective (past participle) meaning development of (*-fication*) a lichen and converted into (*-fied*) a lichen. Thickening of the skin and increase of its markings by agmination of papules are the implications.

lichenoid, lichenoides [lī′kə-noid, lī′kən-oid; lī′kə-noi′dēz, lī′kən-oi′dēz] are respectively an English and a New Latin adjective meaning like (*-oid, -oides*) a lichen. The classicized form appears in titles like *parapsoriasis lichenoides, pityriasis lichenoides* and *tuberculosis cutis lichenoides*.

liminal, liminaris [lĭm′ĭ-nəl, -ə-n'l; lĭm′ĭ-nā′rĭs, -nä′rĭs, när′ĭs] are respectively an English adjective and the masculine or feminine singular of a Latin adjective meaning pertaining to a threshold, border or limit. *Liminal* is a neglected word that could well be rehabilitated and used instead of *minimal*, which is so overworked nowadays in such clichés as *minimal itching*. When one wants to suggest the barely perceptible, *liminal* is far better than *minimal.* The Latin adjective appears in the title *alopecia liminaris frontalis* (feminine).

linea [lĭn′ē-ə] is a direct borrowing of the Latin word for a line.

linea alba (albicans) [ăl′bə, (ăl′bĭ-kănz)] means white (*alba*) line (*linea*) or a line growing white (*albicans*). The phrases are descriptive of the linear scars that run opposite the lines of cleavage of the skin and occur apparently as the result of ruptures in the corium. The effects are seen commonly in obesity, pregnancy and endocrinopathy. The plural form is *lineae albae* (*albicantes*) [lĭn′ē-ē, -ī ăl′bē, -bĭ (ăl′bĭ-kăn′tēz)]. *Striae distensae* is alternate.

linea nigra [nī′grə] describes a stripe of intense pigmentation (*nigra*, black) that sometimes develops during pregnancy and runs from pubes to umbilicus.

linear [lĭn′ē-ər, -ēr], derived from Latin *linearis,* meaning of or belonging to a line, means on or along a line.

linear focal elastosis elastotic striae.

linear IgA bullous dermatosis is perhaps better known as chronic bullous dermatosis of childhood. A bullous eruption seen in children often indistinguishable from bullous pemphigoid except that it is a self-limited condition. Can also occur in adults.

linear nevus [nē′vəs] describes a structural anomaly of embryogenic or hereditable nature (*nevus*) that is in the form of a line or stripe.

linear scleroderma [sklē′rō-dûr′mə] describes a hardened condition of the skin (*scleroderma*) in the form of a depressed line or stripe. *Sclérodermie en coup de sabre* is an alternate title in French.

lines of cleavage [līnz ōv klēv′ĭj, -əj] refers to formative directions determined by the position of collagen bundles and elastic fibers relative to which incisions parallel to them result in cut edges that fall together, or relative to which, incisions at right angles to them result in cut edges that gape. These lines are important in minor surgical and plastic procedures on the skin and in the localization of some dermatoses (e.g., pityriasis rosea).

lingua [lĭng′gwə] is the Latin word for tongue. It is used in classicized titles such as the following:

lingua geographica [jē′ō-grăf′ĭ-kə]. See *geographic tongue.*

lingua nigra [nī′grə]. See *black (hairy) tongue.*

lingua plicata [plĭ-kā′tə, -kä′tə], meaning furrowed (*plicata*) tongue, is an alternate title for *scrotal tongue.*

lingua scrotalis [skrō-tā′lĭs, -tä′lĭs, -tăl′ĭs]. See *scrotal tongue.*

liniment [lĭn′ə-mĕnt] derives from a Late Latin word *linimentum* meaning a material (*-mentum*, noun ending) that is smeared or rubbed on (*lini-*).

lip- and **lipo-** [lĭp, lĭp′ō, lī′pō] are combining forms from Greek *lipos*, fat.

lipid(e) [lĭp′ĭd, lī′pĭd, lĭp′īd] is both a noun meaning a fatty (*lip-*) material (*id, -ide*) and an adjective meaning relating or pertaining to (*-id*) fat (*lip-*).

lipo-. See *lip-*.

lipodystrophy [lī′pō-, lĭp′ō-dĭs′trə-fē,-fĭ] means any faulty (*-dys-*) development (*-trophy*) of fat (*lipo-*).

lipoid [lĭp′oid, lī′poid] is an adjective meaning like (*-oid*) fat (*lip-*).

lipoid proteinosis [prō′tē-ĭ-nō′sĭs]. Urbach-Wiethe disease, hyalinosis cutis at mucosae, autosomal recessive trait. Appears to be a lysomal storage disease marked by nodules, particularly of the skin of the face and in the mouth, oropharynx and larynx. Collagen production is altered and abnormally hydrolyzed in the dermis. There appears to be an increase in the production of basement membrane collagen and it also affects fibroblasts by a decreased synthesis of altered fibrous collagen. (*Andrews' Diseases of the Skin*, 8th Ed. Arnold/Odom/James, W.B. Saunders)

lipoidica [lĭ-poi′dĭ-kə] is a classicized adjective that is equivalent to English *lipoid*. It appears in the title *necrobiosis lipoidica diabeticorum*.

lipoidosis [lĭp′oi-dō′sĭs] means any condition (*-osis*) in which fatty material (*lipoid-*) is abnormally involved.

lipoma [lĭ-pō′mə] is a New Latin formation meaning a massing or over-development (*-ma, -oma*) of fat (*lipo-, lip-*) tissue.

lipomatosus [lĭ-pŏm′ə-, lĭ-pō′mə-tō′səs] is a New Latin adjectival formation from *lipoma* and means full of (*-osus*) fat. It appears in the title *nevus lipomatosus*.

Liponyssus [lĭp′ō-nĭ′səs] designates a genus of mites that are epizootic on rats. One species (*L. bacoti*) is facultatively capable of infesting humans. The word means fat- (*lipo-*) piercing (*-nyssus*).

liposarcoma [lī′pō-, lĭp′ō-sär-kō′mə] describes a malignant development of fat (*lipo-*) tissue as a fleshy (*sarc-*) mass (*-oma*).

liquefaction degeneration [lĭk′wə-făk′shən dĭ-, də-, dē-jĕn′ēr-ā′shən] describes disintegration or poor delineation of the basal-cell layer of the epidermis as a "washing-out" of substance.

Such a dissolution is seen in lichen planus and some other conditions like lupus erythematosus.

livedo [lī-, lĭ-vē′dō] is a direct borrowing from Latin of the word for blueness produced by blows. We do not use the word in the original sense of blueness from contusion but merely for blueness from venous congestions.

livedo racemosa [răs′ē-mō′sə] describes blueness of skin in terms of the pattern of a bunch of grapes (*racemosa*).

livedo reticularis [rĕ-, rē-tĭk′ū-lā′rĭs, -lä′rĭs, -lăr′ĭs] describes a blueness of the skin in terms of a netted or webbed (*reticularis*) pattern.

liver spot [lĭv′ĕr, ər spŏt] is a lay term for pigmentation that is taken to be caused by abnormal function of the liver. It is, of course, not a useful term in modern times. We have profounder ways of saying as little about pigmentary anomalies.

livid, lividity [lĭv′ĭd; lĭ-vĭd′ə-tē, -tĭ] are respectively an adjective and a noun deriving from Latin via French and meaning, respectively, of bluish color and a condition of bluish color.

Loa loa [lō′ə] names a particular filaria that is notable for predilection to infest the eye and the region thereabouts, causing tumefactions (see *Calabar swellings*). The word *loa* is Congolese for eye worm; *Loa loa* is old terminology for *Filaria loa*.

lo(ai)asis [lō′(ə-ī′)ə-sĭs] is the condition (-*iasis*) of infestation with the filaria that is named *Loa loa* or *Filaria loa*.

localized [lō′k'l-īzd] is an adjective (past participle) applied descriptively to changes that are limited or confined to an area.

localized neurodermatitis [nŏō′-, nū′rō-dûr′mə-tī′tĭs, -tē′tĭs] is used by some for *lichen chronicus simplex* and solitary patches of atopic dermatitis. See strictures under *neurodermatitis*.

localized scleroderma [sklĕ′-, sklē′rō-dūr′mə] is used by some for morphea or linear forms of scleroderma.

loose anagen syndrome, a distinctive new hair condition, features anagen hairs that are loosely anchored and easily pulled from the scalp. Majority of patients are blond girls. The easily pulled hairs are misshapen anagen hairs without external root sheaths.

These children have sparse scalp hair that does not grow long and seldom requires cutting. May also occur in adults. No known associated abnormalities. The appearance of the hair improves with time. (Price)

Longitudinal melanonychia (melanonychia striata) is the striking condition manifested by longitudinal hyperpigmented streaking of the nail. Subungual melanoma must be considered in the differential diagnosis. Presence of blood or chromogens may also produce this finding. A biopsy may be necessary to establish the diagnosis. (Baran & Kechijian)

lotion [lō′shən] derives from Latin *lotio,* a washing. In dermatologic pharmaceutics, the word designates a liquid preparation that is applied to the skin as a painter (artist) applies a wash.

Louis-Bar syndrome [loōē′; bär]. See *ataxia telangiectasia.*

louse [lous], deriving from Anglo-Saxon, designates, in purely technical but not expletive contexts, either of the two pediculi (*Pediculus capitis,* the scalp louse, and *Pediculus corporis vel vestimentorum,* the body or clothes louse) and also *Phthir (i)us pubis,* the pubic or crab louse.

Loxosceles reclusa [lŏk-sŏs′ə-lēz rē-klōō′sə] names a species of spiders whose bite is severely sickening. The words describe the creature as slant- (*loxos-*) -legged (*-celes*) and shyly retiring (*reclusa*).

lucidum [loō′sĭ-dəm, -doōm] is the neuter singular of a Latin adjective meaning clear. It appears in the designation *stratum lucidum.*

Lucio leprosy [loō′sē-ō lĕp′rō-, lĕp′rə-sē] is eponymic (of a Mexican physician) for a form of leprosy marked by intensely erythematous plaques that tend to ulcerate.

Ludwig's angina [loōd′vĭg]. Stomatitis and pharyngitis that occur in agranulocytic states.

lues [loō′ēz] is a direct borrowing of the Latin word for plague. The word has so long been used by physicians in the presence of patients as a disguised designation for syphilis that by now many think the word is an original synonym for *syphilis.* The more learned would write and say *lues syphilitica.*

luetic [loō-ĕt′ĭk] is the adjective from *lues* meaning relating or pertaining literally to a plague but actually to syphilis by inevitable extension of meaning.

lunula [loō′nyə-, loō′nū-lə] is a direct borrowing of a Latin word meaning a little (*-ula*) moon (*lun-*). We use the word to designate the exposed or visible portion of nail matrix, which does indeed have the appearance of a tiny (half or quarter) moon.

lunula, diffusion of the. See *diffusion of the lunula.*

lupoid [loō′poid] is an adjective from *lupus* meaning like (*-oid*) that condition.

lupoid sycosis [sī-kō′sĭs] designates a pyodermatous or fugous infection whose clinical appearance is described by the words in their literal senses as a condition (-*osis*) that looks like gnawed (*lupoid*) figs (*syc*-). The condition is so named because it clinically resembles granulomatous processes, particularly those of tuberculosis cutis, and most particularly lupus vulgaris.

luposa, lupous [loo-pō′sə, loo′pəs] are respectively a New Latin and an English adjective meaning relating or pertaining to lupus in the sense of a tuberculous process that is eroded or ulcerated. The Latin adjective appears in the title *tuberculosis cutis luposa.*

lupus erythematosus [loo′pəs, -poos ĕr′ə-, ĕr′ĭ-thĕm′ə-tō′səs] is an inflammatory disease of unknown etiology characterized by involvement of many different organ systems; the skin is affected in some more than 90% of the cases. There is the production of antibodies reactive with nuclear, cytoplasmic and cell membrane antigens.

It is especially associated with fever, rash, photosensitivity, arthritis, anemia, chest pain, proteinuria and in rare but dramatic cases psychosis.

Immunofluorescent studies are of crucial importance in diagnosis. Involved skin shows immunoglobulins, IgG and IgM and complement in more than 90% of cases.

The test for antinuclear antibodies (ANA) represents the most sensitive laboratory test for systemic lupus erythematosus.

lupus erythematosus hypertrophicus [hī′pĕr-trŏf′ĭ′kəs] is descriptive of lesions of lupus erythematosus that are distinctive by being overgrown upward (*hypertrophicus*).

lupus erythematosus profundus [prō-fŭn′dəs, -foon′doos] is descriptive of lesions of lupus erythematosus that are distinctive by being deep (*profundus*).

lupus miliaris disseminatus faciei [mĭl′ĭ-ā′rĭs, -ä′rĭs, -är′ĭs dĭ-sĕm′ĭ-nā′təs, -nä′toos fā′shĭ-ē-ī, -shē-ē-ī] names a condition of the class of lupus that is specified to be spread (*disseminatus*) on the face (*faciei*) in the form of (-*aris*) millet- (*mili*-) -like papules. The condition is thought by some to be a tuberculoderm because the histologic appearance is that of tuberculoid structures and because the tuberculin reaction is negative at a time when one would expect it to be positive.

lupus pernio [pûr′nĭ-ō, pĕr′nē-ō] describes a process within the class of lupus as a frostbite (*pernio*). The condition is thought by many to be a form of sarcoidosis.

lupus vulgaris [vûl-gā′rĭs, - gä′rĭs, -gär′ĭs] names that common (*vulgaris*) form of cutaneous tuberculosis whose lesions have a gnawed or eroded quality (*lupus*) in the form of intermingled scarring and active, tumid inflammatory papules.

lycopenemia. See *carotinemia.*

Lyell's disease [lī′əl]. Toxic epidermal necrolysis.

lymph- [lĭmf] and **lympho-** [lĭm′fō] are combining forms from Latin *lympha,* a poetic word for water, especially clear water or spring water. (This word flowed, so to speak, from the Greek noun *nymphe,* meaning a bride or young woman, but designating especially minor female divinities who lived in seas, rivers, fountains, trees or mountains, i.e., the nymphs of nature. The change of *n* in the Greek *nymphe* to the *l* of the Latin *lympha* is an illustration of the linguistic phenomenon known as *alternation* or *dissimilation;* for further comments on this topic see under *cancer.*)

In New Latin and modern medical terminology *lymph* (*o*)-, with a slight change of sense, is applied to body fluids that are relatively clear, i.e., sparse of cells and other particulate matter, e.g., the liquid within lymphatic vessels, intercellular and ascitic fluid, etc.

lymphadenitis [lĭm-făd′ə-, lĭm-făd′ē-nī′tĭs, -nē′tĭs] designates any inflammatory condition (*-itis*) of a lymph node (*-aden-,* literally gland). This too is a generic word to which specifications can be added, e.g., *tuberculous, syphilitic, pyogenic,* etc.

lymphadenoma, lymphadenomatosis [lĭm′făd-ə-nō′mə, lĭm′făd-ə-nō′mə-tō′sĭs] mean, respectively, a tumorous swelling (*-oma*) of a lymph node and a generalized condition of such enlargements (*-omatosis*). The words are generic and can be applied to conditions like Hodgkin's disease, the leukemias, etc., until specific diagnostic resolution can be made.

lymphadenopathy [lĭm′făd-, lĭm-făd′ə-nŏp′ə-thē, -thī] designates any abnormal condition (*-pathy*) of a lymph node (*lymphadeno-,* literally lymph gland). Clinically means enlargements of lymph nodes.

lymphadenosis cutis benigna [lĭm′făd-, lĭm-făd′ə-nō′sĭs kū′tĭs bə-, bē-nĭg′nə] names a harmless (*benigna*) condition (*-osis*) of the skin (*cutis*) in which something like lymph node (*lymphaden-,* literally lymph gland) structures appear. Alternate titles are *follicular lymphoma* and *lymphocytoma cutis,* which are simpler but otherwise not much better in nosologic distinctiveness. The possibility that what looks benign by way of lymphomatosis may be deceptive, and occasional transition to indubitable malignancy make any title of this sort shaky, and employable only with reservations.

lymphangiectasia, or **-ectasis** [lĭm′făn-jē-, lĭm-făn′jĭ-ĕk-tā′zhē-ə, -zē-ə, -zhə; -ĕk-tā′sĭs], designates abnormal dilatation (*-ectasia, -ectasis*) of lymph vessels (*lymphangi-*). *Lymphangioma* is nearly synonymous; *lymphangiectasia,* or *-ectasis,* may be suggestive of a more diffuse process with a clinical counterpart that is vaguer in outline of tumefaction than lymphangioma generally is.

lymphangioma [lĭm′făn-, lĭm-făn′jē-ō′mə, -jĭ-ō′mə] designates an overdevelopment or massing (*-ma, -oma*) of lymph vessels (*lymphangio-*). The clinical mark of the condition is a more or less sharply circumscribed swelling with no change of color, unlike a hemangioma, which is better outlined and of high red or purple color.

lymphedema [lĭm′fē-, lĭm′fə-dē′mə] designates swelling (*-edema*) of a part resulting from obstruction to proper circulation of lymph. The clinical mark of the condition is enlargeum by brawny induration from constant, usually irreversible, accmulation of intercellular fluid, unlike ordinary edema, which is pitting and, other things being equal, transient and usually reversible.

lympho-. See *lymph-.*

lymphoblastoma [lĭm′fō-blăs-tō′mə] is a generic term for any neoplastic process (*-oma*) resulting from malignant replication (*blast-,* literally, budding) of cells of the lymphocytic series. Diseases of the class have more clinical and histologic specification in titles like *mycosis fungoides, Hodgkin's disease* and *leukemia.* Immaturity of cell types is implied by *blast-.*

lymphocytic infiltration of the skin (Jessner) [lĭm′fō-sĭt′ĭk ĭn′fĭl-trā′shən ŏv thə skĭn] refers to abnormal accumulations within the dermis of lymphocytes without germinal centers. The clinical mark of the process is an indifferent-looking plaque, commonly on the face, neck and thereabouts.

lymphocytoma cutis [lĭm′fō-sī-tō′mə kū′tĭs] designates abnormal lymphocytic infiltration of the skin (*cutis*) in which arrangements of the cells are about germinal centers much in the manner of the structure of ordinary lymph nodes. The clinical mark of the process is not more distinctive than that of lymphocytic infiltration of the skin. See *lymphadenosis cutis benigna.*

lymphogranuloma inguinale, or **venereum** [lĭm′fō-grăn′ū-lō′mə ĭng′gwĭ-nā′lē, -nä′lē, -năl′ē; vē-nēr′ē-əm, və-, vē-nēr′ē-ōōm], names a tumid and nodular process (*granuloma*) involving the lymph nodes of the groin (*inguinale*) that results from infection with an organism of the *Chlamydia trachomatis* incurred in sexual intercourse (*venereum*, related to Venus, Goddess of Love in the lustful sense).

lymphogranulomatosis [lĭm′fō-grăn′ū-lō′mə-tō′sĭs] literally designates any tumid and nodular process (*-granulomatosis*) of the lymph nodes. Hodgkin's disease is meant when *lymphogranulomatosis* is modified by *maligna*, but when it is modified by *benigna*, *sarcoidosis* is meant.

lymphoma [lĭm-fō′mə] is not to be interpreted literally. The word is used generically like *lymphoblastoma* for any neoplastic development involving the lymphocytic series of cells; maturity of cell types is implied. As for lymphoblastoma more clinical and histologic specification is given by titles like *Hodgkin's disease, leukemia, mycosis fungoides*, etc.

lymphomatoid granulomatosis is a systemic disease with characteristics of both inflammatory and neoplastic processes. Marked by a polymorphous cellular infiltrate that is both angiocentric and angiodestructive. The predominant organs of involvement are the lungs, skin, central nervous system and the kidneys.

Skin lesions may be papules, nodules, tumors, ulcerations, annular plaques with central clearing, vesicles, ichthyosis, alopecia and necrobiosis lipoidica-like lesions. It is regarded as a T-cell lymphoma. (C. Camisa, J. Am. Acad. Dermatol Vol. 20, No. 4.) (Lever)

lymphomatoid papulosis [lĭm-fō′mə-toid păp′ū-lō′sĭs] is a term for a papular dermatosis that clinically resembles parapsoriasis acuta et varioliformis and, histologically at some stage of evolution, a malignant lymphoma like mycosis fungoides. Most cases follow a benign course; an occasional one progresses to malignant lymphomatosis. It is moot that the entity is appropriately descriptive if, in one instance, the clinical course proves the disease to be benign like parapsoriasis acuta et varioliformis; and, in another, malignant like mycosis fungoides. The word *lymphomatoid* beclouds the issue in implying "something like (malignant) lymphoma." (See *pseudolymphoma, for more on the point.) The essence of the matter is that histologic interpretation of benign or malignant nature cannot be certain for some lymphomatoses and definitive diagnosis must almost always await the clinical outcome.*

lymphopathia venerea [lĭm′fō-păth′ē-ə vē-nĕr′ē-ə, və-, vĕ-nĕr′ē-ĕ] is an alternate title for *lymphogranuloma inguinale*, or *venereum*, and literally means abnormality (*-pathia*) of the lymphatic system resulting from infection incurred in venery.

-lysis [lĭ′sĭs, lə′səs] is a combining form from Greek meaning loosing, loosening, separation, dissolution or rupture. The plural form is *-lyses* [lĭ′sēz, lə′sēz]. The form *-lysis* appears in words like *dermatolysis, desmolysis* and *electrolysis* (all of which see) among others. It is amusing to find that *Lysistrata*, the name of the eponymous heroine of the play by Aristophanes, means she (*-a*, feminine ending) who shakes loose (*lysis-*) the soldiers from the army (*-strat-*). One may say Lysistrata also shook them up.

lysosome. Cytoplasmic granules that contain a variety of potent hydrolytic enzymes found in a latent form. These enzymes are capable of hydrolyzing a wide variety of both natural and synthetic substances and can digest all intra- and extracellular macromolecules if they are released from their membranes. Certain forms of cellular injury either inside or outside of the cell may release the lysome from the organelles. They are most active at an acid pH. (F.M. Abboud, *Cecil Textbook of Medicine*, 18th Ed. Wyngaarden & Smith, Editors, Saunders)

M

-ma [mə] is a common Greek suffix that means an action, usually the result of an action, as in *derma*, literally the result of flaying and in *trauma*, the result of hurting or wounding. In many English words it appears as *-me* as in *rhizome* (a rooting) and in *theme* (a setting forth of a topic for discussing) or *-m* as in *diaphragm* (an enclosing) and in *poem* (a creating).

Our special purpose in entering *-ma* as a separate item is to call attention to two well-established, odd developments upon it. First, at some time, long after ancient Greek times, the suffix of many Greek words ending in *-ma* was taken, perhaps by mistake, perhaps by design, to be *-oma* if an omega (ω) or an omicron (ο) or an omega changed to omicron in composition preceded *-ma*. Second, a meaning of tumor, particularly malignant tumor, was ascribed to *-oma*, which was thereafter frequently used as a terminal element in that sense in the formation of new words.

Only in modern formations like *paraffinoma* and *cementoma* is it absolutely clear that the tumorous meaning of *-oma* was intended when they were formed.

See *-oma*.

macerate, maceration [măs′ĕr-āt, măs′ə-rāt; măs′ə-rā′-, măs′ĕr-ā′shən] derive from the Latin verb *macerare*, meaning to soak, steep, soften, weaken and waste away. In medicine the derived words are used to refer to the action and result of softening or disintegrating tissue by wetting. In dermatology particularly, the words find common use because effects on the skin of prolonged wetting (excessive sweating in intertriginous places, urine in diapers, frequent and prolonged bathing, etc.) are so plainly visible, first in the form of softening of keratin, then redness and oozing and eventually scaling.

macro- [mak′rō] is a combining form from the Greek adjective *makros*, large. In medicine the element is used to denote enlargement and is antonymous to *micro-*, small. Following are some uses of *macro-* that are of dermatologic interest.

macrocheilia [măk′rō-kī′lē-ə, -lĭ-ə] is New Latin from Greek word elements meaning a condition (*-ia*) of enlarged (*macro-*) oral lips (*-cheil-*). See *macrolabia*.

macrocheiria, -chiria [măk′rō-kī′rē-ə, -ĭ-ə; -kĭr′ē-ə] is New Latin from Greek word elements meaning a condition (-*ia*) of unusually large (*macro-*) hands (-*cheir-*, -*chir-*).

macrodactylia [măk′rō-dăk-tĭl′ē-ə, -ĭ-ē] is New Latin from Greek word elements meaning a condition (-*ia*) of enlarged (*macro-*) fingers (-*dactyl-*).

macroglossia [măk′rō-glŏs′ē-ə, -ĭ-ə] is New Latin from Greek word elements meaning a condition (-*ia*) of an unduly enlarged (*macro-*) tongue (-*gloss-*).

macrolabia [măk′rō-lā′bē-ə, -bĭ-ə] is New Latin from Greek and Latin word elements meaning a condition (-*ia*) of unduly enlarged (*macro-*) oral or genital lips (-*lab-*).

macromelia [măk′rō-mē′lē-ə, -ĭ-ə] is New Latin from Greek word elements meaning a condition (-*ia*) of unusually large (*macro-*) limbs (-*mel-*).

macronychia [măk′rō-nĭk′ē-ə, -ĭ-ə] is New Latin from Greek word elements meaning a condition (-*ia*) of unusually large (*macro-*) nails (-*onych-*).

macula, macule [măk′ū-lə; măk′ūl]. *Macula* is the classical Latin word for a spot, stain, blemish or blot. The English word *macule* derives from it through French. In dermatology we define a macule as a perceptible change in color on, in or of the skin that is not visibly or palpably raised above or depressed below the surrounding general level of the skin. The suffix -*ule* is a diminutive and, therefore, the size of what is to be called a macule cannot be very large within the frame of common, everyday references. We would say that discolorations of the skin up to about one centimeter in diameter could be reasonably called macules; beyond that figure, larger areas of changed color of skin require a less restrictive word like *patch*.

macula c(a)erulea [sē-rōō′lē-ə] means a sky-blue (*cerulea*) spot (*macula*). This picturesque phrase, usually in plural form (*maculae ceruleae*), is applied to bluish macules and patches that are sometimes seen on the bodies of persons infested with *Plthir (i)us pubis* (the pubic or crab louse).

macular [măk′ū-lĕr, -lər] is the adjective from *macule* meaning pertaining to or marked by spots.

macular atrophy [ăt′rō-, ăt′rə-fē] bespeaks spots of underdevelopment or of diminution of tissue. Many conditions, some of known and some of unknown cause and ranging from acne to zona, may produce macules of atrophy. The use of this title may be forgiven even if some such atrophic lesions are slightly raised or depressed, but when change in level is considerable, then words less restrictive than *macule*, like *cicatrix* or *scar* or phrases like *depressed scars* or *hypertrophic scarring* must be used.

macular and **maculo-anesthetic leprosy** [ăn′əs-thĕt′ĭk lĕp′rə-sē] are designations of that clinical form of leprosy in which the lesions are flat and insenitive to touch, pain and heat. Such lesions occur in what is otherwise designated as *tuberculoid leprosy*.

maculo(-)papular [măk′ū-lō-păp′ū-lĕr, -lər] is an adjectival formation that is ambiguous and needs clarification of meaning and standardization of spelling. In a common phrase like "a maculo(-)papular eruption" does it mean consisting of macules and papules or does it mean that the lesions of the eruption are not flat enough to be purely macular nor yet raised enough to be distinctly papular? It strikes us that the second meaning is more verbally logical. The same issues arise with ambiguous combinations like *papulo (-)vesicular, papulo (-)pustular* and *vesiculo (-)pustular*. In these instances too, is one specifying lesions of two types or is one indicating that one is not sure of the quality of the lesions? In some contexts, a sense of rapid evolution of one type of lesion into another seems to be the connotation of the words. In brief, we would counsel avoidance of words of this structure unless by context or in some other way the intended meaning is made clear. Returning to the matter of *maculo (-)papular*, we would say that if it is to be used at all, it should be used to convey a meaning of uncertainty as to the macular or papular character of lesions or to suggest rapid transition from the macular to the papular condition. It should be written with a hyphen, i.e., *maculo-papular*. For instances where both types of lesions co-exist let one speak of an eruption of macules and papules.

Madura foot [mə-do͞or′ə, măd′ū-rə fo͞ot] is another of those parochially eponymic designations, this time for fungous infections on the feet characterized by tumid, granulomatous processes from which any of many species of fungi may be recovered. Madura is a town in Southern India, one of numberless places where barefoot poverty, among other deprivations, is promotional of deep fungous infections in addition to many another more pedestrian difficulty.

maduromycosis [mə-do͞or′ō-mī-kō′sĭs] is the formalized designation for Madura foot. *Mycetoma* is alternate.

Maffucci's syndrome [măf-foo′chē]. Chondrodysplasia, angiomatosis, and cutaneous dyscromia.

Majocchi's disease, granuloma [mä-yūk′ē]. Purpura annularis telangiectodes; deep infection with *Trichophyton rubrum*, resembling a pyogenic abscess.

makro- [măk′rō]. See *macro*. The spelling with *k* is closer to the original Greek but that with *c* is more commonly used.

Malassezia furfur [măl′ă-sā′zē-ă, măl′ə-sē′zē-ə, -zhē-ə, -zhə fûr′fēr] is the botanical designation for the organism that causes tinea versicolor. Like many terms in nomenclature and taxonomy, it is a strange formulation. *Malassezia* is eponymic for the genus of which apparently there is but one species, designated as *furfur*, and that species is thus described as branny. More likely *furfur* relates to the clinical characteristic of fine scaling when lesions of the clinical condition are gently scratched. The organism is *Pityrosporon orbiculare*. In any event, Malassez, after whom the fungus was originally named, was a Frenchman, and we have given two pronunciations for the genus in order to satisfy both Francophiles and Anglophiles.

mal de Meleda [măl′ də mĕ-lā′dä] is a parochial title (hybrid in pronunciation) literally meaning illness of Meleda. In French literature, the title appears as *maladie de Méléda*. Meleda (ancient Melita, Serbian Mljet), is an island in the Adriatic Sea off the Dalmatian coast of Jugoslavia. Many denizens of that island are afflicted by a genodermatosis that is characterized by constant hyperkeratosis of the palms and soles that is far beyond normal or beyond what is evoked by average friction and pressure. Formal, classicized titles for the condition are *keratosis palmaris et plantaris* and *keratoderma (-dermia) palmare (palmaris) et plantare (plantaris)*.

male-pattern baldness, or **alopecia** [māl-păt′ərn bôld′nĕs, ăl′ō-pē′shē-ə, -shĭ-ə, -shə], is a formulation intended to encompass all the common designs of gene-determined loss of scalp hair in males, to wit, frontal recession, recession at the temporo-parietal junctions (creating "philosopher's nooks" or "widow's peak"), loss beginning at the vertex and progressing to a temporo-occipital fringe, etc. See *alopecia*.

Malherbe, calcifying epithelioma of, [măl̆ĕrb′]. Pilomatrixoma.

Malherbe's epithelioma [măl̆ĕrbz′ ĕp′ĭ-thē′lē-ō′mə]. See *pilomatrixoma*.

malignancy, malignant [mə-lĭg′nən-sē; mə-lĭg′nənt] derive from the Latin verbs *malignare* or *malignari*, meaning to contrive mischief. The elements of these verbs are the same as those of *malignus*, evil or mischievous, formed from *malus*, bad, and *gen-*, the root of the Latin verb meaning to give birth. The English noun, therefore, means something badly born or a bad kind of thing, and the adjective describes what has inborn bad quality. In medicine we apply the words particularly to cancers, but also to any condition that develops an unexpectedly and rapidly grave course.

malignant papillomatosis (of Degos) [păp′ĭ-lō′mə-tō′sĭs (ôv dəgəs′, -gūs′)]. See *papulose atrophiante maligne*. Degos's original article in French is entitled "Dermatite papulosquameuse atrophiante," which translates as atrophying papulosquamous dermatitis.

malum perforans [mā′ləm, mä′lōōm pûr′fō-rănz] is Latin, literally meaning an evil (*malum*) that is boring through (*perforans*). The phrase is applied to the type of ulcer that occurs in certain neuropathies like syringomyelia. The sole of the foot is the common location, and continuous, painless loss of substance is the event.

mange [mānj] derives ultimately from the Latin verbs *mandere* and *manducare*, meaning to eat, to chew, via French *mangier*, older form of modern *manger*, to eat, and Middle East *manjewe*, appetite, itching. The word is used by veterinarians and the laity mainly for pilary diseases of animals caused by infestation with mites. The commonest forms of such diseases are a *demodicidosis* (demodectic mange) and animal scabies (sarcoptic mange); see entries for both these forms of mange. An impression of loss of hair in a ragged sort of way, as though chewed, is probably what led to the choice of the word. *Mangy* is an adjective that can be used in plain description but it is commonly used pejoratively.

Mantoux test [män-tōō]. Response of the skin to intradermal deposits of tuberculin.

manus, manuum [mā′nəs, mä′nōōs; mā′nū-əm, mä′nōō-ōōm] are respectively the nominative and genitive singular and genitive plural of the Latin word for hand. The words are used in titles of classicized form, to specify the region, e.g., *keratolysis exfoliativa areata manuum*.

marble skin [mär′b'l skĭn] is straightforward English for *cutis marmorata*. Not all kinds of marble, only pinkish varieties laced with black or bluish streaks (Tennessee marble), are apt in description of skin that is somewhat cyanotic and veined.

Marfan's syndrome [märfäng′] Arachnodactyly, ectopia lentis, cardiopathy, long limbs, skeletal anomalies, and related symptoms.

marginatum [mär′jĭ-nā′təm, -nä′tōͦom] is the neuter singular form of a Latin adjective meaning sharply bordered, enclosed with a margin. It appears in the title *erythema marginatum*.

Marjolin's ulcer [märzhōläng′]. Ulceration within an old scar, often leads to malignant degeneration.

marmorization [mär′mēr-ĭ-zā′shən, -ĭ-zā′shən] derives from Latin *marmor*, marble. The word is used to convey the idea of development of superficial veining of skin that gives it a resemblance to certain pink, streaked marbles. See *cutis marmorata* and *marble skin*.

mast cell [măst, mäst sĕl]. *Mast* in this instance comes from Anglo-Saxon and German words that relate to good nourishment. The mast cell, then, is that rotund and robust unit seemingly so well-nourished with its packed granules. Mast cells are normally found widely and sparsely dispersed in tissues; or abnormally, aggregated, principally in the skin, in urticaria pigmentosa.

mastocyte [măs′tō-sīt′] is another way of saying *mast cell*.

mastocytosis [măs′tō-sī-tō′sĭs] designates a condition (*-osis*) in which mastocytes are abnormally abundant. Urticaria pigmentosa, is, of course, a mastocytosis but the word is mostly applied when infiltrates of mast cells are found in tissues and organs other than skin, e.g., bone, bone marrow, liver, spleen, blood, etc.

matrix [mā′trĭks, măt′rĭks] derives from Greek and Latin words (G. *metra*, womb; L. *mater*, mother). The word also existed as such in ancient Latin and referred to a brood mother of animals; in ecclesiastical Latin it means source, origin and cause. The English word has come to mean a source from which development takes place, a parental stem. Thus, the matrix of the nail is that area, seen in part as the lunula, from which the nail plate keeps growing.

measles [mē′z'lz], or **rubeola**, is derived from Middle English *masel* (pl. *maseles*), a spot or excrescence. The modern plural is considered as a singular and the word designates the well-known exanthematous disease of children that is characterized by a maculo-papular eruption (see *maculo-papular*) associated with constitutional signs of fever and malaise and involvement of other organs in the form of conjunctivitis and coryza. Due to the RNA measles virus, diagnosis is established by the presence of high fever, Koplik's spots (on the buccal mucosa nearest to the upper molars clusters of white papules on an erythematous base) are pathognomonic together with coryza and typical rash. (Andrews)

RNA virus paramyxovirus group. Incubation period 10 to 12 days, prodrome of fever, malaise, coryza, conjunctivitis, cough. Rash occurs on 4th day. Exanthem, macules and papules; downward progression from face: brown pigmentation during resolution. Enanthem, Koplik's spots (blue-white spots on erythematous bases); appear on the buccal mucosa before exanthem. May have associated otitis media or bronchopneumonia. Both a live-attenuated and killed measles vaccine have resulted in more than 90% decrease in the incidence of the disease. (Bialecki et al., JAA Derm Vol. 21, No. 5)

meatus [mē-ā′təs] is a classical Latin word for a passage. The Latin plural is also *meatus* (with a long *u*) but we had better use the English *meatuses* or we will never get out of the singular passage. In the skin there is an aural and a urinary meatus.

medicamentosa [mĕd′ĭk-ə-mĕn-tō′sə] is the feminine singular of a New Latin adjectival formation meaning full of (*-osa*) medicament. It appears in the title *dermatitis medicamentosa*.

Mee's lines [mēz līnz] is eponymic for striations in nail plates sometimes seen in leprosy. Mee's lines are whitish striations that are seen in acute arsenical poisoning also seen in renal failure and other disease states. In acute arsenical poisoning, horizontal striations in the nails.

meg(a)-, megal(o), -megaly [mĕg′ə-; mĕg′ə-lō; mĕg′ə-lē, -lĭ] are combining forms from Greek *megas*, stem *megalo-*, great, large, powerful. The third, *-megaly*, is a compound form consisting of *megal-* and *-y*, a condition (coming from Greek and Latin *-ia*), and means a condition of enlargement. It is frequently misspelled with two *l*'s in words like *hepatomegaly* and *splenomegaly*.

megalonychia [mĕg′ə-lō-nĭk′ē-ə, -ĭ-ə] means a condition (*-ia*) in which the nails (*-onych-*) are unusually large (*megal-*).

melanin [mĕl′ə-nĭn] is the word for colored protein complexes (*-in*, a material) that are formed in many organisms by specialized cells. In humans the common colors of melanin are shades of tan and brown to black and the material results from a polymerization of tyrosine and desoxyphenylalanine under the influence of tyrosinase, an enzyme containing or requiring copper for its catalytic action.

melan(o)- [mĕl′ə-nō] is a combining form from *melan-*, the stem of the Greek word *melas*, black, dark.

melanoblast [mə-lăn′ō-, mĕl′ə-nō-blăst] is a cell that is in the line of development (*-blast*, a shoot or sprout) of those units that in maturity (melanocytes) produce melanin.

melanocarcinoma [(mĕl′ə-nō-kär′sĭ-nō′mə] designates malignant neoplasia (-*carcinoma*) of those cells that produce melanin (melanocytes). Ordinarily the tumor and its metastases are indeed black (*melano-*).

melanocyte [mĕl′ə-nō-sīt′, mə-lăn′ō-sīt] designates a mature cell (-*cyte*) that produces melanin.

melanoderm(i)a [mĕl′ə-nō-dûr′mə; -mē-ə] designates a condition of the skin (-*derma*, -*dermia*) which is characterized by abnormal darkening for any reason or by any material. Not only melanin but silver and iron can darken the skin, so that argyria and hemochromatosis or hemosiderosis can properly be designated melanoderm-(i)as.

melanogenesis [mĕl′ə-nō-gĕn′ə-sĭs] means the production or development (-*genesis*) of melanin.

melanohidrosis [mĕl′ə-nō-hĭ-drō′sĭs] means a condition (-*osis*) in which sweat (-*hidr-*) is dark or black (*melano-*) in color.

melanoma [mĕl′ə-nō′mə] in the generic sense means a dark or black (*melan-*) mass (-*oma*). In loose talk the connotation of malignancy is too readily assumed but that quality is not inherent in the word and should be specified if applicable. Juvenile melanoma is an instance in which the malignant connotation does not apply, and so much so that recent writers have taken to writing *benign juvenile melanoma*.

melanoma warning signs. Any nevus which shows varied color, irregular shape or outline, irregular surface, change in size, unusual sensation, change in surrounding skin or development of new pigmented lesions. Biopsy should be performed.

melanomatosis [mĕl′ə-nō-mə-tō′sĭs] means a condition (-*osis*) in which darkening or blackening (*melan-*) is developing or has developed (-*omat-*). Strictly speaking, argyria, hemosiderosis and tanning from sunburn or other causes of melanogenesis are all melanomatoses. See *melanosis*.

melanomatous [mĕl′ə-nō′mə-, mĕl′ə-nŏm′ə-təs] is an adjective meaning characterized by, pertaining or relating to melanoma.

melanonychia [mĕl′ə-nō-nĭk′ē-ə] means a condition (-*ia*) in which the nails (-*onych-*) are unusually dark in color (*melan-*).

melanonychia striata refers to the striking dark streak seen in long axis of the nail. Common in Blacks and Asians but the sudden appearance in Caucasians is cause for concern. A biopsy would be necessary to rule out acral lentiginous melanoma. (Kopf & Waldo)

melanophage [mĕl′ə-nō-fāj′, mə-lăn′ə-fāj] designates a cell that engulfs (-*phage*, eater) melanin. See *melanophor*.

melanophor [mĕl′ə-nō-fōr′, -fôr′, mə-lăn′ō-fōr, -fôr] designates a cell that carries (-*phor*) melanin. See *melanophage*.

melanosis [mĕl′ə-nō′sĭs] means a condition (-*osis*) in which darkening or blackening has occurred. The word is nearly equal to *melanomatosis* or, if there is a subtle difference, *melanosis* specifies the accomplished fact and *melanomatosis* the still developing event.

melanosis diffusa congenita a pigmentary disorder. A generalized hyperpigmentation develops from birth, diffuse in most areas but mottled in some. There is hyperpigmentation of the stratum basale. Many melanophages are located in the papillary layer of the dermis. (Oomen et al)

melanosome [mel′ə-nō-sōm′, mə-lăn′-ə-sōm] is the specialized epidermal melanin-bearing organelle responsible for the color variation of human skin. Tanning results from increased amounts of epidermal melanin stimulated by ultraviolet light. (Fitzpatrick)

melanotic [mĕl′ə-nŏt′ĭk] is the adjective from *melanosis* meaning pertaining to or relating to a darkened or blackened condition.

melanotic freckle of Hutchinson [frĕk′′l ŏv hŭtch′ĭn-sŭn] names a characteristic development of melanomatous changes of malignant quality in what had long appeared to be a seborrheic keratosis or a lentigo. The condition is commonest on the face in the elderly and as malignant melanoma goes, it is not that serious.

melanotic whitlow [hwĭt′lō] names a subungual melanoma. In this case malignancy is of the worst quality. The origin of *whitlow* is dubious but nevertheless an etymologist's delight. It may derive from *quick* (the living nail matrix) and *flaw* (i.e., abnormality) or from *white* and *flaw*. Some suggest a resemblance to a Dutch word *vijt* or *fijt*, whitlow.

melasma [mə-, mē-lăz′mə] is a direct borrowing from Greek (found in Hippocrates) and means a black spot.

melasma (chloasma faciei). Extremely common hyperpigmentation, the well-known mask of pregnancy. Macular hyperpigmentation occurs over prominent portions of the face. May also involve the nipples and genitalia. Even at times found in the male.

melioidosis [mĕl′ē-, mĕl′ĭ-oi-dō′sĭs] names a glanders- (*meli-*, from *melis*, "a distemper of asses," according to Artistotle) -like (-*oid-*) disease (-*osis*) caused by a glanders-like bacillus (*Malleomyces pseudomallei*). On the skin, ulcers and sinuses are the mark of the infection in its chronic form.

Melkersson-Rosenthal syndrome [mĕl′kĕr-sôn′; rō′zĕn-täl]. Cheilitis granulomatosa. Recurrent facial palsy, edema of the face and lips particularly, and scrotal tongue. Recurrent orofacial edema, recurrent facial nerve palsy and lingua plicata. Biopsy of the usually present swollen lip shows the characteristic granulomatous cheilitis. Cause unknown.

menstrual acne. See *acne, menstrual*.

mentagrophytes [mĕn-tā′grō-, mĕn-tăg′rō-fī′tēz] names a species of the genus *Trichophyton*. The word literally means plant life (*-phytes*) that is related to a painful (*-agro-*, literally a seizure) condition of the chin (*ment-*). Probably recovery of the fungus from a severe case of sycosis barbae prompted the queer coinage.

merocrine [mĕr′ō-krīn, -krēn, -krĭn, -ə-krən] means separating (*-crine*) in part (*mero-*).

merocrine gland is a term sometimes applied to apocrine glands because the product of these glands consists of some of their cellular material which, after chemical alteration, separates and is shed as part of the entire product of the gland. Compare *eccrine* and *holocrine*.

mesoderm [mē′sō-, mĕs′ō-, mĕz′ə-, mĕz′ō-dûrm] literally means the middle (*meso-*) skin (*-derm*). *Skin* in such a context seems to mean a separable layer. What is actually meant by *mesoderm* is the embryonal layer between ectoderm and endoderm that gives rise to connective tissue, muscles, the urogenital system, the vascular system and the epithelial lining of the coelom, the embryonal cavity that eventually differentiates into pericardium, pleura and peritoneum.

mesodermal dysplasia [mĕz′ō-dûr′məl dĭs-plā′zhē-ə, -zē-ə, -zhə], or **nevus** [nē′vəs], names any faulty development of elements that derive from the mesoderm.

meta- [mĕt′ə] is a versatile Greek prefix with meanings of between, beyond, changed, advanced and similar subtleties.

metachromasia [mĕt′ə-krō-mā′zhē-ə] literally means a condition (*-sia*) in which there has been changed (*meta-*) color (*-chroma-*). The word is applied in histologic processing to tinctorial distinctions achieved by certain stains, particularly in the staining of mast cells.

metaplasia [mĕt′ə-plā′zhē-ə, -zē-ə, -zhə] means a condition (*-ia*) in which there has been a change (*meta-*) in development (*-plas-*). For example, ossification in muscle is a metaplasia.

metastasis [mĕ-, mē-, mə-tăs′tə-sĭs] is a Late Latin noun formed from Greek word elements meaning set or placed (-*stasis*) in different or change (*meta-*) position.

Metazoa [mĕt′ə-zō′ə] is New Latin formed from Greek elements meaning more highly organized, i.e., multicellular (extended meaning from *meta-*, changed or different) living things (-*zoa*). Contrast *Protozoa*.

Mibelli, porokeratosis of. See *porokeratosis.*

Mibelli's diseases [mĭ-bĕl′lē]. Angiokeratoma, porokeratosis.

micr(o)- [mī′krō] is a combining form from Greek *mikros*, small. Smallness as a quantity or quality can be relative; a scale of reference or a parameter must be understood. In a word like *microscope* the meaning is visualizing (-*scope*) the ordinarily invisibly small (*micro-*) or enlarging the small to visibility. On the other hand, in a word like *microcosm*, a world (-*cosm*) is named that may be small (*micro-*) only when compared to geologic or astronomic dimensions.

micro-abscess [mī′krō-ăb′sĕs] means a small (*micro-*) abscess. In this word smallness in the sense of invisible by ordinary viewing is meant. See under *abscess* for types.

micronychia [mī′krō-nĭk′ē-ə] is New Latin from Greek elements meaning a condition (-*ia*) of unusually small (*micr-*) nails (-*onych-*). Here smallness is of a quite visible order of magnitude and the reference is to the ordinary size of anatomic nails.

micro-papular tuberculid(e) [mī′krō-păp′ū-lĕr tū-bûr′kū-lĭd, -lĭd] names a condition within the family (-*ide*) of tuberculous processes that is characterized by clinical lesions that are exceedingly small (*micro-*), but still visible, papules. The condition is said to be commonest in blacks and by some is held to be a lichenoid form of sarcoidosis.

Microsporon, -um [mī′krō-spō′rŏn, spôr′ŏn; -əm, -ŭm, -ōōm], formed from Greek elements, designates a genus of fungi that is characterized by small (*micro-*) spores (-*sporon*, -*um*, seed). The -*on* ending is transliterated from Greek; the -*um* is a Latinization. Both forms are neuter. Modifying designations of species have forms that depend on what characteristic is being stated, e.g., *audouini* [ō-dōō′ĭ-nī], of Audouin (eponymic); *canis* [kā′nĭs], of the dog; *felis* [fē′lĭs], of the cat; *ferrugineum* [fĕr′ū-jĭn′ē-əm], rusty, containing iron; *fulvum* [fŭl′vəm], tawny or brown; *furfur* [fûr′fĕr], branny; *gypseum* [jĭp′sē-əm], chalky; *lanosum* [lă-, lə-nō′səm], woolly; *minutissimum* [mī′nū-tĭs′ĭ-məm], very small (smallest).

microsporosis [mī′krō-spō-rō′sĭs, -spô-rō′sĭs, mī′krə-spə-rō′sĭs] is a New Latin formation that names a condition (-osis) caused by a species of *Microsporon* (or *Microsporum*).

midline lethal granuloma [mĭd′lĭn′ lē′thəl grăn′ū-lō′mə] is descriptive of an infiltrative process in which the cellular mass localizes in the middle of the face, in and around the nose, and in which death is a near inevitable consequence. The condition is thought to be a necrotizing angiitis related to Wegener's granulomatosis (which see).

Miescher's cheilitis granulomatosa an idiopathic swelling of the lips which on biopsy show granulomatous cheilitis. See Melkersson-Rosenthal syndrome.

Miescher's granuloma (granulomatosis disciformis chronica et progressiva). Appears like necrobiosis lipoidica but appears on the head and neck, hands, or forearms, commonly in middle-aged, nondiabetic women. (*Andrews' Diseases of the Skin*, 8th Ed., Arnold, Odom, James. W.B. Saunders Co.)

Mehregan states Miescher's granuloma of the face is a variant of the necrobiosis lipoidica-granuloma annulare spectrum.

migrans [mī′grănz] is a Latin present participle meaning departing, going from one place to another. It appears in the titles *larva migrans* and *ulcus migrans*.

mikro- [mī′krō]. See *micro-*. The spelling with *k* is closer to the original Greek but that with *c* is more commonly used.

Mikulicz's disease. Benign swelling of the lacrimal and salivary glands in consequence of an infiltration of and replacement of the normal gland structure by lymphoid tissue. Also called Mikulicz-Sjögren syndrome.

miliaria [mĭl′ĭ-ā′rē-ə, -ä′rĭ-ə, -ē-ăr′ē-ə] is a New Latin formation that designates a condition (-ia) characterized (-ar-) by lesions of millet seed (*mili-*) size. *Prickly heat* is a common, more homely but more expressive, alternate title for that disorder which is characterized by a distinctive pruritus that is like a needling and by smallish papules of vesicles that are situated on and around the sweat pores. *Miliaria* is sometimes modified by another descriptive word like *alba* [ăl′bə] (white); *crystallina* [krĭs′tə-lī′nə] (clear); *profunda* [prō-fūn′də] (deep); *pustulosa* [pŭs′tū-lō′sə] (purulent); *rubra* [rōō′brə] (red); and *tropica* [trŏp′ĭ-, trō′pĭ-kə] (of the warmest climates). Modifying adjectives are in the feminine singular to agree with *miliaria*, which is a feminine singular noun.

miliaris [mĭl′ĭ-ā′rĭs, -ä′rĭs, -ē-ăr′ĭs] is the masculine or feminine singular of a New Latin adjective meaning miliary (which see). It is found in the titles *lupus miliaris disseminatus faciei* (masculine) and *acne miliaris* (feminine).

miliary [mĭl′ē-ĕr′ē, -ĕr′ĭ, mĭl′yə-rē, -rĭ] is an adjective used in medicine to denote a size of the order of a millet seed. If we can trust our parakeet, that size is of the order of 0.5 to 1.5 mm.

miliary acne [ăk′nē] is applied to that form of acne in which abundant comedones appear like milia. See also *acne, miliaris,* or *miliary acne.*

miliary tuberculosis [tōō-, tū-bûr′kū-lō′sĭs] is descriptive of tuberculous process in which tiny lesions like millet seeds have appeared. It is usually a fatal complication of pulmonary tuberculosis.

milium [mĭl′ĭ-əm, -ē-ōōm] is a direct borrowing of Latin *milium,* millet. The word is applied to those white papules that occur commonly and apparently spontaneously on the face, and frequently elsewhere after healing of blisters. In microscopic section they consist of whorls of keratinized epidermal cells whose origin is adnexal. *Whitehead* is a vernacular alternate.

milker's nodules [mĭl′kĕrz nŏd′ūlz, nōj′ōōlz] is the homely title for lesions in humans caused by a paravaccinia virus that afflicts cattle. The occupation of the victim and something of the clinical characteristics of the disease are told by the title.

Milroy's disease [mĭl′roiz dĭ, də-zēz′] is eponymic for a form of elephantiasis that is hereditary, frequently congenital and usually bilateral. Chronic hereditary lymphedema.

minimal [mĭn′ə-məl] is currently a popular, vogue word in medical talk and writing that makes nonsense. It actually means constituting the least possible of something but is used as though it meant very little, as in phrases like "minimal itching" and "minimal erythema." For qualities like itching and erythema, minimal would be zero. In most instances where *minimal* is used, *liminal* would be better because, in such instances, the speaker or writer intends to say "barely appreciable" rather than "the least possible."

mite [mīt]. In Old English *mite* meant a small insect. Later it became the name of a small coin (as in "the widow's mite"). Now it means a small or tiny arachnid. In keeping with the idea of smallness *mite* now also means a small bit of anything, a small creature, object or person.

mitis [mī′tĭs, mē′tĭs, mĭt′ĭs] is a Latin adjective meaning mild. It appears in a title like *prurigo mitis.* Its opposite is *immitis.*

Mitsuda [mĭ-tso͞o′də] **antigen, reaction, test.** The "antigen" is material crudely processed from lepromatous (bacillary-rich) tissues. The test is performed by intracutaneous deposition of a small amount. The reaction, when positive, consists of erythema and infiltration at the test site which develops weeks (four or more) after injection of the "antigen." Positive reactions are common in, and deemed diagnostic of, so-called tuberculoid leprosy; negative reactions are usual in lepromatous leprosy. A tuberculin-like reaction developing weeks after injection of a crudely processed material from lepromatous tissue in a patient with tuberculoid leprosy.

mixed connective tissue disease, a typical clinical pattern, presents with Raynaud's phenomenon, polyarthralgia, swelling of the hands leading to a sausage appearance and sclerodactyly of the fingers, esophageal hypomotility, inflammatory proximal myopathy and pulmonary disease. Lab findings are high titers of serum antibodies to an extractable nuclear antigen and epidermal nuclear staining of normal-appearing skin on direct immunofluorescence. (Sharp & Anderson)

mixed leprosy [mĭkst lĕp′rə-sē] designates a clinical and histologic form of leprosy in which lesions of both lepromatous and tuberculoid nature are simultaneously present.

Mohs's chemosurgery and fresh-tissue technique [mōz]. Methods of near certain, complete extirpation of cutaneous malignancies by serial excisions of thin slices of presumably affected tissue, chemically fixed in vivo or fresh, immediate staining and microscopic examination of each successive slice until a surely negative specimen is achieved.

moisturizer [mois′chĕr-, mois′tū-rī′zĕr]. See *humectant.*

mold, or **mould** [mōld], as a noun designating certain botanical formations that are slimy, derives from Middle English *mowle* and *mowlde,* which have the same meaning. The *d* is believed to have come into the word as an altered form of *mowle* through confusion with another Middle English word, *mold* (*e*), meaning earth. *Mould* is the preferred British spelling.

mole [mōl] derives from the Anglo-Saxon word *mol,* a congenital spot. The word is used, more by lay persons, to designate pigmented nevi, particularly on the face.

molle [mŏl′ē] is the neuter singular of a Latin adjective meaning soft. It occurs in a title like *fibroma molle.*

molluscum [mə-lŭs′-, mŏl-ŭs′kəm] is a Latin word for a fungus that grows on the maple tree (according to Pliny). The word derives from *mollis*, soft, and one would think that it should be used to designate things that are of soft quality. However, in the illustrative titles below that carry the word, softness is not the fact.

molluscum contagiosum [kŏn-tā′jĭ-ō′səm, -jē-ō′səm] names a disease that is characterized by firm, scattered, papular units. The condition is caused by a pox virus; nuclei contain DNA, both contagious and auto-inoculable. Itching is a symptom, extirpation a cure, i.e., curettage or freeze with liquid nitrogen. The histiopathology is characeristic, clusters of balloon viral cells.

molluscum fibrosum [fī-, fĭ-brō′səm] is descriptive of a protuberant mass that is firm in a fibrous way.

molluscum sebaceum [sē-bā′shē-əm, -sē-əm, -shəm] is an obsolete title for kerato-acanthoma, which is also a hard lesion.

Mondor's disease [môngdôr′]. Phlebitis of veins of the chest and epigastrium.

This is a superficial thrombophlebitis due to a secondary hypercoagulable state. It occurs mainly in women, 3:1 ratio over men. There may be a history of trauma or surgery near the affected veins which are the thoracoepigastric, lateral thoracic, or the superior epigastric vein. Rarely may occur bilaterally.

Presents as a red linear cord running down the chest wall to the abdominal wall. Sometimes tender and sometimes not. Usually just a few millimeters in width and often short, a few centimeters, but can be very extended. A benign condition. (Rook/James)

Mongolian spot [mŏng-gō′lĭ-ən, -lē-ən, -lyən spŏt] designates a bluish discoloration of the skin, commonly on the small of the back, that is caused by collections of mesodermal melanocytes. Common in infants, frequently in association with other anomalies, there is a strong tendency for the macules and patches of pigmentation to disappear in time. Asiatic children exhibit the phenomenon very frequently.

monilethrix [mō-nĭl′ē-thrĭks, mə-nĭl′ə-thrĭks] literally means a necklace (*monile-*) of hair (*-thrix*). *Beaded hair* is a good translation and describes the anomaly of hair shafts in which nodosities or points of thickening alternate with normal or less than normal girth. It is a congenital defect.

Monilia [mō-nĭl′ē-ə, -ĭ-ə], in classical Latin, is the plural of *monile*, a noun of neuter gender meaning a necklace. However, as a New Latin noun with a new, metaphorical meaning, *Monilia* is treated as a feminine singular on analogy with other neuter plural nouns (all neuter plurals end in *a* in Latin) which were treated as feminine singulars in Late and Medieval Latin because of confusion with feminine nouns of the first declension, all of which end in *a* in the singular. Modifying Latin adjectives must therefore be in corresponding number, e.g., *albicans*. *Monilia* is applied to a common genus of fungi, one of whose characteristics is string-of-bead arrangements of cellular elements.

Monilia albicans [ăl′bĭ-kănz] is the commonest facultative pathogen of the genus *Monilia*. See *albicans*.

Moniliaceae [mō-nĭl′ē-ā′sē-ē, -ĭ-ā′sē-ē] is the name of that family of the *Thallophyta* that includes the dermatropic genera *Microsporon*, *Trichophyton*, *Candida*, *Epidermophyton*, *Sporotrichon*, *Blastomyces* and *Cryptococcus*.

moniliasas [mō′nĭl-ĭ′ə-sĭs] designates any condition (*-iasis*) caused by a pathogenic member of the genus *Monilia*.

moniliform [mō-nĭl′ĭ-fôrm, mə-nĭl′ə-fôrm] and **moniliformis** [-fôr′mĭs] are respectively an English adjective and the masculine and feminine singular of a New Latin adjective meaning in the shape (*-form, -formis*) of a necklace (*monili-*). The New Latin form appears in the title *lichen ruber moniliformis*.

moniliid [mə-, mō-nĭl′ē-ĭd] should mean any lesion within the class (*-id*) or possibilities of *moniliasis*. See *-id* and under *zosteriform*.

mono- [mŏn′ō, mō′nō] is a combining form from Greek *monos*, one, single.

monomorphous [mō′nō-, mŏn′ō-môr′fəs] is said of lesions and other things that are of but one (*mono-*) form or shape (*-morphous*).

moon facies [mo͞on fā′shĭ-ēz, -shē-ēz, -shēz] is the picturesque designation of the rounding of the face that supervenes when a large enough dose of adrenocorticosteroids is administered for a long enough time and seen in Cushing's disease.

morbilli [môr-bĭl′ī] is a plural diminutive coined in Medieval Latin from classical Latin *morbus*, disease. It is restricted to mean measles.

morbilliform [môr-bĭl′ĭ-fôrm] means resembling or in the shape of (*-form*) the lesions of measles (*morbilli-*).

morbus [môr′bəs] is a direct borrowing of the Latin word for disease, illness. In some writing, particularly German, eponymic formations are made by simply adding the name of a relevant individual after *morbus*, e.g., *morbus Darier*, Darier's disease.

Morgan's line [môr′gənz līn] is an eponymic designation for a secondary crease commonly seen in the lower eyelids of patients with atopic dermatitis. Dennie is said to have been the first to call attention to the appearance. We amend this eponym to the *Dennie-Morgan sign.*

morphe [môr′fē] derives from the Greek word for form, figure or structure.

morphea [môr′fē-ə] appears in Medieval Latin. Its precise origin is unknown but it seems likely that it derives from Greek *morphe*, form or figure. Nowadays the word is applied to characteristic patches of what is otherwise termed *localized or circumscribed scleroderma.* Five types: guttate, plaque, linear, segmental, and generalized (combination of the four types).

morpho- [môr′fō] is the combining form from Greek *morphe*, form, figure or structure. The *o* is a link vowel; see under *zosteriform.*

morphology [môr-fŏl′ō-jē, -ə-jē, -jī] is the study or science (*-logy*) of form or structure (*morpho-*).

mosaic [mō-zā′ĭk] derives via Late Latin, Middle English, Medieval Latin, French and Italian ultimately from a Greek word meaning belonging to the Muses, hence artistic. The word is applied to a patterned arrangement of small pieces of ceramic, glass, stone or similar substances, or to anything resembling such a pattern, e.g., "a mosaic of light and shade," "a mosaic of society."

mosaic fungus [fŭng′gəs] refers to a finding in keratolysis exfoliativa areata manuum, which is a condition of unknown cause and surely not mycotic at that. The term was suggested by the appearance under the microscope of scales from the condition processed with potassium hydroxide in the common manner of examination for fungi. That appearance is a sort of mosaic that was mistakenly thought to be composed of fungal elements.

mosaic wart(s) [wôrt(s)] describes the appearance of warts on the sole of the foot when multiple units are agminated in a circumscribed area that then looks like a mosaic.

mossy foot [mŏs′-, môs′ē, -ĭ fŏŏt] is a homely designation for maceration of the skin of the feet as might occur from prolonged wetting of the feet in marshes (from Anglo-Saxon *mos*, a marshy place; akin to *meos*, moss, and Latin *mucus*).

"moth-eaten" alopecia. See *alopecia, "moth-eaten."*

mottled [mŏt′′ld] and **mottling** [mŏt′lĭng] are words that are probably derived from Middle English *mote*, a speck, and are related to spotty coloration. *Mottled* means marked with spots; and *mottling*, as a noun, means an appearance like that of being marked with colored spots. The words are apt in description of poikilodermatous conditions of the skin. *Motley*, as an adjective, means spotted like a jester's or clown's wear.

mould. See *mold*.

moxa [mŏk′sə] and **moxibustion** [mŏk′sĭ-bŭs′chən]. The first word is derived from Japanese (*moe kusa, mokusa* or *mogusa*, for "burning herb") and the second from the first plus the last elements of *combustion. Moxa* designates vegetable substance, particularly leaves from plants of the genus *Artemisia* (wormwoods and mugworts) cut or fashioned into short cylinders which, when ignited, burn without fusing. Punks such as were used to fire ancient cannons, and are still used to ignite firecrackers, are comparable. *Moxibustion* refers to a practice in China and Japan of applying the flaming material to the skin as a cautery or counterirritant. It is in the class of cupping in the arts of folk medicine and not very much different from modern practices of counterirritation by applications of hot wet dressings and rubefacients, and by diathermy. Some acupuncturists even now practice moxibustion in connection with their needling. They pass the burning moxa over the "points" from which they have removed the needles; that is supposed to enhance the therapeutic effect.

muc-, muco- [mŭk; mū-kō] are combining forms from Latin *mucus*, snivel, mucus of the nose, hence, meaning of a slimy nature.

Mucha-Habermann disease [moo̅′khä-hä′bēr-mŏn dĭ-, də-zēz′] is eponymic for *pityriasis lichenoides et varioliformis acuta*. Also known as PLEVA.

mucin [mū′sĭn] means a material (*-in*) that derives from or is of the nature of mucus. Mucin is a glycoprotein. In dermatohistopathology the word is applied to collagen and ground substance that has undergone degeneration and consequently a tinctorial change from pink to light blue after staining with hematoxylin and eosin.

mucinoid [mū′sĭn-oid] is an adjective meaning resembling (*-oid*) mucin.

mucinosa [mū′sĭ-nō′sə] is the feminine singular of a New Latin adjective meaning full of (*-osa*) mucus. It appears in the title *alopecia mucinosa*.

mucinosis [mū′sĭ-nō′sĭs] means a condition (*-osis*) in which mucin is present as an abnormal constituent or in abnormal amount.

mucinous [mū′sĭn-əs] is an adjective meaning pertaining, relating to or containing mucin.

muco-. See *muc-*.

mucocele [mū′kō-sēl]. See *ranula* and *retention cyst.*

mucocutaneous [mū′kō-kū-tā′nē-əs] refers to both mucous membrane and skin, particularly the line of meeting of those tissues.

mucocutaneous lymph node syndrome. See *Kawasaki's disease.*

mucoid [mū′koid] is an adjective meaning like (*-oid*) mucus.

mucopolysaccharid(e)s [mū-kō-pŏl′ĭ-săk′ə-rīdz, -rĭdz] are complexes of sugars and protein that make up much of connective tissue.

mucormycosis [mū′kĕr-mĭ-kō′sĭs] is a New Latin noun formation meaning a condition (*-osis*) caused by infection with a mold of the genus *Mucor.*

mucosa [mū-kō′sə] and **mucosae** [mū-kō′sē]. The first word is the nominative singular and the second is the genitive singular or nominative plural of a New Latin noun meaning respectively the mucous membrane and either of the mucous membrane or the mucous membranes. The noun *mucosa* is derived from the classical adjective *mucosa*, meaning slimy, mucous.

mucosum [mū-kō′səm] is the neuter singular of a Latin adjective meaning mucous. It appears in the title *stratum mucosum.*

mucous [mū′kəs] is an adjective meaning pertaining or relating to mucus.

mucous cyst. See *ranula* and *retention cyst.*

mucous membrane(s) [mĕm′brān(z)] designates the epithelial coverings of the nose, sinuses, mouth, pharynx, larynx, lungs, gut, urethra, vagina, bladder, etc.

mucous-membrane pemphigoid. See *ocular pemphigus* and *cicatricial pemphigoid.*

mucus [mū′kəs] is the secretion of mucous cells, slimy material that is largely glycoprotein. The word is found in Celsus, and in Catullus, Poem 23, where he presents a clinical picture of a certain Furius, whom he considers healthy because he is free from sweat, saliva, snivel and troublesome nasal catarrh: *A te sudor abest, abest saliva,/mucusque et mala pituita nasi.*

Muir-Torre syndrome is a finding of keratoacanthomas and sebaceous neoplasms associated with visceral neoplasms. (Muir et al)

multicentric reticulohistiocytosis. See *reticulohistiocytoma.*

multiforme [mŭl′tĭ-, -tē-, mŭl-′tĭ-fôr′mē] is the neuter singular of a Latin adjective meaning of many (*multi-*) shapes (*-forme*). It appears in the title *erythema multiforme* (*exudativum* or *bullosum*).

multigemini [mŭl′tĭ-, -tē-, mŭl′tĭ-jĕm′ĭ-nī, -ə-nĭ, -nē] is a New Latin formation meaning many-, (*multi-*) -paired (*-gemini*, twins).

multiple [mŭl′tĭ-p'l, -tə-p'l], derived from Latin *multiplex* (which see), manifold, means consisting of more than one part, including more than one, many, various, complex. It can be used to modify either a singular or a plural noun according to the particular sense: plural, *multiple contusions*; singular, as in the following entries.

multiple benign cystic epithelioma. See *epithelioma adenoides cysticum.*

multiple hereditary hemorrhagic telangiectasis. See *Osler's disease.*

multiple idiopathic hemorrhagic sarcoma. See under *sarcoma.*

multiple myeloma (plasma cell myeloma, myelomatosis) [mī′ə-lō′mə] is a disseminated, malignant disease in which a clone of transformed plasma cells proliferates in the bone marrow, disrupting its normal functions as well as invading adjacent bone. The disease is frequently associated with extensive skeletal destruction, hypercalcemia, anemia, impaired renal function, immunodeficiency, and increased susceptibility to infection. Amyloidosis, clotting disorders, and other protein abnormalities are occasional associations. The neoplastic plasma cells usually produce and secrete M-component immunoglobulin, the amount of which in any given case varies proportionally with the total body tumor burden. (Sydney E. Salmon)

A malignant lymphoma may show itself on the skin as urticaria. Very elevated serum total protein is due to increase in globulins (with decreased A/G ratio) in one-half to two-thirds of patients. Serum protein immunoelectrophoresis reveals abnormal proteins in eighty percent of patients. Sixty percent of patients show IgG myeloma protein; twenty percent of patients show IgA myeloma; while ten to twenty percent of patients show Bence Jones protein only. Bence Jones proteinuria occurs in thirty-five to fifty percent of patients. Urinary electrophoresis is positive in fifty percent of patients. Electrophoresis of serum or urine or both is abnormal in almost all patients. If only serum electrophoresis is performed, kappa and some lambda light-chain myelomas will be missed. Bone marrow aspiration usually shows twenty to fifty percent plasma cells or myeloma cells; multiple sites may be required. Anemia (normocytic, normochromic) occurs in sixty percent of patients. Rouleaux formation (due to serum protein changes). Increased ESR is seen in ninety percent of patients. Laboratory findings of repeated bacterial infections, especially those due to *Diplococcus pneumoniae, Staphylococcus aureus,* and *Escherichia coli.* Renal failure is usually present when there is a marked increase of Bence Jones protein in the blood. Presymptomatic phase (may last up to many years) may show only unexplained, persistent proteinuria, increased ESR, myeloma protein in serum or urine. Repeated bacterial infections, especially pneumonias. Amyloidosis may develop. (Wallach, *Interpretation of Diagnostic Tests*, 3rd Ed., Little, Brown)

multiplex [mŭl'tĭ-plĕks] is a Latin adjective of manifold meanings, including many, numerous, various. Literally *multiplex* means having many (*multi-*) folds (*-plex*, as in *complex*) i.e., having many parts, like *multiple*. It appears in a title like *osteitis tuberculosa cystica multiplex.*

Munro's abscess [mŭn'rōz ăb'sĕs]. See under *abscess, micro-*. Intraepidermal microabscess of psoriasis.

mutilating keratoderma of Vohwinkel is a palmoplantar hyperkeratosis of the honeycomb type, associated with starfish-like keratoses on the backs of the hands and feet, linear keratoses of the elbows and knees, and annular constriction (pseudoainhum) of the digits, which may progress to autoamputation. (*Andrews' Diseases of the Skin*, 8th Ed., Arnold, Odom, James, eds. W.B. Saunders Co. 1990)

myc-, myco- [mīk; mī'kō] are combining forms via New Latin from the Greek word *mykes*, mushroom, and relate to fungus and mushroom.

mycelium [mī-sē'lĭ-əm, -lē-əm] is a New Latin formation from Greek *mykes*, mushroom or fungus. Words of this origin are etymologically related to *mucus* as something slimy. In any event, *mycelium* is applied to an aggregate of hyphae or the aerial crown of a fungus.

mycetoma [mī'sē-tō'mə, -sə-tō'mə] is another New Latin formation from Greek *mykes*, fungus. The literal meaning is a swelling or tumor (*-oma*) caused by a fungus (*mycet-*). Specifically, kerionic fungous infections, particularly the tumid processes caused by the *Phialophora* and *Hormodendra* are called mycetomas.

Maduromycosis, Madura foot, a fungal disease due to actinomycetoma (produced by Actinomycetes) and eumycetoma (true fungi). Present are draining sinuses, tumors and granules (seen with KOH). Bone involvement shows on x-ray.

mycid [mī′sĭd] is a comprehensive word that can mean any process in the class or family (-id) of fungous infections. It encompasses dermatophytid moniliid, trichophytid, etc.

myco-. See *myc-*.

Mycobacterium [mī′kō-băk′tē′rĭ-əm, -rē-əm] names the genus that includes the bacilli that cause tuberculosis and leprosy. The kinship with fungi or the cultural characteristic that is fungal (*myco-*) for organisms of the genus is told by the combining form affixed to the beginning of the word.

mycology [mī-kŏl′ō-jē, ə-jī] is that branch of microbiology and botany that deals with fungi (*myco-*).

mycosis [mī-kō′sĭs] is a New Latin formation from Greek elements and designates a condition (-osis) caused by a fungus (*myc-*).

mycosis fungoides [fŭng-goi′dēz] literally means a fungous infection (*mycosis*) that is lush and exuberant in growth like (-oides) a mushroom (*fung-*). The real thing is, of course, nothing of the sort. The title is given to that lymphoma cell disorder that starts out indifferently as a pruritic erythroderma, a vague eczematous process or a parapsoriasis, particularly parapsoriasis en plaques, and then eventuates in tumors. When well developed, histopathology becomes fairly characteristic in terms of subepidermal, pleomorphic cellular infiltrate and intra-epidermal micro-abscesses.

mycosis fungoides d'emblée [dängblā′] is that form of the disease in which the "pre-mycotic" phase, i.e., the early "nonspecific" events do not appear—but suddenly and at once (*d'emblée*) there are tumors! Emendation: The complete French phase is *mycosis fundoides aux tumeurs d'emblée*.

mycotic [mī-kŏt′ĭk] is an adjective meaning pertaining, related to or characteristic of mycosis.

myeloma [mī′ə-lō′mə] means a mass (-oma) of plasma cells in bone marrow (*myel-*).

myiasis [mī′yə-sĭs, mī-ī′ə-sĭs] is a New Latin formation from Greek word elements that mean a condition (-iasis) caused by flies (*my-*). The common event is deposition of ova by flies in open wounds and development of larvae therein. The condition is more hazardous to the aesthetic sense than to health.

myo- [mī′ō] is a combining form from Greek *mys*, which means both muscle and mouse. The older meaning is mouse and the attribution of the word to muscle arises from playful imagination that contraction of a muscle is a rippling as though a mouse were running under the skin.

myoblastoma [mī′ō-blăs-tō′mə] means a tumor (-oma) composed of muscle (myo-)-derived elements (-blast-, literally offshoots or spouts).

myoblastoma, granular-cell. See under granular-cell myoblastoma.

myo(-)epithelium [mī′ō-ĕp′ĭ-thē′lĭ-əm, -ē-thē′lē-əm] names a lining (epithelium) which consists of cells that somehow resemble muscle (myo-) cells. The coil of the sweat gland contain such cells.

myoma [mī-ō′mə] means a mass or tumor (-oma) of muscle (my-) cells or cells of muscle origin.

myrmecia [mûr-mē′shē-ə, -sē-ə, -shə] and **myrmekiasm** [mûr-mē′kē-ăz′′m] mean "wartiness." The words derive from Greek myrmeks, ant, and myrmekia, ant hill or wart. The lively imagination of ancient writers pictured warts to be like ants running about in an ant hill on the skin.

myx-, myxo- [mĭk′sō] are combining forms from Greek myxa, mucus, slime (of fish and snails in ancient Greek writings).

myxedema [mĭk′sē-dē′mə, -sə-dē′mə] literally means swelling (-edema) caused by some form of mucoid (myx-) degeneration.

myxedema, circumscribed, generalized, pretibial [prē-tĭb′ē-əl]. These terms are obviously descriptive of amount, form or distribution. It happens too that the circumscribed and pretibial varieties occur in hyperthyroidism and the generalized form in hypothyroidism.

myxoid cyst [mĭk′soid sĭst] describes a circumscribed, walled structure that contains mucoid (myxoid) material.

myxoma [mĭk-sō′mə] is a tumorous development (-oma) of material that has properties like those of mucus (myx-).

N

naevoid [nē′void]. See *nevoid*.

naevus [nē′vəs]. See *nevus*.

nail [nāl] derives from Old English *næg (e)l* and names the plates of dense keratin on the dorsal surfaces of the distal phalanges of the fingers and toes. See also *clavus* and *hangnail*.

  nail matrix. A specialized germinative epithelium that lies beneath the proximal nail fold and cuticle and gives rise to the nail plate. (Baran & Kechijian)

  nail-patella-elbow syndrome [nāl pə-tĕl′ə ĕl′bō sĭn′drōm] is a title like hand-foot-mouth disease that is elegant in its homely English. Unlike the latter, it has a ponderous Latinized title too, namely, *osteo-onycho-dysplasia*. By either, a dyscrasia of bones, particularly absence or hypoplasia of the patellae and underdevelopment of nails, is proclaimed. Webbing of the elbows, ocular anomalies, and scattered maldevelopment of other bones may also occur in the syndrome.

naked tubercle [tōō′-, tū′bĕr-k'l] describes a characteristic bunching of epithelioid cells with few or no small round cells intermixed or surrounding. Such a histologic appearance is seen in sarcoidosis, and the qualification of "naked" is in contrast to the more common tubercles of tuberculosis, which are "dressed" by considerable admixture and surrounding with small round cells.

naris [nā′rĭs, nä′rĭs], **narium** [nā′rĭ-əm, năr-, nä′rē-ōōm]. The first word is the nominative and genitive singular of the Latin word for nostril; the second word is the genitive plural, meaning of the nostrils. They find uses in classicized titles of processes on the nostrils, e.g., *folliculitis narium* (or *naris*) *perforans*.

nasi [nā′sī, nä′sē] is the genitive singular of the Latin word *nasus*, nose. It is found in classicized titles, e.g., *granulosis rubra nasi*.

native, or **natural, anergy.** See *anergy, native,* or *natural*.

necrobiosis [nĕk′rō-bī-ō′sĭs] is one of those words that carry an etymological contradiction or paradox. Obviously, it does not mean a matter or condition (-*osis*) of life (-*bio-*) and death (*necro-*) in ordinary connotation. The word is used by dermatohistopathologists to describe simultaneous or concurrent death of tissue and replacement thereof by living elements. Such a phenomenon is said to occur in granuloma annulare and in the following condition:

necrobiosis lipoidica (diabeticorum) [lĭ-poi′dĭ-kə (dĭ′ə-bĕt′ĭ-kō′rəm, -bē′tĭ-kôr′əm], in which fat tissue (*lipoidica*) is heavily involved in the simultaneously destructive and reparative process. Diabetic subjects are particularly, but not exclusively, liable to develop this abnormality.

A rare but troublesome complication of diabetes. Seen three times more frequently in women than in men. Occurs in approximately 3/1000 diabetics. Characterized by well-circumscribed, indurated, waxy, yellow-brown atrophic areas on the skin of patients who may have diabetes. (Andrews. *Diseases of the Skin*, 8th ed., Arnold, Odom, James, eds. Saunders)

necrogenic tubercle [nĕk′rō-jĕn′ĭk too′-, tū′bĕr-k′l] refers to tuberculosis cutis, usually tuberculosis cutis verrucosa, acquired from a corpse or carcass (*necrogenic*). Such an event may occur during autopsies on tuberculous corpses in morgues, embalming and other preparation for burial of bodies harboring tubercle bacilli, and from slaughter of tuberculous animals in abattoirs. The requirement is an individual with established sensitivity to tuberculin from previous adequate exposure to, or actual infection with, tubercle bacilli and chance re-inoculation in the skin, usually of a finger, with viable tubercle bacilli from a dead body. The result is Koch's phenomenon, i.e., a local and localized re-institution of tuberculous activity whose character is determined by the immunologic complex obtaining at the time of reinoculation. *Anatomic* and *prosector's wart* are alternate terms for *necrogenic tubercle*, a term for which *necrogenous tubercle* (see *-genic* and *-genous*) would be still better.

necrolysis [nĕk-rŏl′ĭ-sĭs], from its Greek word elements, means separation (-*lysis*) of tissue caused by death (*necro-*) thereof. It appears in the title *toxic epidermal necrolysis.*

necrolytic migratory erythema (glucagonoma syndrome). Malignant pancreatic tumors that secrete glucagon. Blistering skin lesions develop which are gyrate and circinate. An erosive erythema develops on the limbs. Intertrigo and stomatitis also ensue. This is often mistaken for psoriasis or mucocutaneous moniliasis. (Fitzpatrick) Histology is quite specific.

necrosis [nə-, nĕ-krō′sĭs] literally means a condition (-*osis*) of death (*necro-*). We apply the word in a gross or microscopic frame of reference to death of parts or bits of parts, not total death.

necrotic [nǝ-, nĕ-krŏt′ĭk] and **necrotica** [nǝ-, nĕ-, nē-krō′tĭ-kǝ] are respectively an English adjective and the feminine singular of a New Latin adjective formed from Greek word elements and meaning causing death, dying or dead, and relates to death of bits or parts of tissue (see *necrosis*). The classicized form appears in a title like *acne necrotica*.

necrotizing [nĕk′rō-tī′zĭng] means death-dealing.

necrotizing angiitis, vasculitis [ăn′jē-ī′tĭs, -ē′tĭs; văs′kū-lī′tĭs, -lē′tĭs], describe an inflammatory condition of blood vessels (*angiitis, vasculitis*) that results in or is attended by death of tissue in the region of the damage to blood vessels.

necrotizing fasciitis is a rare soft tissue infection characterized by widespread fascial necrosis with relative sparing of the underlying muscle. It is frequently associated with severe systemic toxicity and is usually rapidly fatal unless recognized quickly and treated aggressively. Cultures from involved tissue are usually positive for multiple aerobic and anaerobic bacteria as well as for fungi. (Umbert et al., *JAAD*, May 1989; 20:774-781.)

negative [nĕg′ǝ-tĭv] in medical contexts means nonreactive, productive of nothing readable or meaningful, or absent.

negative nevus. See *nevus, negative*.

negative reaction [rē-ăk′shǝn] is a terminological paradox. It says a something (*reaction*) is nothing (*negative*). It is one of those paradoxes that is livable with. We mean by it that something that may occur did not.

negative Schick [shĭk] **test.** The negative Schick test is an allergic or immunologic event, i.e., it is failure to react to a substance to which one is naturally sensitive because immunologic development has resulted in antibodies that neutralize a naturally irritative substance.

neo- [nē′ō] is a combining form from Greek *neos*, new, recent.

neoformans [nē′ō-fôr′mănz] is a New Latin adjective formed from the Greek word element *neo-*, new, and the present participle of the Latin verb *formare*, to fashion, shape, form. The word therefore means literally "new-forming" or "forming new." It was used at the turn of the century by Francesco Sanfelice as part of the designation *Saccharomyces neoformans*, which is now designated *Cryptococcus neoformans* (which see). *Neo-* may also have an implication of being different or unusual, like *novus*, the Latin word corresponding to Greek *neos*, of which *neo-* is a combining form; the

English words *novel,* when used as an adjective, and *novelty* illustrate this sense.

We get the impression from Sanfelice's account in Italian that he intended by *neoformans* to mean granulomatous or tumorous lesions in animal hosts infected with that pathogenic species of *Cryptococcus* which he called *Saccharomyces neoformans.*

neonatorum [nē′ō-nə-tō′rəm, -nä-tôr′əm, -ōōm, -nä-tôr′əm] is the masculine genitive plural of a New Latin adjective meaning of the new- (*neo-*) -born (*-natorum*). It appears in titles like *acne neonatorum, edema neonatorum* and *sclerema neonatorum.*

neoplasm [nē′ō-plăz′′m] is a New Latin formulation from Greek word elements that mean a new (*neo-*) formation (*-plas-,* from a verb meaning to mold, shape or form, plus *-m,* short for *-ma,* the result of the action). The usual definition is "new growth" and the usual implication is of something gravely abnormal and tumorous. The latter connotations are not inherent in the word, and for best use special character should be specified.

Netherton's syndrome [nĕth′ĕr-tŏn] A form of congenital ichthyosiform erythroderma further characterized by bamboo hairs.

nettle rash [nĕt′′l răsh] is an old folk-designation for urticaria. The nettle is a plant of the genus *Urtica.* Apparently there is a primary urticariogenic principle in the plant.

Nettleship's disease [nĕt′′l-shĭp]. Urticaria pigmentosa.

neural leprosy and **neuro-leprosy** describe leprosy as it affects nerves. See *leprosy.*

neuri- (neuro-)lemmoma [nū′rī, nū′rō-lēm-ō′mə] is seen in either spelling (the middle vowels *i* and *o* are linkages) and is a more revealing term than the eponymous synonym *schwannoma* for a neoplasm (*-oma*) of a nerve (*neuri-, neuro-*) sheath (*-lemm-*). The clinical lesion is an indifferent nodule usually on a limb, and histologically it is much like a neurofibroma.

neurodermatitic [nōō′-, nū′rō-dûr′mə-tī′tĭk, -tĭt′ĭk] is the adjective from *neurodermatitis* that is even more objectionable than the parent word. See *dermatitic* and *neurodermatitis.*

neurodermatitis [nōō-, nū′rō-dûr′mə-tī′tĭs, -tē′tĭs] is one of those controversial words that badly need agreement on meaning or agreement to drop. The word comes into English via French *névrodermatite.* The implication in the French word is inflammation of the skin arising from disturbance at the neurovascular junction, a vague but still reasonably neutral concept. The English word carries psychosomatic connotations to most people and the tendentiousness of psychosomatic explanations is what makes the word objectionable to some. The two conditions to which *neurodermatitis* is usually applied, with modification either by *circumscribed* or *disseminated*, have alternate titles, namely *lichen chronicus simplex* and *atopic dermatitis*. In our opinion it would be better for everybody's nerves to settle for the latter and drop *neurodermatitis* entirely.

neurodermatitis, circumscribed. See *circumscribed neurodermatitis*.

neurodermatitis, disseminated. See *disseminated dermatitis*.

neurofibroma [no͞o'-, nū'rō-fī-brō'mə] bespeaks a tumorous (*-oma*) lesion that is a mixture of fibrous and nervous tissue, i.e., fibroblasts and their product and nerve elements, all in abundance.

neurofibromatosis [no͞o'-, nū'rō-fī-brō'mə-tō'sĭs] names a condition (*-osis*) characterized by neurofibromata. The best-known example is that bearing the eponymous title *von Recklinghausen's disease* (which see).

neurolemmoma. See *neurilemmoma*.

neuroma [no͞o-rō'mə] as a word means neoplastic hyperplasia (*-oma*, in the sense of tumor) of neural (*neur-*) tissue. True neuromas, unmixed with other tissues, are said to be rare in skin. A characteristic lesion, however, is the plantar neuroma, which is further said to be commoner in men; to cause a metatarsalgia, usually in the third metatarsal space; and to be devoid of cholinesterase activity.

neurotic excoriation(s) [no͞o-, nū-rŏt'ĭk ĕk-skō'rē- ĕks-kôr'ē-ā'shən(z)] names lesions self-induced on the skin with fingernails or more deadly weapons by emotionally disturbed individuals. It is well to note that the psyche itself is the impelling agency; very common important clinical problem.

nevoid [nē'void] is the adjective from *nevus* meaning like whatever *nevus* (which see) means.

nevoid hyperkeratosis of nipple and areola may start at puberty or pregnancy. Seen in both men and women. There is both hyperkeratosis and papillomatosis. Various mild destructive therapies may be successful.

nevoxantho-endothelioma [nē'vō-zăn'thō-ĕn'dō-thē'lē-ō'mə, -lĭ-ō'mə] names a fairly characteristic clinical and histologic entity that is yellowish (*-xantho-*), papular or nodular (*-oma* in the tumorous sense) and related to faulty embryonal (*nevo-*) development of endothelium. There is a tendency now, among histopathologists, to change the name of this condition to something like *lipogranuloma* in order to get away from some of the implications of *-xantho-* and confusion of relationship to the "yellowing dermatoses." The condition is notable for a relatively benign course to eventual disappearance of the lesions.

nevus [nē′vəs] is a word that needs subtle understanding. Ordinary dictionaries give it a restricted definition of a spot, particularly a pigmented spot, on the skin—a birthmark. The root of the word is *-gna* in Sanskrit and *-gen* in Latin and basically refers to birth. Words related by derivation from this root are *nativity, nation, agnate,* etc. The widest implication of *nevus*, then, is anything, especially anything odd, abnormal or faulty, that is related to conception, gestation and postnatal development and stems from hereditable or embryogenic fault, abnormality or oddity. The most noticeable oddities of this order (rather than abnormalities or faults, *sensu strictu*) are those common pigmented spots or papules of which everyone has some. Lay persons call them *moles*; physicians say *nevi*, which they are indeed but that is not all there is to the deep sense of the word *nevus*. It is this commonness of moles that tends to make *nevus* secondarily and restrictively synonymous with *pigmented spot*. That is well enough if the wider implications of *nevus* are not excluded. It is like restricting the word *salt* to mean sodium chloride and forgetting the generic chemical sense of a salt. Supernumerary digits and nipples are nevi too; surely they are not merely pigmented spots. The inadequacy of restricting the word *nevus* to a pigmented spot on the skin becomes apparent in some of the following entries.

nevus anemicus [ə-nē′mĭ-kəs], from its Latin and Greek elements, means a spot or genetic abnormality (*nevus*) that is bloodless (*anemicus*). The clinical condition is a macule of lighter color than normal surrounding skin because it is histologically marked by deficiency or absence of small blood vessels, which defect removes the red component from the complex of skin color. Here one notices that *nevus* does not mean a pigmented spot; if anything it is a relatively unpigmented spot.

nevus araneus [ə-rā′nē-əs], from its Latin word elements, means a spot or genetic abnormality (*nevus*) that is like a spider or its web (*araneus*). The clinical condition is a hemangioma that appears as a central red punctum from which radiate small blood vessels. Often seen in high estrogen conditions, e.g., pregnancy and liver cirrhosis.

nevus, basal-cell [bā′s′l-, bā′z′l-sĕl] is a rare neoplastic and dysplastic genetic anomaly (*nevus*) which takes the form of multiple basal-cell epitheliomata in association with dentigerous cysts, possibly dysplasias of other organs, punctate dyskeratoses of the palms, anomalies of parathyroid function, etc. The complex constitutes a syndrome.

nevus, blue. *Blue nevus* is descriptive by color of a macule or flattish papule that consists histologically of melanocytes situated deep in the dermis. These melanocytes are believed to be mesodermal in origin, i.e., not of the same lineage as those ectodermal melanocytes found in and about the basal cells of the epidermis. Their product is ordinary melanin but the deep position of the pigment makes for a blue, rather than brown or black, color because of the physics of light dispersion (Tyndall effect).

nevus comedonicus [kŏm′ē-dō′nĭ-kəs, -ə-dŏn′ĭ-kəs], from its Latin word elements, means a congenital abnormality (*nevus*) consisting of comedones (*comedonicus*). The clinical condition is a conglomerate of blackheads appearing at wrong ages (infancy, childhood) and sometimes in wrong places (outside the acne areas).

nevus, compound [kŏm′pound] is the title applied to the common pigmented mole (*nevus*) when it consists histologically of thèques of melanocytes situated in both the dermo-epidermal and intracutaneous position.

nevus, connective tissue [kə-nĕk′tĭv tĭsh′ōō] is a general term for any genetic anomaly (*nevus*) that involves connective tissue. Notice how inadequate is *nevus* in the restricted sense of a spot.

nevus, epithelial [ĕp′ĭ-thē′lē-əl] describes abnormal overdevelopment of the epidermal portion of the skin as a genetic (*nevus*) fault.

nevus fibrosus [fī-, fĭ-brō′səs] is descriptive of a common mole (*nevus*) that is hard because it consists in great part of dense fibrous tissue.

nevus flammeus [flăm′ē-əs] is applied to an angiomatosis that is flat and of fiery (*flammeus*) color. The real thing is not so hot. Commonly on the face, the condition is a patch of red to purple which is clearly caused by blood vessels. *Port-wine mark,* or *stain,* is an alternate title.

nevus fusco-c(a)eruleus (ophthalmo-maxillaris) [fŭs′kō-sē-rōō′lē-əs ŏf-thăl′mō-măk′sĭ-lā′rĭs] is a title of the order of *nevus flammeus.* It describes a melanocytic infiltration that produces a dark brown (*fusco-*) and dark blue (*ceruleus*) patch in the region of the eye (*ophthalmo-*) and upper jaw (-*maxillaris*). The condition is also known by the eponym *Ota.*

nevus, halo [hā′lō] is an alternate title for *leukoderma acquisitum centrifugum.* It is picturesquely descriptive of the leukodermatous

development in the form of a halo around a pre-existing nevus but
it is unsatisfactory in suggesting that the entire process is an anomaly related to birth processes. As in vitiligo the depigmentation
takes place by the loss of melanocytes.

nevus, intracutaneous, intradermal, intra-epidermal [ĭn′trə-kū-
tā′nē-əs, ĭn′trə-dûr′məl, ĭn′trə-ĕp′ĭ-dûr′məl]. The adjectives specify
positions of melanocytes which in conglomeration produce a pigmented mole.

nevus, junction(al). See *junction (al) nevus.*

nevus, linear [lĭn′ē-ər] is descriptive of a genetic process (*nevus*) in
which cellular reduplication takes the form of a stripe (*linear*).

nevus lipomatosus [lĭ-pŏm′ə-, lĭ-pō′mə-tō′səs] means a genetic
anomaly (*nevus*) composed of fat tissue (*lipomatosus*, New Latin
adjective). More than a mere lipoma but a diffuse dysplasia of fat
tissue is implied.

nevus, negative [nĕg′ə-tĭv] bespeaks a congenital anomaly (*nevus*)
in which a structural part of an organ is absent (*negative*), e.g.,
phocomelia.

nevus, nevus-cell. *Nevus-cell nevus* is a question-begging title that
has gained great, uncritical popularity. It has to be interpreted as a
common mole (restricted meaning of *nevus*) that consists of cells
such as one finds in moles. One might ask what one expects to find
in a mole if not cells characteristic of it. Those cells are melanin-
producing. Why not therefore *melanocytic nevus*? Proponents of
the title *nevus-cell nevus* then object that some common moles consist of elements that are modified Schwann cells rather than those
of neuro-ectodermal origin. Both, nevertheless, are melanin-producing, i.e., melanocytes, even if of different lineage. Moreover, the title *nevus-cell nevus* does not make more distinction than *melanocytic nevus* does. Another sense that can be read into the title is first
the broader meaning of *nevus* (any genetic anomaly or dysplasia)
with modification that, for the matter in point, the cellular composition is set as a certain type of cell, which, now termed *nevus-cell*,
is designated by the restricted meaning of *nevus*. The title becomes
more ridiculous if one translates it as "spot-cell spot."

Nevus of Ito. Nevus fuscoceruleus acromiodeltoideus.

nevus pigmentosus (et pilosus) [pĭg′mĕn-tō′səs (ĕt pĭ-lō′səs)] is a
classicized title for a common mole that describes it, in short form,
as pigmented (with melanin, no doubt) and, in long form, as hairy
(*pilosus*) too.

nevus sebaceus [sē-bā′shē-əs, -sē-əs, -shəs] designates a genetic anomaly or dysplasia (*nevus*) involving the sebaceous glands, particularly a characteristic process of that sort on the scalp.

nevus spilus [spī′ləs] literally means a genetic anomaly (*nevus*) that is spotty (*spilus*). Here the understanding has to be a macule or patch of melanization that is further marked by still smaller macules or patches of still darker color.

nevus syringocystadenomatosus papilliferus [sī-rĭng′gō-sĭst-ăd′ē-nō′mə-tō′səs păp′ĭ-lĭf′ér-əs] is a classicized title that describes a genetic anomaly or dysplasia (*nevus*) of a portion of the sweat apparatus *syringo-* from *syrinx*, a tube) in terms of dilatation (*-cyst-*), acinargland-like structure (*-adenomatosus*) and nipple-like formation (*papilliferus*). The description refers to histology, not to gross clinical appearance.

nevus, systematized [sĭs′tə-mə-tīzd′] designates a genetic anomaly or dysplasia (*nevus*) that is widespread on the skin and in some suggestively meaningful arrangement.

nevus tardus [tär′dəs, -düs] denotes a genetic anomaly (*nevus*) in which the abnormal development comes on relatively late (*tardus*) in life, i.e., in adolescence or adulthood, rather than early, i.e., in infancy or childhood.

nevus unius lateris [ōō-, ū-nī′əs, ū′nĭ-əs lä-, lā′tér-ĭs, lăt′ə-rĭs] describes a genetic anomaly or dysplasia (*nevus*) that is located on but one (*unius*) side (*lateris*). The title is frequently miswritten with *lateralis,* which means relating to a side. The special sense of *unius lateris* (literally, of one side) is that the location on one side is more than chance and that this process occupies a considerable portion of the side affected.

nevus verrucosus [vér′ōō-kō′səs] describes a genetic anomaly or dysplasia (*nevus*) in terms of warty (*verrucosus*) surface character.

nigra [nī′grə] is the feminine singular of a Latin adjective meaning black. It appears in a title like *lingua nigra.*

nigricans [nĭg′rĭ-, nī′grĭ-kănz] is the present participle of the classical Latin verb *nigricare,* to be black, to turn black. *Nigricans* therefore literally means blackening or being black, i.e., blackish, swarthy. It appears in titles like *acanthosis nigricans.*

Nikolsky's sign [nyĭ-kōl′skē]. Production or enlargement of blisters by pressure with torque on skin in pemphigus foliaceus and vulgaris and some other blistering diseases.

nit [nĭt] derives from Anglo-Saxon *hnitu,* the egg of a louse or other insect or the insect itself when young, especially as an encased embryo.

nitidus [nĭt′ĭ-dəs] is the masculine singular of a Latin adjective meaning gleamy, glistening, shiny. It appears in the title *lichen nitidus.*

Nocardia [nō-kär′dē-ə, -dĭ-ə] is an eponymic designation for a genus of fungi named after a French biologist and veterinarian (Edmond I. E. Nocard, 1850–1902).

nocardiosis [nō-kär′dĭ-ō′sĭs, -dē-ō′sĭs] is a comprehensive designation for any condition (*-osis*) caused by any species of *Nocardia.*

node [nōd] derives from Latin *nodus,* a knot. The word is most commonly applied to the well-known masses of lymphocytic tissue of the lymphatic system, but also to other "knots" or conglomerations in the nervous and vascular systems or to abnormal knobby developments like osteomas (e.g., Heberden's nodes).

nodosa [nō-dō′sə], **nodose** [nō′dōs, nō-dōs′], and **nodosum** [nō-dō′səm] are respectively the feminine singular of a Latin adjective, an English adjective and the neuter singular of the Latin adjective meaning full of (*-osa, -ose, -osum*) knots (*nod-*). The Latin adjectives appear in titles like *periarteritis nodosa* and *erythema nodosum.*

nodosity [nō-dŏs′ə-tē, -tĭ] may mean simply a node or a nodose condition (*-ity*).

nodular [nŏj′o͞o-, nŏd′ū-lĕr, -lər] and **nodularis** [nŏd′ū-lā′rĭs, -lä′rĭs, -lär′ĭs] are respectively an English adjective and the masculine and feminine singular of a Latin adjective meaning pertaining to (*-ar, -aris*) a small (*-ul-,* from *-ulus*) node (*nod-,* from *nodus*). The Latin adjective appears in a title like *prurigo nodularis.*

nodular fasciitis [nŏd′ū-lĕr fă′shē-ī′tĭs] designates a characteristic clinical picture of somewhat tender nodules in multiplicity on the upper extremities and a histologic picture that resembles sarcomatous neoplasia. The condition is, however, benign and is thus also designated *pseudosarcomatous fasciitis. Fascia* is a Latin word for a band or bandage. It is applied in anatomy to the layer of condensed fibrous tissue beneath the panniculus adiposus (superficial fascia), to the sheaths of muscles, and to the investments of deep structures (deep fascia). The idea of inflammation (*-itis*) in *fasciitis* seems ill-founded. *Nodular fasciosis,* meaning nonspecifically an abnormal condition of fascia, might have been a better term.

nodular leprosy [lĕp′rə-sē] describes lepromatous leprosy in its common clinical form of tumid lepromas.

nodular vasculitis [văs′kū-lī′tĭs, -lē′tĭs] describes an inflammation of blood vessels (*vasculitis*) that is attended by swellings.

nodule [nŏd′ūl, nŏj′o͞ol] is derived from *nodulus*, diminutive of *nodus*, and means a small (*-ule*) node.

nodule, cutaneous. See *cutaneous nodule.*

nodule, rheumatic. See *rheumatic nodule.*

nodulus [nŏd′ū-lo͞os, nō′dū-ləs] is a Latin word, the diminutive of *nodus*, a knot, and hence means a small (*-ulus*) node.

nodulus cutaneus [ko͞o-tä′-, kū-tā′nē-əs] literally means a small node in the skin. The lesion is clinically of fair stereotypy in the form of a hard, pea-sized (i.e., smallish) mass on legs or arms with equally fair histologic stereotypy in the form of dense accumulation of histiocytes. *Dermatofibroma, histiocytoma* and *sclerosing hemangioma* are alternate designations.

noma [nō′mə] is New Latin from the Greek word *nome,* a feeding. The word, then, brings to mind a picture of something eaten, devoured or consumed and is applied to certain gangrenous processes on the face, particularly around the mouth, and on the genitalia, especially of the labia majora. *Cancrum oris* and *gangrenous stomatitis* are alternate titles for the condition on the face around the mouth.

North American blastomycosis. See under *blastomycosis.*

Norwegian scabies. see *scabies, Norwegian* and *Boeck's scabies.*

nos(o)- [nŏs; nō′sō] is a combining form from Greek *nosos,* disease.

nosocomial infection is a hospital-acquired infectious disease. Nosocomial is derived from the Greek word for hospital.

nostras [nŏs′trăs, nō′străs] is an uncommon Latin adjective related to *noster,* our. It has the stronger specific sense of "native, of our country, our very own." It appears in the title *elephantiasis nostras.*

noxa [nŏk′sə] and **noxae** [nŏk′sē, -sī] are respectively the nominative singular and the nominative plural of a New Latin word with many meanings of badness, to wit, evil, harm, hurt, ill, injury, offence, sickness, and the like.

nuchae [no͞o′-, nū′kē] is the genitive singular of the Late Latin word *nucha,* back of the neck, nape. The Latin word is derived from the Arabic word for spine marrow. It appears in the title *erythema nuchae.*

nummular [nŭm′ū-lēr] derives from Latin *nummularius* meaning like a little coin (*nummulus,* diminutive of *nummus,* a coin).

nummular eczema [ĕk′sə-mə] is the title given to a highly characteristic eruption of vesicles in coin-sized and -shaped configurations. The condition is of unknown cause, commoner in the wintertime, pruritic, self-resolving and recurrent and usually on hands, arms and legs. *Orbicular eczema* is an alternate title.

O

obliterans [ŏb-lĭt′ĕr-ănz] is a Latin present participle meaning wiping out, obliterating. It appears in the title *balanitis xerotica obliterans*.

"occipital forelock." See under *forelock*.

ochronosis [ō′krō-nō′sĭs, ō-krŏn′ō-sĭs, -ə-sĭs] is New Latin from Greek word elements meaning a pale yellow (*ochro-*) condition (*-osis*; the *n* may be an insert for euphony or it appears as an influence from *nosos*, disease). The gross clinical fact, however, is a gray, blue, brown or black discoloration of skin, mucous membranes and cartilage (as seen through the skin in the ears and possibly the nose). In histologic processing, selections of cartilage and viscera, viewed under the microscope, may have more of a yellowish hue. When the phenomenon is caused by an inborn error of metabolism, the defect lies in failure of further degradation of homogentisic acid (metabolite of phenylalanine and tyrosine) from deficiency of homogentisic acid oxidase. Homogentisic acid concentrated in tissues imparts color of gray-blue-brown-black character and as it is passed in urine turns urine black when oxidized after standing awhile. The latter effect is called alkaptonuria, *alkapton* being an old term for oxidation product of homogentisic acid. Phenomena similar to ochronosis and alkaptonuria are caused by chemical toxicoses (phenol poisoning for example) but not, of course, on the same biochemical bases.

oculocerebral syndrome of Cross and McKusick. Universal albinism, autosomal recessive disorder "moon children." Near total or total absence of pigment in skin, hair and eyes. Nystagmus is a major finding. There is a genetically determined deficiency of tyrosinase in melanocytes and mental retardation. (Fitzpatrick)

ode, odes, oid, oides [ōd; ō′dēz; oid; oi′dēz] are combining forms derived from Greek, all meaning like or in the form of. Although there is no doubt about their meaning, a complication arises about their etymology because philologists, especially lexicographers, are not in agreement about the relationship of *-ode* and *-odes* to the other two. According to some authorities, *-odes* (anglicized as *-ode*) was originally a Greek word element meaning smelling, from the Greek verb *ozein*, to smell, to whose root are related *odor* and *ozone.* The explanation here is that in the Greek compound word *euodes*, fragrant, "well" or sweet smelling, the final element *-odes* had its original meaning of smelling, but that when it was used to form other words, it lost its primary, specific meaning and acquired extended, general meanings of full of (like Latin *-osus*), or (more often) like, in the form of.

A similar phenomenon is cited in the history of the English endings *-ly* and *-like* from Old English *lic*, body. The ending *-ode* appears in words like *geode*, something like earth, and *sarcode*, something like flesh, protoplasm of animal rather than vegetable origin. Other authorities, however, consider *-ode* and *-odes* as having the same origin as *oid* and *-oides*, but all agree that the latter derive from the Greek combining form *-eides* meaning having the form (*eidos*) or quality of, resembling, in the shape of. The letter *o* appears either as part of the word entering into combination with *-eides* or as a mere connective insert, giving *-o-eides* or *oeides*, which finally become *-oides* in classical and *-oid* in anglicized form. (For more on connective inserts see under *zosteriform.*) The classicized elements are found in old titles like *pemphigus erythematodes* (*erythematosus*), *lupus erythematodes* (*erythematosus*), and in a word like *pemphigoides* when it is used to designate a dermatosis that resembles, but is not quite, phemphigus. In fact, the anglicization *pemphigoid* is now a popular title by itself. Finally, *-oid* is a most widely used English terminal word element in dermatologic formulations, e.g., *discoid, lichenoid,* etc.

"oid-oid" disease [oid′oid′ dĭ-, də-zēz′] is a faintly humorous and slightly mnemonic designation for *distinctive exudative discoid and lichenoid chronic dermatosis* (which see).

oil acne is another of those titles that tell something of clinical characteristics and occupational cause. See *acne.*

"old-man's pemphigus" [ōld mănz pĕm′fi-gəs] is a homely term for what is now burdensomely called bullous pemphigoid. In some ways it is a better designation than the tautologic formal term for that blistering process of unknown cause that sometimes afflicts aged individuals. Since it also afflicts women, perhaps it would be better still to call it "old-person's pemphigus."

oligo- [ŏl′ĭ-gō] is a combining form from Greek *oligos*, few, little, scanty, slight, small.

oligohidria [ŏl′ĭ-gō-hĭd′rē-ə, -rĭ-ə] and **oligohidrosis** [ŏl′ĭ-gō-hĭ-drō′sĭs] mean a condition (*-ia, -osis*) of diminished, little or scanty (*oligo-*) sweat or sweating (*-hidr-*).

Olmstead's syndrome. Congenital, sharply marginated palmoplantar keratoderma, constriction of the digits, linear keratotic streaks on the flexural aspects of the wrists, onychodystrophy and periorificial keratoses. (Poulin et al)

-oma [ō′mə]. Let it be repeated here (as noted under *-ma*) that *-oma* is not an original Greek suffix meaning tumor. The true Greek suffix is *-ma* meaning the result of whatever action is specified by the preceding word element. Many words ending in *-ma*, but not all, have an *-o-* (representing in Greek an omega, an omicron or an omicron lengthened to omega in composition) preceding *-ma* and frequently, but not always, such words describe something tumid. As a result either an error of taking *-oma* to be a true and original suffix meaning tumor was made or a willful creation of a new element was made.

    -Oma is by now an accepted suffix meaning tumor in neologisms coined with that meaning in mind. However, that meaning may not always be read into original Greek or English words derived from Greek elements and ending in *-(o)ma*. Into some of these words it does no harm to read a sense of tumor or cancer but as a generality the tumorous sense does not apply at all. The plural of nouns ending in *-(o)ma*—to put it as a rule of thumb—is formed by adding *-ta* in the Greek fashion or *-s* in the English manner, e.g., *sarcomata*, *sarcomas*.

    See *-ma*; also comments on *-oma* under *zosteriform*.

Omenn's syndrome. Familial reticuloendotheliosis with eosinophilia.

-on [ŏn, ən] is a Greek neuter singular ending of some nouns, pronouns and adjectives, and is equivalent to the Latin ending *-um*. The plural form of such Greek and Latin (or New Latin) endings is *-a*, e.g., Greek *phylon, phyla*, Latin *phylum, phyla*. However, often this fine point of philologic morphology is brushed aside by forming the plural in the English manner, e.g., (Greek) *dendron, dendra* or *dendrons*; (Latin) *serum, sera* or *serums*.

Onc(h)ocerca [ŏng′kō-sûr′kə] is a New Latin formation from Greek word elements that mean barbed (*onco-*) tail (*-cerca*). The Greek word *onkos* means both barb and mass. The appearance of the *h* in some spellings is inexplicable. Nevertheless the word in one spelling or the other is applied to a zoologic genus, two species of which, namely, *O. caecutiens* (blinding) and *O. volvulus* (a twisting) can invade the skin.

    onchocerca volvulus. Filarial parasite causes onchocerciosis resulting in eye (river blindness) and skin lesions. The blackfly bites and transmits infective larvae. In several months these become adult worms. These coil into bundles in the subcutaneous tissues and deeper fascial planes forming onchocercomata, fibrous subcutaneous nodules containing adult worms. (Bruce M. Green, *Cecil Textbook of Medicine* 18th edition, Wyngaarden & Smith Eds., Saunders)

onchocerciasis. Parasitic infection, very rare in the USA. Vector is the black fly which inoculate infective larvae of onchocerca into the skin. These mature to the adult form which become subcutaneous nodules called onchocercomas. Adult filaria produce myriads of microfilaria which live in the dermis and the aqueous humor of the eye. These cause an apparent delayed hypersensitivity-type of reaction resulting in onchocercal dermatitis, iritis and often blindness. On biopsy of the skin lesions, adult filaria may be seen in sections. (Lever)

onc(h)ocerciasis, -cercosis [ŏng′kō-sûr-sī′ə-sĭs; -sûr-kō′sĭs] name the condition (*-iasis, -osis*) caused by infestation with a species of *Onc (h)ocerca.*

oncology [ŏng-kŏl′ō-jē, -ə-jĭ] derives from Greek elements meaning the study (*-logy*) of tumors (*onco-*).

ongles en raquette [ŏng′glə äng, zäng, răkĕt′] is French for *racket nails* (which see).

onych-, and **onycho-** [ŏn′ĭk; ŏn′ĭ-kō, ŏn-ĭk′ō] are combining forms from Greek *onyx*, nail, *onychos*, of (a, the) nail. A list that is not exhaustive of useful formations with *onych (o)-* as the first element of the word follows. There are also many formations with *-onyx* or *-onychia* in terminal position.

onychatrophy [ŏn′ĭ-kăt′rō-fē, -rə-fĭ] means defective (*-a-*, alpha privative) development (*-trophy*, literally nourishment) of nail (*onych-*). Congenital and acquired conditions of underdeveloped nails may be so designated.

onychauxis [ŏn′ĭ-kôk′sĭs] means over- or excessive development (*-auxis*) of nail (*onych-*). Very large through normal, or abnormally thickened nails may take the word.

onychia [ō-nĭk′ē-ə, -ĭ-ə] means a pathologic condition (*-ia*) of nail (*onych-*).

onycho-. See *onych-.*

onychodystrophy [ŏn′ĭ-kō-dĭs′trə-fē] means a condition (*-y*) of mal- (*-dys-*) development (*-troph-*, literally nourishment) of nail (*onycho-*).

onychogryp(h)osis [ŏn′ĭ-kō-grĭ-pō′sĭs, -grĭ-pō′sĭs; -grĭf-ō′sĭs] is New Latin from Greek word elements meaning a condition (*-osis*) of curved (*-gryp-*, *-gryph-*) or claw-like nails (*onycho-*).

onychoheterotopia [ŏn′ĭ-kō-hĕt′ĕr-ō-tō′pē-ə, -ə-tō′pĭ-ə] means a condition (*-ia*) of dis- (*-hetero-*, different) -placed (*-top-*) nails (*onycho-*).

onycholysis [ŏn′ĭ-kŏl′ĭ-sĭs] means separation or loosening (*-lysis*) of nail (*onycho-*) plate from nail bed. Compare *onychomadesis*.

onychomadesis [ŏn′ĭ-kō-mə-dē′sĭs] means a shedding (*-madesis*) of nail (*onycho-*). The phenomenon is different from onycholysis (compare), in which the plate separates in entirety from free edge toward matrix whereas in onychomadesis the separation is in the form of fragmentation from lunula toward free edge.

onychomalacia [ŏn′ĭ-kō-mə-lā′shē-ə, -sē-ə, -shə] means a condition (*-ia*) of softness (*-malac-*) of nail (*onycho-*).

onychophagia [ŏn′ĭ-kō-fā′jə, -je-ə, -jĭ-ə] means nail- (*onycho-*) biting (*-phagia*, eating).

onychorrhexis [ŏn′ĭ-kō-rĕk′sĭs] means breakage (*-rrhexis*) of nail (*onycho-*). Compare *onychoschizia*.

onychoschizia [ŏn′ĭ-kō-skĭ(t)z′ē-ə, -ĭ-ə] means splitting (*-schizia*) of nail (*onycho-*). Compare *onychorrhexis*. If there is any difference between onychoschizia and onychorrhexis, the latter is weaker and refers to fragmentation and horizontal separation in lamellae at the free edge whereas the former applies to all sorts of cleavages including the longitudinal.

onychotillomania [ŏn′ĭ-kō-tĭl′ō-mā′nē-ə, -nĭ-ə, -nyə] means a violent compulsion (*-mania*) to tear at (*-tillo-*) nails (*onycho-*). Like onychophagia, onychotillomania is a neurosis representing a minor indulgence of masochism.

oozing [o͞oz′ĭng] is both a noun and also the present participle of the verb *ooze*. The word derives from Anglo-Saxon *wos*, juice, and thus carries senses of the fact or continuing process of exudation of juicy fluid. The word refers to serous discharge on or from the skin.

ophiasis [ō-fī′ə-sĭs] is a word used by Galen for a type of baldness. Literally, the word means a snaky (*oph-*) condition (*iasis*). Nowadays it is applied to that form of alopecia areata in which loss of hair snakes along the temples, parietes and occiput.

ophryogenes [ŏf'rĭ-, ŏf'rē-ŏj'ə-nēz, -ē-nēz] is a New Latin formation from Greek word elements meaning arising (-*genes*) on the eyebrow (*ophryo-*). It appears in the title *ulerythema ophryogenes*.

oral hairy leukoplakia occurs almost exclusively in persons infected with human immunodeficiency virus (HIV), and is highly predictive for the development of AIDS. The leukoplakia is the result of pervasive infection of epethelial cells by Epstein-Barr virus (EBV). (Herbst et al)

orbicular [ôr-bĭk'ū-lêr] and **orbiculare** [ôr-bĭk'ū-lā'rē, -lä'rē, -lär'ē] are respectively an English and a neuter singular Latin adjective which mean resembling (-*ar*, -*are*) a small (-*cul-*) disc (*orbi-*), hence annular, circular or round. The classical form appears in *Pityrosporon orbiculare*.

orbicular eczema is an alternate designation for *nummular eczema*.

ordinal designation of the exanthemata. After Duke described the exanthem that he labelled *fourth disease*, measles (rubeola) came to be thought of as *first disease*, scarlet fever (scarlatina) as *second disease* and German measles (rubella) as *third disease*. Later, newly observed exanthemata like erythema infectiosum and roseola infantum (exanthema subitum) were numbered *fifth* and *sixth disease* respectively. Note that only the macular, erythematous exanthemata are numbered; chicken pox and smallpox, which are papular, then vesicular and pustular, are not assigned numbers.

orf [ôrf] is of obscure origin, possibly from English dialectal *hurf* and Old Norse *hrufa*, crust, scab. It may be related to the -*ruff* of *dandruff*. In any event, the word is applied to a viral disease, epizootic in sheep and communicable to humans. It shows as papulo-vesicles or bullae that may umbilicate in the manner of other viral infections that are dermatotropic. Fingers, hands, wrist and face are common sites. Constitutional effects are absent or minor; self-limitation and immunity are usual. *Ecthyma infectiosum* is a more formal title.

oriental sore [ôr'ĭ-, ôr'ē-ĕn't'l sôr] is another of those parochial designations for the chancriform lesion (primary complex) of cutaneous leishmaniasis. See *button* for strictures on use.

orificial [ŏr'ĭ-fĭsh'əl], **orificialis** [ō'rĭ-, ôr'ĭ-fĭsh'ĭ-ā'lĭs, -fĭsh- ä'lĭs, -ē- äl'ĭs] are respectively an English adjective and the masculine and feminine singular of a New Latin adjective meaning pertaining to an orifice, i.e., the oral, genital or anal. The classicized form appears in a title like *tuberculosis cutis orificialis* (feminine).

oris [ō′rĭs, ôr′ĭs] is the genitive singular of the Latin word *os*, mouth, and means of the mouth. It appears in a title like *leukokeratosis oris.*

orthokeratinization [ôr′thō-kĕr′ə-tĭn′ĭ-zā′shən, -ĭ-zā′shən] means normal, correct or proper (*ortho-*) formation (*-ization*) of keratin.

-osis [ō′sĭs] is a Greek suffix meaning a condition. In medical connotations, an abnormal or pathological condition, a disease, in short, is meant.

Osler's disease [ōs′lĕrz dĭ-, də-zēz′], or **Rendu-Osler-Weber** [räng-dōō′-ōs′lĕr-vā′bĕr, -wĕb′ĕr] **disease,** is eponymic for a condition marked by development in skin and mucous membranes of telangiectasias that tend to rupture and bleed. See hereditary hemorrhagic telangiectasia.

Osler's nodes are painful, urticaria-like nodules in the pulp of the fingers and toes in subacute bacterial endocarditis caused by viridans and group D streptococci. Also seen are purpuric macules of the acral areas (Janeway's lesions) and subungual splinter hemorrhages. Petechiae may also occur in crops on the skin or on the mucosae of the conjunctiva or palate. (Fitzpatrick)

osmidrosis [ōz′mĭ-drō′sĭs] means foul (*osm-*) sweating (*-idrosis*). It is synonymous with *bromhidrosis,* which is more commonly said.

osteoma cutis [ŏs′tē-ō′mə kū′tĭs] is a classicized title (in which the first word is composed of Greek word elements and the second is Latin) meaning a bony (*oste-*) formation (*-oma*) in the skin (*cutis*).

osteomatosis [ŏs′tē-ō′mə-tō′sĭs] is a New Latin formation from Greek word elements meaning a condition (*-osis*) of bone (*osteo-*) formation (*-mat-*). The implication of the word is formation of bone in places where bone does not normally belong.

ostium [ŏs′tĭ-əm, -tē-əm] is a Latin word meaning an opening, such as a door, entrance or mouth.

ostraceous [ŏs-trā′shəs] derives from Greek and Latin words that relate to oyster. It is used to describe heaped-up scaling such as sometimes occurs in lesions of psoriasis and reminds one of the external surface of an oyster's shell. It is frequently misunderstood to mean rupial. Ostraceous scales may appear filthy but the words *ostraceous* and *rupial* are not synonyms.

-osus [ō′səs, ō′sōōs] is a Latin adjectival ending meaning full of, having the characteristics of. It appears in English adjectives as *-ous* and *-ose,* e.g., *eczematous, nodose.*

Ota's nevus [ō′tä] a congenital facial melanocytic lesion may involve the forehead, cheek, nose and sclerae and other structures of the eye. Patients are at risk for developing open-angle or angle-closure glaucoma. New thoughts are to regard this as two disorders rather than one, i.e., mainly superficial and deep pigment. (Charles Taylor, *Yearbook of Dermatology 1990* Mosby, Year Book, Inc.)

ovale [ō-vā′lē, -vä′lē, -vāl′ē] is the neuter singular of a Latin adjective meaning oval. It appears in the designation *Pityrosporon ovale.*

Oxyuris [ŏk′sē-, ŏk′sĭ-ū′rĭs] is an old name for a genus of nematodes which is now displaced by *Enterobius* (which see). The word means sharp- (*oxy-*) -tailed (*-uris*).

P

pach- and **pachy-** [păk; păk′ĭ, -ē] are combining forms from Greek *pachys* meaning thick.

pachonychia [păk′ō-nĭk′ē-ə, -ĭ-ə]. See *pachyonychia.*

pachyderma, -mia [păk′ĭ-dûr′mə; -dûr′mē-ə, -mĭ-ə] is New Latin from Greek word elements meaning an exceedingly thick (*pachy-*) condition of the skin (*-derma, -dermia*). The word is generic but is heard most often in connection with acromegaly and elephantiasis.

pachydermatocele [păk′ĭ-dûr′mə-tō-sēl′, -dēr-măt′ō-sēl], deriving from Greek elements, literally means thick (*pachy-*) swelling (*-cele*) of the skin (*-dermato-*). What is referred to is that massiveness which is imparted to exceedingly loose skin as it folds. *Cutis laxa, chalazoderma* and *dermatolysis* are alternate terms.

pachydermoperiostosis [păk′ĭ-dûr′mō-pěr′ĭ-ŏs-tō′sĭs, -ē-ŏs-tō′səs] names a rare condition (*-osis*) in which the skin (*-dermo-*) and the periostia of bones are markedly thickened (*pachy-*). May be associated with underlying malignancy.
Idiopathic hypertrophic osteoarthritis; idiopathic clubbing and periostosis.

pachyonychia [păk′ĭ-ō-nĭk′ē-ə, -ĭ-ə] is New Latin from Greek word elements meaning a condition (*-ia*) of excessively thick (*pachy-*) nails (*-onych-*). The word is generic, but the title which follows is specific.

pachyonychia congenita [kŏn-jĕn′ĭ-tə] is the title of a genodermatosis apparent from birth (*congenita*) in which excessively thick nails (*pachyonychia*) are the least of it. Other abnormalities of the skin in the form of bullae and papular hyperkeratoses, and of the mucous membranes in the form of leukokeratoses may occur and are more distressing.

Paget's disease, extramammary [păj′ĕt]. A histologically characteristic malignant degeneration of the skin of the vulva, lips, penis, scrotum, perineum, and axillae, akin in Paget's disease of the nipples.

painful piezogenic pedal papules [păn′f′l pī-ē′zō-jĕn′ĭk pĕd′′l păp′ūlz] is one of those playfully conceived, alliterative titles that can be amusing when not erroneous. The error in this one lies in the choice of *piezogenic* (which means, from its Greek elements, producing [*-genic*] pressure [*piezo-*]) instead of *piezogenous* (which exactly means produced by [*-genous*] pressure [*piezo-*]). Nevertheless, the intent of the title is to name a condition of the feet characterized by papules about the heels that are tender. The lesions are said to be caused by small herniations of fat into the dermis.

paint, as a pharmaceutical form, describes a preparation of an active ingredient in a vehicle which, upon evaporation, leaves a hard film.

pallida [păl′ĭ-də] and **pallidum** [păl′ĭ-dəm] are respectively the feminine singular and the neuter singular of a Latin adjective meaning pale. They appear in the titles *Spirocheta pallida* (feminine) and *Treponema pallidum* (neuter).

palmer, palmare, palmaris [păm′ĕr, -ər; păl-mā′rē, -mä′rĕ, -mär′ē; păl-mā′rĭs, -mä′rĭs, -mär′ĭs] are respectively an English adjective and the neuter singular and masculine or feminine singular of a Latin adjective (in a New Latin usage) meaning of the palm of the hand. In classical Latin *palmaris* denoted a hand's-breadth or meant full of palms, i.e., the trees. In modern anatomy, the palm is taken to be the region between the wrist and the bases of the fingers on the ventral surface of the hand. Some thrifty editors object to the phrases *palm* (*s*) *of the hand* (*s*) and *sole* (*s*) *of the foot* (*feet*). However, there are contexts in which specification of *hand* (*s*) or *foot* (*feet*) is wise, because, it may be recalled, there are also botanical palms and ichthyologic soles. The last part of the second sentence of this entry is an illustration.

palmoplantar pustulosis refers to the recalcitrant pustular eruptions of the hands and feet. These are chronic relapsing eruptions limited to the palms and soles and characterized by numerous sterile, yellow, deep-seated, small pustules that evolve into dusky-red macules. (Fitzpatrick et al)

They include acrodermatitis continua (dermatitis repens), pustular psoriasis of the hands and feet and pustular bacterid. These are often examples of inverse psoriasis, so look elsewhere for that disorder and seek complete family history.

palpable purpura, formerly known as "allergic" vasculitis, is characterized by symmetrical red papules ("palpable purpura"), usually on the lower extremities. The purpuric lesions frequently develop into bullae and infarcts and may be associated with arthralgia, abdominal pain, melena and neuropathy. Red cell casts may be present in the urine sediment. Biopsy of the purpuric papules shows a necrotizing angiitis involving the venules of the dermal vascular plexus. (Fitzpatrick)

panaritium [păn′ə-rĭsh′ĭ-əm, -ē-əm] is ultimately derived from the Greek word *paronychia*, a condition (*-ia*) near or next to (*par-* = *para-*) a nail (*-onych-*). Latin adopted the Greek word intact but also adapted it to a form with a neuter ending, *paronychium*. Then, in Late Latin, further changes, including an apparent metathesis of *r* and *n*, preference for *a* to *o*, and an extension of the new ending by substitution of *-ic* for *-ych*, whereby the *-onych-* element was entirely lost, resulted in *panaricium* and *panaritium*. The latter word is still used sometimes synonymously with *paronychia* to designate those well-known bacterial and mycotic infections of the soft tissues around nails.

panniculitis [pə-nĭk′ū-lī′tĭs, -lē′tĭs] is New Latin literally meaning inflammation (*-itis*) of the little cloth (*pannicul-*, diminutive of *pannus*, a cloth). Of course, that "little cloth" is *panniculus adiposus* (which see).

panniculus adiposus [pə-nĭk′ū-ləs ăd′ĭ-pō′səs] is New Latin literally meaning the little cloth (*panniculus*) that is full of (*-osus*) fat (*adip-*). The entire subcutaneous layer of fat tissue, an organ that is large and heavy as things go, is so designated.

papilla [pə-pĭl′ə] is a Latin word for nipple or teat and also a pimple. The word is not applied to the mammary nipples but rather to what is like a mammary nipple in miniature.

papillaris, papillary [păp′ĭ-, pā′pĭ-lā′rĭs, -lä′rĭs, -lär′ĭs; păp′ə-, păp′ĭ-lĕr′ē, -ĭ, pə-pĭl′ə-rē, -rĭ] are respectively a Latin and an English adjective meaning pertaining to a nipple or characterized by nipple formation. Thus, the upper portion of the cutis whose surface is mammillated or studded with papillae is called the *pars papillaris* or *papillary part*.

papilliferum [păp′ə-, păp′ĭ-lĭf′ĕr-əm, -ĕr-əm, -ə-rəm] is the neuter singular of a New Latin adjectival formation meaning bearing papillae. It appears in the title *syringocystadenoma papilliferum*. *Papilliferus*, the masculine singular form of the adjective, appears in *nevus syringocystadenomatosus papilliferus*, which is alternate.

papilloma [păp′ĭ-lō′mə, -ə-lō′mə] is a New Latin formation meaning a swelling or tumor (*-oma*) that looks like or is shaped like a nipple (*papill-*). The word suits a cutaneous tag and other small tumors, particularly the benign, that have a broad pedicle or otherwise resemble a nipple.

papillomatosis [păp ĭ-lō′mə-tō′sĭs] means a condition (-osis) marked by tumor formation (-omat-) that consists of many nipple-like (papill-) lesions. The word is generic but acquires specificity in a title like the following:

papillomatosis, malignant [mə-lĭg′nənt] **(of Degos)** [dəgəs′, -gŭs′]. See *papulose atrophiante maligne*.

Papillon-Lefèvre syndrome [päpēyông′; ləfèvrə′]. Hyperkeratosis of the palms and soles together with dyscrasia of the periodontal bone.

papular [păp′ū-lĕr, -lər] is an adjective meaning pertaining or related to a papule, characterized by or consisting of papules.

papular mucinosis [mū′sĭ-nō′sĭs] describes a condition (-osis) in which mucin is present in abnormal amount (as histologically determined), and in which the clinical appearance is an aggregate of papules.

papular urticaria [ûr′tĭ-kâr′-ē-ə, -rĭ-ə, -kā′rē-ə, -rĭ-ə] describes a condition (-ia) in which wheals (urticar-) are of the size of papules. Insect bites, cholinergic urticaria and variants of atopic dermatitis cause such a picture.

papulation [păp′ū-lā′shən] means development of papules as a process accomplished.

papule [păp′ūl] derives from Latin *papula*, which is akin to *papilla*, and means a small swelling. In modern dermatologic sense, a lesion that is solid and raised above the level of the skin is termed a *papule*. Since the word has a suffix (-ule) that is diminutive, a lesion of small size within an everyday frame of reference, something, say, up to pea-size, is described. For larger, solid, elevated lesions, *nodule* and *tumor* are more suitable designations.

papuloerythroderma consists of pruritus, widespread red-brown, flat-topped papules that spare the skin creases, the so-called deck-chair sign, the striping effect seen in obese subjects sunbathing on deck chairs, eosinophilia, and profound lymphopenia. Appears to be a new clinical entity. Histopathologic examination rules out cutaneous lymphoma. Reported to respond to photochemotherapy. (Wabeel et al, *Archives Dermatology*, v. 127, January 1991)

papulo(-)necrotic tuberculid(e) [păp′ū-lō-nĕ-krŏt′ĭk tōō-, tū-bû-r′kū-lĭd, -lēd] describes a special form of cutaneous tuberculosis which is clinically notable for small, solid, elevated lesions (papules) that evolve into equally small, crust-covered, necrotizing ulcers and heal with varioliform scars. The extensor surfaces of the arms are common sites.

papulo(-)pustular [păp′ū-lō-pŭs′tū-lẽr, -lər] and **papulo(-) vesicular**
[vĕ-sĭk′ū-lẽr, -lər] are words like *maculo* (-) *papular*. The same considerations apply again. The words in point ought to be used to
suggest difficulty in deciding upon the papular, pustular or vesicular nature of a lesion or to suggest rapid transition from papulation
to pustulation or vesiculation and not simultaneous presence of
papules and pustules or papules and vesicles.

papulo(-)pustule [păp′ū-lō-pŭs′tūl] and **papulo(-)vesicle** [vĕs′ĭ-k'l].
Do we mean lesions that are simultaneously a papule and a pustule
and a papule and a vesicle? In line with what we have written
above, we suggest that the words are evasions because we cannot
decide whether we are dealing with papules, pustules or vesicles.

papulosa [păp′ū-lō′sə] is the feminine singular of a New Latin adjective meaning full of papules. It appears in the titles *acne papulosa*
and *dermatitis papulosa nigra*.

papulose atrophiante maligne [păpo͞olōz′ ătrŭfyängt′ mălĕny′ə] is
Degos' title for the rare disorder which he described as malignant
(*maligne*) in the sense that it may be fatal because the papular condition (*papulose*) tends to ulceration and atrophy (*atrophiante*),
and in the intestinal portion is serious even if not so in cutaneous
location. See *malignant papillomatosis (of Degos)*.

papulosis [păp′ū-lō′sĭs] is a generic word describing a condition characterized by numerous papules.

papulosis atrophicans maligna [ə-trŏf′ĭ-kănz, -trō′fĭ-kănz măl-
ĭg′nə] is the classicized title for *papulose atrophiante maligne*.

papulo(-)vesicle. See *papulo (-)pustule*.

papulo(-)vesicular. See *papulo (-)pustular*.

par(a)- [păr′ə] is a Greek prefix of many and diverse meanings, e.g.,
besides, alongside of, beyond, aside from, amiss, etc. In some medical contexts the element implies abnormality and in others resemblance to what is deemed a true form, as is evident in many entries
following.

paracoccidioidomycosis [păr′ə-kŏk-sĭd′ĭ-oid′ō-mī-kō′sĭs] is the term
for infection with an organism that is named *Paracoccidioides brasiliensis*. The disease is also known by the parochial designation
South American blastomycosis. *Paracoccidioidomycosis* and *Paracoccidioides brasiliensis* suggest that both the disease and the causative
organism greatly resemble coccidioidomycosis and *Coccidioides immitis*.

paraffinoma [păr′ə-fĭ-nō′mə] is a formation from *paraffin* and *-oma* to denote a lumpiness that ensues sometimes and some time after injection of paraffin into living tissues for cosmetic purposes. The practice of injecting paraffin is largely abandoned by now. It may be of passing interest to note that the Greek prefix *para-* is not involved in the etymology of *paraffin*, a word coined in 1830 by Reichenbach from the Latin words *parum* (too little, barely) and *affinis* (related to, having affinity with or attraction for) to designate a material that has small chemical attraction for or to other material.

parakeratosis [păr′ə-kĕr′ə-tō′sĭs] literally means a condition (*-osis*) of abnormal (*para-*) cornification (*-kerato-*). The clinical mark of the condition is scaling; the histologic mark is imperfectly keratinized epithelial cells that still possess nuclei as they rise to the position of stratum corneum.

parameter [pə-răm′ə-tẽr, păr-ăm′ĕ-tẽr] is a popular vogue word in current medical writing. We doubt that it will last long there because, when not used in its strict mathematical sense, it is also a vague word. The mathematical sense of the word, difficult enough to understand, is that of a "variable constant," i.e., a changing factor which, in each change, characterizes a ratio or relationship between members of a system of, for example, curves. As near as we can make out when we see the word in medical contexts, usually in the plural, what is meant is something like *characteristic elements, constant factors, variables, limits* or *frames of reference.* If someone says: "Alopecia has been studied in all its parameters," which of the above meanings, or what other meaning, applies?

However, a reasonable use of *parameter* in a medical context would be in a statement like, "There are parameters between obesity and diet, endocrine function, psychic condition, and heredity." The misuse of this word goes on as thoughtlessly as ever.

paraphimosis. See *phimosis.*

parapsoriasis [păr′ə-sə-rī′ə-sĭs] literally means a condition that resembles (*para-*) psoriasis. Critically examined, the clinical resemblance is not great, course is quite different, cause, to be sure, is equally unknown and, but for the arbitrary names, the conditions have nothing in common. Then, of parapsoriasis alone, there are more or less stereotypic variants bearing that name with many modifying adjectives and, as before, not related to each other any more than nominally. A few of numerous titles are given following.

parapsoriasis acuta (et varioliformis) [ə-kū′tə ĕt văr′ē-, văr′ĭ-ō-lĭ-fôr′mĭs] is the title for a process that hardly resembles psoriasis, but takes the form of rapidly developing (*acuta*) papules that become necrotic and eventuate in scars that resemble those of smallpox (*varioliformis*) in recovery. The process is thought to be in the class of the necrotizing angiitides.

parapsoriasis en gouttes [äng go͞ot′], a title in French, specifies a process somewhat like psoriasis but in the form of scaly, drop-sized (*en gouttes*) lesions. See *parapsoriasis guttata.*

parapsoriasis en plaques (disseminées) [äng plăk′ dēsĕmēnā′], a title in French, describes a process, of all the parapsoriases, most reminiscent of psoriasis in the form of finely scaling, discoid (*en plaques*) lesions scattered (*disseminées*) on the body.

parapsoriasis guttata [gŭ-tā′tə] is a classicized alternate for *parapsoriasis en gouttes* and means the same thing, namely, the disease with lesions in drop (*guttata*) form.

parapsoriasis lichenoides [lī′kə-noi′dēz] is alternate for *parapsoriasis acuta* (*et varioliformis*). With *chronica* in the title *parapsoriasis guttata* is meant.

parapsoriasis variegata [vā′rĭ-, văr′ĭ-ē-gā′tə, -ē-gä′tə] designates process of that class of things that vaguely resembles (*para-*) psoriasis but in this instance the scatter of lesions is variable and their scaliness more.

parasitaria [păr′ə-sĭ-tā′rē-ə, -tä′rĭ-ə, -tăr′ē-ə] and **parasitica** [păr′ə-sĭt′ĭ-kə] are the feminine singular of New Latin adjectival formations meaning relating to parasites. The words appear in the title *achromia parasitaria* (or *parasitica*).

para-ungual [păr′ə-ŭng′gwəl] means near or next to (*para-*) a nail (-*ungu-*, plus -*al*, adjectival ending).

paronychia [păr′ō-nĭk′ē-ə, -ĭ-ə], from its Greek elements, means a condition (-*ia*) near or next to (*par-*) a nail (-*onych-*). Inflammatory conditions of the soft parts around the nails (folds, eponychium, etc.) of any cause can be designated by the word. See *panaritium* for an alternate word.

pars [părz] is a Latin word for part or portion.

pars papillaris [păp′ĭ-lā′rĭs, -lä′rĭs, -lăr′ĭs] designates that portion (*pars*) of the corium, the upper third, that is characterized by papillae (*papillaris*). See *papilla* and *papillaris.*

pars reticularis [rĕ-, rē-tĭk′ū-lā′rĭs, -lä′rĭs, -lăr′ĭs] designates that portion (*pars*) of the corium, the lower two-thirds, that appears like a network (*reticularis*) under microscopy.

partial combined immunodeficiency disorder. Immunodeficiency with thrombocytopenia and eczema (Wiskott-Aldrich syndrome). This X-linked, recessive syndrome is characterized by the triad of eczema, thrombocytopenic purpura and undue susceptibility to infection. (*Cecil Textbook of Medicine*, 18th Edition, W.B. Saunders Co., Wyngaarden & Smith, eds.)

Pasini and Pierini, atrophoderma of [pä-sē′nē; pyĕ-rē′nē]. Progressive idiopathic atrophoderma.

passage. See *burrow*.

patch [păch] derives from a Middle English word of uncertain origin, and means, among other things, an area of difference upon a large background of sameness. The word has a use in descriptive morphology to designate a change of color of skin that is flat and largish, i.e., larger than *macule* would suggest.

patch test refers to a method of determining sensitivity by placing suspect allergens in contact with bare, unbroken skin and covering for 48 hours more or less hermetically. The procedure is most useful in allergic contact dermatitis. The allergens are simple chemicals (i.e., inorganic or organic but of less than protein complexity) in concentrations and vehicles that are known not to be primary irritants. Reading is done in 24-48-96 hours; forty-eight hours is average. Positive reactions appear as erythema and vesiculation; negative reactions show no change. This may show evidence of delayed hypersensitivity which is T cell mediated.

Pautrier's abscess [pōtrēāz′ ăb′sĕs]. See under *abscess, micro-*. Intraepidermal microabscess in mycosis fungoides.

peau de chagrin [pō də shăgräng′] is French for *shagreen skin*. *Chagrin* as well as *shagreen* developed from Turkish *cagri*, or *saghri*, rump of a horse. *Shagreen* denotes leather processed in a characteristic way, namely, embossed by pressing upon pellets during tanning and then colored greenish. This gives the finished product a knobbed surface. The skins of certain sharks are that way naturally and some of the skin changes in epiloia, neurofibromatosis and Hurler's disease have a vague similarity to shagreen.

The English word *chagrin* [shă-, shə-grĭn′] meaning acute annoyance, distress, sorrow or vexation from failure is a metaphoric change from the idea of "rough skin" to "gnawing trouble." Another explanation for the sad meanings of *chagrin* is that the word developed from Old French *grain*. The latter word goes back to another of Germanic origin, *gram*, which is still used in German to mean vexation and sorrow. Finally, an old pejorative prefix was added and the spelling at one time became *sagrin*. This too affected the spelling and meaning of the word for leather. All in all, the skin is rubbed the wrong way.

Pediculoides ventricosus [pĕ-, pə-, pē-dĭk′ū-loi′dēz vĕn′trĭ-kō′səs] designates a species of mites that is described by the words as being louse-like (*Pediculoides*) and full of belly (*ventricosus*). The gravid female is, indeed, amazingly so. Mites of this species are parasitic on some insects but, failing what they prefer, will infest flesh. Human beings may become infested from harvesting, storing or processing grain. *Pyemotes ventricosus* is a more modern designation.

pediculosis [pĕ-, pə-, pē-dĭk′ū-lō′sĭs] means infestation (-*osis*, condition) with lice (*pedicul-*).

pediculosis capitis [kăp′ə-, kăp′ĭ-tĭs] means infestation (-*osis*) of the head (*capitis*) with lice (*pedicul-*).

pediculosis corporis vel vestimentorum [kôr′pō-rĭs, -pô-rĭs vĕl vĕs′tĭ-mĕn-tō′rəm, -tôr′əm] means infestation (-*osis*) of the body (*corporis*) or (*vel*) of the clothes (*vestimentorum*) with lice (*pedicul-*). Strictly speaking, the infestation is of the clothes; the louse comes on the body only to feed and does not stay in residence there.

pediculosis pubis [pū′bĭs] means infestation (-*osis*) of the pubes, i.e., the pubic hair (*pubis* is the genitive of *pubes*) with lice (*pedicul-*). Strictly speaking, the condition is not a pediculosis but a phthiriasis because the infesting louse is not a *Pediculus* but a *Phthir* (*i*)*us*, and another peculiarity is that this infestation may reach the hair of the abdomen, chest and axillae in adults and the eyelashes and eyebrows in babies.

Pediculus [pĕ-, pə-, pē-dĭk′ū-ləs] is the name of a genus of lice. There are but two species that affect humans in selected sites and special ways.

Pediculus humanus capitis [hū-mä′-, hū-mā′nəs kăp′ə-, kăp′ĭ-tĭs] is the louse (*pediculus*) that infests the head (*capitis*, of the head) of humans (*humanus*).

Pediculus humanus corporis [kôr′pō-rĭs, -pô-rĭs, -pə-rĭs] is the louse (*pediculus*) that feeds upon the body (*corporis*, of the body) of humans (*humanus*).

pedis [pē′dĭs, pĕd′ĭs] is the genitive singular of the Latin word *pes*, foot, and means of the (a) foot. It appears in the title *tinea pedis*.

pelade [pəläd′] is a French noun meaning alopecia, from the verb *peler*, to strip of hair. The word is used by the French-speaking for *alopecia areata*.

pelage [pĕl′ĭj, pəlazh′] is another French noun, meaning the hairy coat. It is derived ultimately from the Latin noun *pilus*, hair.

pellagra [pə-lăg′rə, -lā′grə, pĕl-ăg′rə]. There are two theories regarding the origin of this word. Either it is directly from Latin *pellis*, skin, and Greek *agra*, a seizure, a pain; or it is from Italian *pelle agra*, rough skin, such as once appeared in Lombardy from the eating, it was thought, of diseased maize. In any event, the modern word is applied to that condition attributable to an inadequate diet and deficiency of nicotinic acid that results in characteristic skin changes in the form of dermatitis of the face, neck, hands, forearms, feet and legs. Neuropathy and deep constitutional disturbance are other consequences.

pellagrin [pə-lăg′rĭn, -lā′grĭn] denotes a sufferer (*-in*) from pellagra.

pellagroid [pə-lăg′roid, -lā′groid] is an adjective meaning like or resembling (*-oid*) pellagra.

pellagrous [pə-lăg′rəs, -lā′grəs, pĕl-ăg′rəs] is an adjective formed from the New Latin adjective *pellagrosus*, literally full of pellagra, and means pertaining, related to or affected with pellagra.

pellicle [pĕl′ĭ-k'l] literally means a fine or little (*-cle*, diminutive) skin (*pelli-*). However, the word is rarely or not at all used like *cuticle*, which means the same thing. Rather, it is applied to skin-like formations, such as films or scums, on the surface of liquids.

pelt [pĕlt] is a word for a raw fur or the skin of an animal with the hair still on, and also for the skins of animals, especially sheep and goats, stripped of hair for tanning. Like *fell* (which see), it derives from Latin *pellis*, ultimately from Greek *pella*, probably via French.

pemphigoid [pĕm′fĭ-goid] is an adjective meaning like (*-oid*) pemphigus. It is also now used by some as a noun to designate a bullous eruption that resembles but is not pemphigus. Called by some "old man's pemphigus." See *bullous pemphigoid*.

pemphigus [pĕm′fĭ-gəs, pĕm-fī′gəs] is New Latin from Greek *pemphix*, genitive *pemphigos*, respectively bubble, of a bubble. The word names, with modifying adjectives, several conditions characterized by severe blistering.

A rare, mucocutaneous blistering disease due to loss of keratocyte cohesion. Immunofluorescent studies show characteristic intercellular antibodies. Pemphigus vulgaris is the most common varient which shows large flaccid bullae on noninflamed skin with mucous membrane involvement present in 90% of cases. (Castle et al) Indirect immunofluorescence shows circulating antibodies which correlates with disease activity and response to treatment.

pemphigus erythematosus [ĕr′ĭ-thĕm′ə-tō′səs] is one of the prognostically grave types of pemphigus, and is clinically marked by lesions that may look like a cross between impetigo, seborrheic dermatitis or lupus erythematosus in its vesiculation and crusting. The condition is histologically marked by acantholysis high in the epidermal stratification. Some place the condition close to pemphigus foliaceus, others, close to pemphigus vulgaris. Some cases do indeed behave like pemphigus foliaceus in chronicity, unresponsiveness to treatment and invariant morphe; other cases change to pemphigus vulgaris and then follow a more fulminating course. The eponym *Senear-Usher* is commonly heard in connection with pemphigus erythematosus.

pemphigus, familial benign chronic. See *familial benign chronic pemphigus.*

pemphigus foliaceus [fō′lĭ-ā′shē-əs, -sē-əs]. *Pemphigus foliaceus* (classicized form) or *foliaceous pemphigus* (anglicized form) is that variant of the prognostically grave type of pemphigus that is of least gravity and greatest chronicity. Clinically, the condition appears as a leaf-like (*foliaceus,* or *foliaceous*) scaliness but histologically, the process can be seen to be an exceedingly superficial acantholysis with formation of bullae so high in the epidermis (subcorneal) that the blisters may not readily be recognized as such.

Fogo selvagem.

pemphigus neonatorum [nē′ō-nə-tō′rəm, -tôr′əm] is still another of those inadequate titles that this time specifies an age of predilection for a pyodermatous process that takes the form of bullae that pustulate. Like butcher's pemphigus it is a matter of superficial infection with staphylococci.

pemphigus, ocular [ŏk′ū-lĕr, -lər]. See *cicatricial pemphigoid.*

pemphigus vegetans [vĕj′ē-tănz] designates that type of pemphigus which is clinically characterized by exuberant overgrowth (*vegetans*) of tissue in and about what is essentially a bullous process. The phenomenon is seen most often when the blistering starts or is confined to intertriginous spaces like the axillae, umbilicus, groin, intergluteal cleft and inframammary regions. Otherwise, the condition behaves or becomes pemphigus vulgaris in eventual appearance and course.

pemphigus vulgaris [vŭl-gā′rĭs, -gä′rĭs, -gär′ĭs] means the ordinary or common (*vulgaris,* of the crowd) variety of that prognostically grave blistering process which untreated is inevitably fatal. Aside from clinical severity, the quintessential histopathology of this type of pemphigus is acantholysis at the level of the basal-cell layer resulting in bullae in which the floor of the blisters is the basal-cell layer and the roof the rest of the epidermis. Diagnosis is confirmed by both direct and indirect immunofluorescent studies.

pendulum [pĕn′dū-ləm] as a Latin adjective in the neuter singular means hanging. It appears in the title *fibroma pendulum*.

penetrans [pĕn′ē-, pĕn′ə-trănz] is the present participle of a Latin verb and means penetrating, boring into. It appears in titles like *hyperkeratosis follicularis et parafollicularis in cutem penetrans* and *Tunga penetrans*.

per- [pĕr, pûr, pĕr, pər] is Latin prefix meaning through. It is often used as an intensive, i.e., with the meaning of thoroughly.

percutaneous [pĕr′kū-tā′nē-əs] is an adjective meaning having the quality or ability (*-aneous*) of passing through (*per-*) the skin (*-cut-*).

perforans [pĕr′-, pûr′fō-rănz, -fə-rănz, -fô-rănz] is a Latin present participle meaning perforating or boring through. It appears in a title like *folliculitis narium perforans*.

peri- [pĕr′ī, -ē] is a Greek prefix meaning around, enclosing, surrounding and nearby.

periarteritis nodosa [pĕr′ī-är-tə-rī′tĭs, -rē′tĭs nō-dō′sə] literally means inflammatory processes (*-itis*) around (*peri-*) arteries (*-arter-*) in the form of many knots (*nodosa*). The title is applied to a grave disease whose symptomatology depends on what organs and combination or succession of organs have the process in sufficient degree. *Polyarteritis nodosa* is the preferred title. Skin involvement occurs in about one quarter of those affected with polyarteritis nodosa. Signs are polymorphic exanthemato-purpuric, urticarial, and multiform in character and severe subcutaneous hemorrhage, resulting from necrotizing arteritis, with secondary gangrene.

periderm [pĕr′ē-, pĕr′ī-dûrm]. See *epitrichium*.

perifolliculitis abscedens et suffodiens. See *folliculitis et perifolliculitis abscedens et suffodiens*.

periodic acid-Schiff stain [pûr′ī-ŏd′ĭk ăs′ĭd shĭf stān]. We enter this item only to remark on the peculiar appearance of the first word and the tendency to mispronounce it because it is written without a hyphen between *per* and *iodic*. As it is, it looks as though it should be pronounced pēr′ĭ-ŏd′ĭk and mean cyclic. If it were written *periodic* the natural tendency would be to pronounce it correctly, pûr′ĭ-ŏd′ĭk, and there would be no mistaking the chemical meaning or relation to H_5IO_6. See *hyphen, uses of.* Useful additional stain to show fungi and natural mucopolysaccharides.

perioral dermatitis [pĕr′ĭ-ō′rəl dûr′mə-tī′tĭs] is indifferent coinage for an eruption of inflammatory papules about the mouth. The condition is spoken of as if it were something startlingly new. Perhaps it is, but it also appears to have resemblances to ancient conditions like follicular pyoderma or moniliasis, seborrheic dermatitis, and rosacea, especially the latter two when it appears about the nose and higher in the center of the face. Some cases seem to respond to a combination of a broad-spectrum antibiotic by mouth and topical application of anti-microbial formulations. Most cases do not respond favorably to adrenocorticosteroid preparations; indeed, many observers think the fluoridated cortisone preparations are exacerbating if not causative.

periporitis [pĕr′ĭ-pō-rī′tĭs, -rē′tĭs] means inflammatory process (-*itis*) around (*peri-*) a pore (-*por-*). *Pore* means a small opening, and, in the skin, the opening of the sweat duct is meant, not that of the pilosebaceous apparatus which is better referred to as the *pilosebaceous ostium*. In any event, periporitis occurs in prickly heat (miliaria rubra) and in primary pyogenic infections of the upper reaches of the eccrine gland structure.

periungual [pĕr′ĭ-ŭng′gwəl] means around or about (*peri-*) a nail (-*ungu-*, -*al*, adjectival ending).

perlèche [pĕrlĕsh′] is a French word that is applied to inflammatory processes at the angles of the mouth. From its elements the word means to lick (-*lèche*) all around (*per-*) or thoroughly (*per-*, intensive). It is likely that the word was chosen because the condition is caused or promoted by a habit of licking the angles of the mouth or because persons afflicted with *perlèche* of any cause do indeed lick the angles of the mouth a great deal to relieve discomfort. *Pourlèche* [poorlesh′] is an alternate word found in French writing.

pernio [pûr′nĭ-ō, pĕr′-, pûr′-, pĕr′nē-ō] is a Latin word found in Pliny meaning chilblain, frostbite or congelation. The plural is *perniones* [pûr′nĭ-ō′nēz, pĕr′-, pûr′-, pĕr′nē-ō′nēz]. The word may be used to designate frostbite in general or in synonymy with *chilblain(s)*.

pernio, lupus. See *lupus pernio.*

persistent pearly penile papules [pĕr-sĭs′tĕnt pûr′lē pē′nĭl păp′ūlz] is still another of those playfully conceived alliterative titles, this time coined to tell of papular fibroplasias on the corona of the glans penis. The histology of the lesions is said to be similar to those of adenoma sebaceum and acrokeratomas.

perspire, perspiration [pĕr-spīr'; pər'spə-, pûr'spĭ-rā'shən] literally mean to breathe through and the action or result of breathing (*-spire, -spiration*) through (*per-*). It must be said immediately, in breathless haste, that the modern words refer to sweating, not breathing.

perstans [pĕr'-, pûr'stănz] is a Latin present participle meaning lasting, persistent. It is found in classicized titles, e.g., *erythema perstans.*

pertenue. See *Treponema pertenue.*

petechia [pĕ-, pē-tē'kē-ə, -kĭ-ə] is a New Latin formation from an Italian word of unknown origin that means a spot, speck or freckle. The modern word is used to designate minute hemorrhages. The plural is *petechiae* [pĕ-tē'kē-ē, -kĭ-ē].

Peutz-Jeghers syndrome [pûts; yā'gĕrz], cutaneous lentiginosis, is eponymic for a condition that is marked by intestinal polyposis and macular pigmentation, particularly on the oral lips, i.e., the pigmentation, polyposis syndrome.

Peyronie's disease [pārŏnē']. Indurato penis plastica.

phacomatosis. See *phakomatosis.*

phagedena [făj'ə-, făj'ē-dē'nə] derives from a Greek word meaning an eaten-out or consuming ulcer. The original word was used by Hippocrates, Galen and other Greek medical writers; the derived word too was once used extensively but in modern times it is rarely heard because precise designation by specific cause of ulceration is frequently possible.

phagedenic [făj'ə-, făj'ē-dĕn'ĭk] is the adjective from *phagedena* meaning relating or pertaining to an eaten-out or consuming ulcer.

phagedenic ulcer [ŭl'sĕr] is a title that is not without some usefulness if one considers that there are ulcers which do not have much of an "eaten-out" or "consuming" quality and that one might want to specify that quality emphatically.

phakomatosis [făk'ō-mə-tō'sĭs] is a word whose special meaning is not derivable from the meaning of its Greek word elements. Literally, the word means a condition (*-osis*) resulting from tumor formation (*-omat-*) of the lens (*phak-*) of the eye. In recent days the word has attained currency to designate conditions that are genetically based on and simultaneously characterized by both cutaneous and neuro-ectodermal, particularly intracranial and ocular, anomalies.

phenotype designates the measurable features of the organism that are expressed by its genotype in conjunction with environmental factors.

Phialophora [fī′ə-lŏf′ə-rə] is a New Latin formation from Greek word elements that mean a bowl (*phialo-*)-bearing (*-phora*) structure. The word is used to designate a genus of fungi, members of which have bowl-like structures bearing spores.

Phialophora verrucosa [vĕr′o͞o-kō′sə] is a species of the genus whose cultural characteristic is wartiness (*verrucosa*). Infection with it causes a form of chromo(blasto)-mycosis.

phimosis [fī-mō′sĭs] is a literal transliteration of a Greek word meaning a muzzling or strangulation. It is applied to stenosis of the preputial orifice. *Paraphimosis* is a correlative word that means strangulation of the glans penis by phimosis so that the foreskin cannot be drawn over it from behind. Neither word has in it any element suggestive of cause; both merely announce the facts. The causes may be congenital anomalies or acquired inflammatory conditions of the prepuce or glans penis. For the latter see *balanitis*, and *balanoposthitis*. Circumcision at elective times is curative.

phleb- [flĕb] is a combining form from the Greek word for a vein.

phlebectasia [flĕb′ĕk-tā′zhē-ə, -zē-ə, -zhə] means abnormal dilatation or extension (*-ectasia*) by reduplication of veins (*phleb-*) and capillaries. Venous anomalies as far apart as common varicosities and rare angiomatoses involving veins may be designated by the word.

phlyctena [flĭk-tē′nə] is a New Latin formation from a Greek word for a vesicle or pustule.

phlyctenular [flĭk-tĕn′ū-lĕr] means relating or pertaining to (*-ar*) a small (*-ul-*) vesicle or pustule (*phlycten-*).

photo- [fō′tō] is a combining form from the Greek word for light. The original sense was of visible light but nowadays we stretch the spectrum a bit to encompass ultraviolet and infrared.

photo-allergy [fō′tō-ăl-ĕr-jē, -jī] is a formation to express specific acquired alteration in the capacity to react (*-allergy*) occasioned by the shine of light (*photo-*). It must be understood that the alteration in reaction is not to light per se but to substances rendered allergenic by electromagnetic energy of wave lengths in the general range of the visible and ultraviolet spectrum.

photodermatitis [fō'tō-dûr'mə-tī'tĭs, -tē'tĭs] is a comprehensive word coined to encompass all inflammatory conditions of the skin (-*dermatitis*) caused in any manner or by any mechanism by the shine of light (*photo-*).

photodynamic [fō'tō-dī-năm'ĭk] means moved, motivated or activated (-*dynamic*) by light (*photo-*).

photo-onycholysis is separation of the nail secondary to drug induced changes of the nail structure. May also occur in photosensitizing diseases such as the porphyrias or may be spontaneous. (Torras et al. JAAD, Vol 21, No. 6)

photopheresis. Treatment for cutaneous T-cell lymphoma (CTCL) (mycosis fungoides) or Sezary syndrome. This is an extracorporeal photomedical therapy that combines ultraviolet light with a photoactivatable drug in a UVA light unit which alters nucleated blood cells. When reinfused, the damaged cells of the malignant clone responsible for CTCL prime the body's immune system to destroy the clone.

photophytodermatitis [fo'tō-fī'tō-dûr'mə tī'tĭs, -tē-tĭs] is a useful formulation to designate an inflammatory condition of the skin (-*dermatitis*) caused by plant (-*phyto-*) products deposited on the skin and activated by the shine of light (*photo-*).

photosensitive, photosensitivity [fō'tō-sĕn'sĭ-tĭv'; ə-tē, -tĭ] are respectively an adjective and a noun implying more than average reactivity to light.

phototoxic, phototoxicity [fō'tō-tŏk'sĭk; -tŏk-sĭs'ĭ-tē, -ə-tĭ] are respectively an adjective meaning relating or pertaining to, and a noun denoting, injury or primary irritancy occasioned by the shine of light. Again it is not light per se but the action of light upon a substance that is ordinarily not irritant becoming so by the action of electromagnetic energy of wave lengths in the general range of the visible and ultraviolet spectrum.

phrynoderm(i)a [frī'nō-dûr'mə, -mē-ə, -mĭ-ə] denotes a condition of the skin (-*derma, -dermia*) that is like that of a toad (*phryno-*). The allusion is to papulation and perifolicular hyperkeratosis such as seen in extreme form in deficiency of vitamin A.

phthiriasis [thī-rī'-, thĭr-ī'ə-sĭs] is a word used by Pliny for infestation with lice. Nowadays we restrict the word to designate infestation with *Phthir (i)us pubis*, a particular species of lice. *Crabs* is a racy alternate expression. See *pediculosis pubis*.

Phthir(i)us [thĭr′əs, thĭr′ē-əs, -ĭ-əs] is New Latin from Greek *phtheir*, a louse. It is used as the name of a genus of lice different from *Pediculus*.

Phthir(i)us pubis [pū′bĭs] is the species of *Phthir (i)us* that infests the pubic region and other hairy outposts up to the axillae (and eyelashes in infants) but not the scalp. *Pubic louse* and *crab louse* are alternate designations.

physical dimensions of the skin. It is a self-serving conceit on the part of dermatologists to claim that the skin is the largest organ of the body. The skin is not the largest organ of the body on any scale of measurement be it area, volume, specific gravity or total weight. In area it is exceeded by the endothelial surface of the entire vascular tree, the pulmonary alveolar surface and the peritoneal surface. In volume it is exceeded by musculature, skeleton, blood and panniculus adiposus. In specific gravity it is exceeded by bone and ligament. In weight it is exceeded by musculature, skeleton, blood and panniculus adiposus. However, if it comforts anyone, the skin exceeds in all respects liver, brain, intestines and spleen and from a relative position in scales of each of the physical quantities, the skin can justly be rated among the large organs of the body. In absolute units, the skin of an adult 170 cm in height and 70 kg in weight has a surface area of about 1.8 m^2 (20 sq. ft.), a volume of about 3000 ml (3 liters or quarts), a specific gravity of about 1.1 (1.3 for hair and nail) and a total weight of about 4 kg (8.8 lbs; $^1/_{16}$ or 6% of body weight). Only in the sense that skin encloses the largest volume is it the greatest.

phytodermatitis [fī′tō-dûr′mə-tī′tĭs, -tē′tĭs] designates an inflammatory condition of the skin (-*dermatitis*) caused by a plant (*phyto-*) principle. Dermatitis caused by poison ivy, for example, could be so designated.

pian [pī′ăn, pyän] as a designation for yaws derives via French from a word for ulcer in the language of an extinct South American tribe (Tupinamba).

piebald [pī′bôld] derives via Middle English from Old French *pie* (Latin *pica*), the magpie, and *bald*, with an early meaning of white, or streaked with white. The developed sense of *piebald* is covered with, or having two colors, black and white or brown and white. *Pied* is another word meaning parti-colored or mottled in two colors, not necessarily black and white. In his poem "The Pied Piper of Hamelin," Robert Browning thus describes the Piper:
And in did come the strangest figure!/His queer long coat from

heel to head / Was half of yellow and half of red. . . . (from Stanza V)

"And people call me the Pied Piper." / (And here they noticed round his neck / A scarf of red and yellow stripe, / To match with his coat of the self-same check. . . .) (from Stanza VI)

piebald skin, as one might expect, is skin that is mottled brown and white or black and white. Vitiligo and partial albinism are such conditions.

piebaldism [pī′bôld-iz'm] designates a condition (*-ism*) of dual coloration, white and black or brown.

piebaldism (patterned leukoderma) dominant disorder. Most have a white forelock.

piedra [pyä′drä] is a Spanish word for stone. It is used dermatologically to designate a trichomycosis which is characterized by formation of hard concretions on extruded hairshafts only. There is a "white" variety caused by *Trichosporum beigeli* and a "black" by *Piedraia hortai.*

pigment, pigmentary, pigmentation [pĭg′mənt′; pĭg′mən- tĕr′ē, -tĕr-ē; pĭg′mən-tā′shən] are respectively a noun, an adjective and a noun meaning, in order, colored material, relating to colored material, and coloration. In the skin that colored material may be melanin (tan to black), hemosiderin (gray, brown), carotene (yellow) and adventitious matter (silver and tattoo materials that are gray, blue red, black, etc.).

pigmented purpuric lichenoid dermatitis [pĭg-mĕn′tĕd, -tĭd, -təd pûr-pū′rĭk lī′kə-noid dûr′mə-tī′tĭs, -tē-tĭs] **(of Gougerot)** [gōōzhərō′] names by some of its characteristics a dermatosis of the legs that is notable for brown-purple papules.

pigmentosa [pĭg′mĕn-tō′sə], **pigmentosum** [pĭg′mĕn-tō′səm], and **pigmentosus** [pĭg′mĕn-tō′səs] are respectively the feminine singular, neuter singular and masculine singular of a New Latin adjective meaning full of color. They appear in titles like *urticaria pigmentosa, xeroderma pigmentosum* and *nevus pigmentosus.*

pil-, pili-, pilo- [pīl, pĭl; pĭl′ĭ, pĭl′ə, pī′lĭ; pĭl′ō, pī′lō] are combining forms from Latin *pilus,* hair.

pilar, pilaris and **pilary** [pī′lĕr, -lər; pī-, pĭ-lā′rĭs, -lä′rĭs, -lăr′ĭs; pī′lə-rē] are respectively an English adjective, the masculine and feminine singular of a New Latin adjective and another English adjective, all three meaning pertaining or related to hair. The Latin adjective appears in a title like *keratosis pilaris.*

pili [pī′lī] is the genitive singular and nominative plural form of Latin *pilus*, hair. *Pilorum* [pī-, pĭ-lō′rəm, -lôr′əm] is the genitive plural. The genitive forms appear in titles like *arrector pili, arrectores pilorum* and *atrophia pilorum propria*. The nominative plural form appears in the titles below.

pili annulati [ăn′ū-lā′tī] means ringed (*annulati*) hairs (*pili*). The phenomenon occurs from an alternation of pigment and depigmentation in bands within hair shafts of the scalp.

pili incarnati [ĭn′kär-nā′tī, -nä′tī, -tē] means ingrown (*incarnati*, enfleshed) hairs (*pili*).

pili multigemini [mo͞ol′tē-, mŭl′tī-, mŭl′tĭ-jĕm′ĭ-nī] means many-paired (*multigemini*) hairs (*pili*), i.e., several hairs exiting from a common follicle.

pili torti [tôr′tī] means twisted (*torti*) hairs (*pili*).

piliform [pĭl′ə-, pī′lĭ-fôrm] means hair- (*pili-*) -shaped (*-form*). *Filiform*, meaning thread-shaped, is more commonly used to denote long, fine structures.

pilomatrixoma [pī′lō-mā′trĭk-sō′mə] is new coinage for neoplasia (*-oma*) of the growing portion (*-matrix-*) of the hair (*pilo-*) apparatus. It remains to be seen if it will displace *calcifying epithelioma of Malherbe*. *Trichomatrioma* is an alternate title. This neologism is peculiar in that it consists of a Latin element (*pilo-*) attached to a Latin noun derived from Greek (*-matrix-*) and finished off by a suffix (*-oma*) that is mistakenly Greek. Some purists have refined it to *pilomatrioma* and others to *pilomatricoma*. The intent of the coinage was to specify the place of origin of the dysplasia.

pilonidal [pī′lō-nī′dəl], formed from Latin word elements, means pertaining to (*-al*) a nest (*-nid-*) of hair (*pilo-*).

pilonidal cyst [sĭst], **fistula** [fĭs′tū-lə], **sinus** [sī′nəs] denote the well-known anomalies in the sacral region that consist of openings and channels in sacculations that contain vestiges of cutaneous adnexa, especially of the hair apparatus.

pilorum. See *pili*.

pilose, pilosus [pī′lōs; pī-, pĭ-lō′səs] are respectively an English adjective and the masculine singular of a Latin adjective meaning full of (*-ose, -osus*) hair (*pil-*), shaggy. The Latin form appears in the title *nevus pigmentosus et pilosus*.

pilosebaceous [pī′lō-sē-bā′shəs] means pertaining or relating to hair and sebaceous gland as an organized apparatus.

pilosebaceous follicle [fŏl′ĭ-k'l], **ostium** [ŏs′tĭ-əm, -tē-əm], refer to those portions of the hair apparatus that are a sac (*follicle*) and an opening (*ostium*).

pilosis [pĭ-lō′sĭs], from Latin, means a condition (-*osis*)—any abnormal condition—of hair (*pil-*). *Trichosis*, from Greek, is equivalent.

pimple [pĭm′p'l] is a word of unknown origin. Whatever its origin, whether Latin, Old English or Middle English as conjectured, *pimple* is a common, homely designation for an ugly papule or pustule.

pink disease [pĭnk dĭ-, də-zēz′] is a simple alternate title for acrodynia, dermatopolyneuritis or erythredema.

Pinkus's tumor [pĭn′kûs]. Fibroepithelioma.

pinta [pĭn′tə] is a Spanish word for a spot or mark and may derive from Latin *pincta*, feminine of *pinctus*, painted. In medical use, the word designates a disease caused by a treponema (*T. carateum*). One mark of the disease is depigmentation of the skin which produces a spotty appearance, something like an abstract painting. *Carate* (which see) is alternate.

pinworm [pĭn′wûrm′]. See *Enterobius vermicularis*.

pit [pĭt] may derive from Latin *puteus*, a well, via Anglo-Saxon and Middle English words meaning a hole. In medical contexts a rather small hole or depression is suggested by the word.

pitted nails [pĭt′ĕd, -ĭd nālz] is descriptive of the tiny depressions one sometimes sees in nail plates, particularly in psoriasis.

pityriasis [pĭt′ĭ-rī′ə-sĭs] is a word that was used by Galen and other ancients for conditions (-*iasis*) that are characterized by branny (*pityr-*) scaling, especially those of the scalp. Several titles bearing the word with modifying adjectives are still current; some are obsolescent.

pityriasis alba [ăl′bə] is the title of a condition (-*iasis*) marked by branny (*pityr-*) scaling that is noticeably white (*alba*). The actual condition so designated is marked by macules or patches of fine scaliness on faintly erythematous bases. The face is a common site of the process. Cause is unknown but some hold that the condition is streptogenous impetigo and others that it is a variant of atopic dermatitis.

pityriasis folliculorum is a facial eruption attributed to Demodex mites and also known as demodicidosis. There is facial erythema and follicular scaling, giving a "frosted" appearance and rough texture. May give the skin a sandpaper-like texture. (Dominey et al; Bernhard)

pityriasis lichenoides [lĭ′kə-noi′dēz] describes a condition (-*iasis*) as branny (*pityr-*) and like (-*oides*) grouped papules (*lichen-*) morphologically. The condition is related to the parapsoriases.

pityriasis lichenoides et varioliformis acuta [văr′ē-, văr′ĭ-ō-lĭ-fôr′mĭs ə-kū′tə] is a designation made up of elements first used by Mucha and later Habermann for the condition more commonly designated as *parapsoriasis acuta et varioliformis* and classed among the necrotizing angiitides. Also known as PLEVA.

pityriasis rosea [rō′zē-ə] is a title meaning a finely scaling condition (*pityriasis*) that is rose-red (*rosea*). It is the title of that common condition that occurs epidemically in spring and fall, starts with a solitary oval or circular macule or patch of erythema and scaling (the herald patch) and evolves over a period of two to three weeks into an exanthem of similar lesions that arrange themselves on the trunk and extremities along the lines of cleavage of the skin. A vague prodrome of malaise may precede eruption, and itching is a common symptom in adults; the condition may be asymptomatic in children. The entire course of the condition is roughly two to three weeks to evolve, two to three weeks to stay and two to three weeks to resolve, but as with other conditions that are exceedingly common, great variations occur. In general the condition clears completely, leaving no sequelae.

pityriasis rubra pilaris [rōō′brə pĭ-lā′rĭs, -lä′rĭs, -lär′ĭs] is the title for a finely scaling condition (*pityriasis*) which is red (*rubra*) and in which the lesions are located around the hair (*pilaris*) follicles. In well-developed cases follicular location is best recognized on the distal phalanges of the fingers. On the body the redness and scaling tend to become confluent and on the palms hyperkeratosis rather than fine scaling is to be seen.

pityriasis sicca [sĭk′ə] describes a condition (-*iasis*) of the scalp as a dry (*sicca*) fine scaling (*pityr-*). It is what lay persons call dandruff. It is an extreme of normal desquamation in which scales are abundant and visible on head and shoulders because they accumulate there.

pityriasis versicolor [vûr′sĭ-kō′lôr, vûr′sĭ-kŭl′ĕr, vər′sə-kəl′ər] means a finely scaling condition (*pityriasis*) which changes color (*versicolor*). The condition is more often referred to as *tinea versicolor* and is that exceedingly superficial fungous infection on the chest and back that appears as tan or brown macules in the spring and as white macules later, after sunning. The change of color is more likely owing to the sun-screening action of the fungous colonies on the skin rather than to inhibition of melanogenesis by some product of the fungus.

Pityrosporon, -un [pĭt′ĭ-rō-spō′rŏn, -spôr′ŏn; -rəm] names a genus of fungi whose spores (*-sporon, -um*) are fine like bran (*pityro-*). The endings *-on* and *-um* are Greek and Latin respectively. Compare *Microsporon, -um.*

Pityrosporon orbiculare [ôr-bĭk′ū-lā′rē, -lä′rĕ, -lär′ē] is the name of a species in which the spores are further described as being like small discs (*orbiculare*). The micro-organisms are thought by some to be the cause of tinea versicolor, which, if true, makes *Malassezia furfur* a superfluous designation.

Pityrosporon ovale [ō-vā′lē, -vä′lĕ, -văl′ē] is the name of a species in which the spores are further described as being egg-shaped (*ovale*). The micro-organisms are thought by some—very few—to be the cause of seborrhea capitis and by most to be saprophytic on the scalp.

planopilaris [plā′nō-pĭ-lā′rĭs, -pĭ-lä′rĭs, -pĭ-lär′ĭs] is a New Latin adjectival formation meaning flat and relating to hair. It appears in the title *lichen planopilaris.*

planta, plantae [plăn′tə; plăn′tē, -tī] are respectively the nominative singular and the genitive singular and nominative plural of a Latin noun meaning respectively the sole of the foot, of the sole of the foot and the soles of the feet. The genitive form is sometimes used in *verruca plantae* (of the sole) instead of *plantaris* (pertaining to the sole).

plantar, plantare, plantaris [plăn′tēr, -tər; plăn-tā′rē, -tä′rĕ, -tär′ē; -tā′rĭs, -tä′rĭs, -tär′ĭs] are respectively an English adjective, the neuter singular and the masculine or feminine singular of a Latin adjective meaning pertaining or relating to the sole of the foot. The Latin forms appear in titles like *keratoderma palmare et plantare* (neuter) and *verruca plantaris* (feminine).

plantar wart [wôrt] specifies a wart on the sole of the foot. Since *plantar* and *planter* sound alike, some persons make the mistake of saying "planter's wort" as though there were something agricultural or occupational about it (an example of folk etymology).

planus [plā′nəs, plä′nōōs] is the masculine singular of a Latin adjective meaning flat. It appears in the title *lichen planus.*

plaque [plăk, pläk] derives via French through Dutch from a word meaning a slab or flat piece of wood. A common mistake in spelling is to insert a *c* in front of the *q*—but, and alas, Webster's Third enters *placque* as an alternate without comment! The Oxford English Dictionary also gives *placque* as a variant without explanation. It was that way in Old French, but is not so in modern French. The Dutch have it as *placke*. At best, *placque* is archaic.

plasmacytoma, plasmocytoma [plăz′mə-sī-tō′mə; plăz′mō-sī-tō′mə] means a massing (*-oma*) or infiltration with plasma cells. The infiltration is not so massive or tumorous as *-oma* usually implies. Such infiltrations are known to occur in extramedullary sites in *multiple myeloma*, in some infectious diseases like syphilis and "idiopathically" on sites like the genitalia.

platyonychia [plăt′ĭ-ō-nĭk′ē-ə, -ĭ-ə] is a New Latin formation from Greek word elements meaning a condition (*-ia*) of excessively broad (*platy-*) nails (*-onych-*).

plexiform neuroma [plĕk′sĭ-fôrm nōō-rō′mə] describes neural hyperplasia (*neuroma*) as an interwoven, intertwined, or plaited (*plexiform*) structure. The term is used to designate subcutaneous neurofibromas that reveal themselves as discrete nodules along peripheral nerves in neurofibromatosis.

Plummer-Vinson syndrome is a combination of microcytic anemia, dysphagia and glossitis, seen almost entirely in middle-aged women. Koilonychia, "spoon-shaped nails," is frequently present. The skin is dry and wrinkled. The syndrome is precancerous (mouth and upper respiratory tract). The dietary deficiency is probably in iron. (Andrews)

pluriorificialis [plōō′rē-ō′rē-, plōōr′ĭ-ō-rī-fĭsh′ĭ-ā-lĭs, -ē-ä′lĭs, -ăl′ĭs] is a New Latin formation meaning relating to (*-alis*) many (*pluri-*) openings (*-orifici-*), i.e., oral, anal, genital, etc. It appears in a title like *ectodermosis erosiva pluriorificialis*.

pock [pŏk] derives from Middle English *pokke*, a pustule. In modern use, the scars of pustules of viral diseases, particularly smallpox and chicken pox, are termed *pocks* or *pock marks*. See *pox* for a related word.

-poesis, -poiesis, -poetic, -poietic [pō-ē′sĭs; poi-ē′sĭs; pō-ĕt′ĭk; poi-ĕt′ĭk] are combining forms from original Greek noun and adjectival elements meaning a making (the first two) and related to making (the last two). The first and third forms have been Latinized by the change of *oi* to *o*. We recommend them as simpler to spell and pronounce. The word *poem* is of the same origin meaning a creation and *poesis*, from which we get *poesy*, was used in former times for *poetry*. Examples of words with the combining forms are *hemopo (i)esis* and *erythropo (i)etic*.

poikiloderm(i)a [poi′kĭ-lō-dûr′mə, -dûr′mē-ə, -mĭ-ə] is a New Latin formation from Greek elements meaning a dappled variegated or multicolored (*poikilo-*) condition of the skin (*-derma, -dermia*).

poikiloderma atrophicans vasculare this is erythema with slight superficial scaling, a mottled pigmentation and telangiectases. Late stages resemble chronic radiodermatitis. This disease can be seen with some genodermatoses, i.e., Bloom's syndrome, dyskeratosis congenita, as an early stage of mycosis fungoides; and in association with dermatomyositis and occasionally with lupus erythematosis. (Lever)

poikiloderma congenitale [kŏn-jĕn′ĭ-tā′lē, -tä′lē, -tăl′ē] bespeaks a condition in which a dappled, variegated or multicolored (*poikilo-*) condition of the skin (*-derma*) appears at or shortly after birth (*congenitale*). The condition is also called *Thompson's syndrome.*

poikiloderm(i)a vasculare (vascularis) atrophicans [vās′kū-lā′rē, -lä′rē, -lär′ē (văs′kū-lā′rĭs) ə-trŏf′ĭ-kănz, -trō′fĭ-kănz] designates a dappled, variegated or multicolored (*poikilo-*) appearance of the skin (*-derma, -dermia*) that results from changes in the small vessels (*vasculare, vascularis*) in the form of dilatations and telangiectasia and tends to atrophy (*atrophicans*) and depigmentation. The condition has a strong resemblance to many other conditions in which small blood vessels are affected in the same way, particularly radiodermatitis. When not clearly any of those other conditions, the eventuation is frequently lymphomatous.

poikilodermatomyositis [poi′kĭ-lō-dûr′mə-tō-mī′ō-sī′tĭs, -sē′tĭs] is a longer title for *dermatomyositis*, which specifies the dappled, variegated or multicolored (*poikilo-*) condition of the skin in that disease.

poison ivy, oak, sumac(h) dermatitis [poi′z'n ī′vē, ōk, sōō′măk dûr′mə-tī′tĭs, -tē′tĭs] are common designations for allergic contact dermatitis caused by sensitization to and evocation by allergenic principles in and on the leaves, stems and roots of the plants all mediated - delayed type hypersensitivity dermatitis. Those principles are of the chemical nature of catechols which are relatively simple, i.e., nonproteinous substances. We advise against titles of this type; we think it is better to use long titles like *allergic contact dermatitis caused by poison ivy, oak or sumac (h)*. Finally, "poison" is a misleading and ineradicable designation that persists even in the botanical terminology of *Rhus toxicodendron*. Nothing in the plants is a primary irritant or an inherent poison in ordinary concentrations.

poliosis [pŏl′ē-, pŏl′ĭ-ō′sĭs] is a New Latin formation from Greek word elements meaning a condition (-*osis*) of grayness (*poli-*). Grayness of the hair is meant.

poliosis circumscripta [sûr′kəm-skrĭp′tə] describes gray hair in a limited area (*circumscripta*) of the scalp.

poly- [pŏl′ĭ, -ē] is a combining form from Greek meaning many, more, much, often, abounding in, very.

polyarteritis nodosa [pŏl′ē-, pŏl′ĭ-är-tə-rī′tĭs, -rē′tĭs nō-dō′sə] is the title of a disease (-*itis*) which is characterized by multiple (*poly-*) knots (*nodosa*) of inflammation in arterial walls. The skin sometimes has palpable nodules but general symptomatology depends on considerable involvement of organs like the kidneys, heart and other visceral organs with small functional reserve. *Periarteritis nodosa* is alternate.

polydactylia [pŏl′ē-, pŏl′ĭ-dăk-tĭl′ē-ə, -ĭ-ə] is a New Latin formation from Greek word elements meaning a condition (-*ia*) of having more (*poly-*) fingers and toes (-*dactyl-*) than normal.

polymastia [pŏl′ē-, pŏl′ĭ-măs′tē-ə, -tĭ-ə] is a New Latin formation from Greek elements meaning a condition (-*ia*) of having more (*poly-*) breasts (-*mast-*) than normal i.e., supernumerary breasts (polymastia).

polymorphic, -ous [pŏl′ē-, pŏl′ĭ-môr′fĭk; -fəs] are adjectives meaning of many (*poly-*) forms (-*morphic, -ous*).

polymorphic, -ous light eruption [līt, ē-rŭp′shən] are designations for a dermatosis that is precipitated by light exposure, particularly sunlight, upon the skin. The implication is that the induced lesions may be of many forms, namely, erythematous, papular, lichenified, plaque-like, vesicular or pigmented. The commonest clinical appearance is much like discoid or disseminated lupus erythematosus but pictures like those of lichen planus and porphyria cutanea tarda are also known. The precise mechanisms by which electromagnetic energy of certain wave lengths incites the cutaneous effects are not settled. Some skin changes seem to be due to conversion of ingested drugs into allergenic materials followed by sensitization to them and then allergic eczematous dermatitis (photo-allergy); others result from conversion of drugs into primary irritant materials with resultant phototoxicity.

polythelia [pŏl′ē, pŏl′ĭ-thē′lē-ə, -lĭ-ə] is a New Latin formation from Greek elements meaning a condition (-*ia*) of having more (*poly-*) nipples (-*thel-*) than normal.

pomade [pō-mād′, pō-mäd′] derives via French and Italian from Latin *pomum*, apple. It has come to mean an elegant, perfumed unguent. Materials to dress the hair of the scalp and grease the lips of the mouth are commonly designated as pomades.

pompholyx [pŏm′fō-līks] derives from a Greek word meaning bubble. The word is now used to designate a vesicular eruption of the hands and sometimes of the feet. The condition is thought to be caused by a fault of sweating. In those instances where the content of the vesicles is acid in reaction, relation to dyshidrosis, which as a word is also used as an alternate designation, is likely. In other instances, where the vesicular content is alkaline in reaction, allergic eczematous dermatitis, dermatophytid, pustular psoriasis and superficial pyoderma are more likely diagnoses.

porcupine disease, boy, man [pôr′kū-pīn dī-, dəzēz′, boi, măn] are lay terms for ichthyosis hystrix and a sufferer therefrom.

pore [pōr, pôr] derives via French from Greek and Latin words meaning a passage. Of the two passages in the skin, the opening of the sweat duct is commonly referred to as the pore whereas the opening of the pilosebaceous apparatus is termed *ostium*.

porokeratosis [pŏr′ō-, pôr′ō-, pō′rō-kĕr′ə-tō′sĭs] literally means a condition (*osis*) marked by cornification (-*kerat*-) around pores. Further distinguished by the eponym *of Mibelli*, a rare atrophy that begins with hyperkeratosis about sweat pores and spreads centrifugally is designated. *Keratoderm (i)a eccentricum (-ca)* are alternate titles.

poroma [pə-, pō-, pô-rō′mə] is a New Latin formation from Greek word elements for epidermal neoplasia (-*oma*) in the region of the eccrine pore. See *eccrine poroma*. *Periporoma* would have been better coinage.

porphyria [pôr-fīr′ē-ə, -ĭ-ə] is generic for conditions (-*ia*) resulting from abnormalities of prophyrin metabolism. This represents a group of metabolic diseases of porphyrin metabolism due to the abnormal accumulation of porphyrins or one of their precursors, i.e., delta-aminolevulinic acid or porphobilinogen, causing neurological and cutaneous tissue damage. There are both hereditary and acquired forms of these important diseases. These must be separated from porphyrinuria which is not pathological. The most commonly encountered skin disease in this group by far is PCT or *porphyria cutanea tarda*.

porphyria cutanea tarda [kū-tā′nē-ə tär′də] designates a characteristic condition of the skin (*cutanea*) that appears late or slowly (*tarda*) and is dependent on abnormality of porphyrin metabolism (*porphyria*). Bullae and their consequences (crusting), sclerodermatous changes, hypertrichosis and hypermelanosis on exposed skin, discoloration of teeth and increased excretion of uroporphyrins are marks of the condition. By far the most common of the porphyrias. Symptomatic porphyria, one of the hepatic porphyrias. Seen mainly in alcoholics and other patients with liver disease. The marked photosensitivity leads to the very characteristic blister formation on the dorsal surface of the hands as these are exposed to light. Blistering may also occur on the feet and elsewhere exposed to light. Milia are commonly seen in areas that have previously blistered. Facial hypertrichosis is common. Due to accumulation of uroporphyrin and coproporphyrins, the urine will fluoresce red with Wood's light.

porphyria, erythropo(i)etic. See *erythropo (i)etic protoporphyria.*

port-wine mark, or **stain** [pôrt-wīn mărk; stān], is a common designation for nevus flammeus in terms of the color of a familiar substance.

positive [pŏz'ə-, pŏz'ĭ-tĭv], in medical contexts, means reactive, productive of something readable and meaningful or definite.

positive reaction [rē-ăk'shən], like *negative reaction,* is a bit of a terminological paradox. We mean by it something that may occur did occur.

posthitis [pŏs-thī'tĭs, -thē'tĭs], from its Greek word elements, means inflammation (-*itis*) of the prepuce (*posth-*).

poultice [pōl'tĭs] goes back to the Latin word *puls* (or its plural, *pultes,* considered as a collective singular) meaning a thick pap or porridge made of meal or pulse, i.e., edible seeds. A poultice, then, is a pap or porridge originally, and perhaps still, made of cooked seeds (like flaxseeds) and more often, in days recently gone by, of bread, bran or other organic material. The preparation was then used not to eat but to heat. Even inorganic materials like clay may be used provided that retention and delivery of heat are insured. However made, a poultice is an old-fashioned material and the method of delivering heat by bagging and laying on a mess is hardly ever practiced when hot water and ancillary gadgets are more freely available. It is well, nevertheless, to recall the ingenuity of therapists of bygone days and to remember it when electic power is blacked out, for then our vaunted modernity reverts to an ice age.

powder [pou'dĕr], as a pharmaceutical agent, designates a material in fine particulate form.

pox [pŏks] is plural in form but singular in modern sense. A condition of pustules terminating in scars is a pox. *Smallpox, chicken pox* and *cowpox* contain the word; syphilis was sometimes called *the great pox*. See *pock.*

P.P.D. is acronymic for purified protein derivative, a tuberculin.

pratensis [prä-, pră-, prə-těn'sĭs] is a Latin adjective meaning found or growing in a meadow. It appears in the title *dermatitis pratensis striata* where it has a special and extended meaning of caused by plants growing in a meadow.

Prausnitz-Kuestner reaction [prows'nĭts; kĭst'něr]. Response of the skin prepared with foreign antibody to deposition of corresponding antigen.

Prausnitz-Kuestner test [prou'snĭts-kōōst'něr těst] is eponymic for passive transfer testing for immediate (urticarial) reactivity.

pre- [prē] derives from *prae, prae-,* a Latin preposition and prefix meaning before, previous, greater and many.

precancer, precancerous [prē-kăn'sěr; prē-kăn'sěr-əs] are convenient neologisms to designate and describe processes that have strong likelihood to turn into malignancies. Severe burn scars, particularly from gamma rays, actinic and senile keratoses and leukoplakia are examples of precancers or precancerous processes.

prematura [prē'mə-tū'rə, -mä-tōō'rə] and **premature** [prě'-, prē'mə-tūr', -chōōr'] are respectively the feminine singular of a Latin adjective (with *prae-* written as *pre-*) and an English adjective meaning before maturity or full growth. The Latin adjective appears in the title *alopecia prematura.*

"pre-mycotic" [prē'mī-kŏt'ĭk] has nothing to do with fungi or fungous infections. For want of better, the skin changes that precede mycosis fungoides (another misleading designation), before that T cell lymphoma can be or has been undisputably diagnosed, are termed "pre-mycotic."

pretibial myxedema [prē-tĭb'ē-əl, -ĭ-əl mĭk'sə-, mĭk'sē-dē'mə]. By this title the common location of the process is specified. See *myxedema, circumscribed.*

prickle [prĭk'l] derives from Anglo-Saxon *pricel,* diminutive of *prica,* a point or dot.

prickle cell is descriptive of some of the morphology of an epidermal cell of the Malpighian layer as seen under the conventional light microscope. The intercellular "bridges" that appear "spinous" suggest prickles.

prickle-cell carcinoma [kär′sĭ-nō′mə], or **epithelioma** [ĕ′pĭ-thē′lē-ō′mə, -lĭ-ō′mə], bespeaks malignant, neoplastic development of prickle cells. *Squamous-cell carcinoma* or *epithelioma* is alternate.

prickly heat [prĭk′lē, -lĭ hēt] is a homely title for miliaria rubra. It has the virtue of calling to mind an important cause (heat) and an important symptom (prickling).

primary [prī′mə-rē, -mĕr-ē, mĕr-ē, -ĭ] means first or initial, but in some contexts acquires shades of meaning of only, sole, idiopathic or *sui generis*. The entries below illustrate the fine differences.

primary atrophy [ăt′rō-, ăt′rə-fē, -fĭ] describes diminution of substance as the first and only discernible manifestation of a process.

primary complex [kŏm′plĕks]. When the skin is the usual portal of entry of certain micro-organisms or is made so although it is not usual, a train of local changes occurs which is termed the *primary complex*. The development of the chancres of syphilis, tuberculosis and cowpox are familiar examples; those of deep mycoses like sporotrichosis and blastomycosis and that of cutaneous leishmaniasis are less familiar but equally representative. The sequence of events is inoculation, incubation period (one to three weeks of no grossly evident change) and then chancre development beginning with erythema at the point of inoculation and more or less rapid transition of edema, papulation, vesiculation, pustulation and ulceration to eventual scarring. The entire process may be a matter of a month for cowpox, two to three to four to six months for syphilis, tuberculosis and the deep mycoses and to a year for cutaneous leishmaniasis.

primary irritant dermatitis. See *dermatitis, primary irritant.*

primary lesion. See *lesion, primary.*

primary syphilis [sĭf′ĭ-lĭs] is applied to the first stage and first discernible signs of the disease, mainly its primary complex (the chancre).

prion (slow viruses). Novel infectious pathogens, i.e., small proteinaceous infectious particles which resist inactivation by procedures that modify nucleic acids. (Prusiner)

pro, pro- [prō] are both a Greek and a Latin preposition and prefix meaning before, in front of, premature, forward, outward, etc. The prefix may also have intensive force.

profunda [prō-fŭn′də, -fōōn′də] and **profundus** [prō-fŭn′dəs, -fōōn′dŭs] are respectively the feminine singular and the masculine singular of a Latin adjective meaning deep. They appear in the titles *miliaria profunda* and *lupus erythematosus profundus*.

progenitalis [prō′jĕn′ĭ-tā′lĭs, -tä′lĭs, -tăl′ĭs] is the masculine or feminine singular of a New Latin adjective meaning on, upon the front, i.e., external (*pro-*) part of the genitalia (*-genitalis*). It appears in a title like *herpes progenitalis.*

progeria [prō-jē′rē-ə, -rĭ-ə] is a New Latin noun formed from Greek word elements meaning a condition (*-ia*) of premature (*pro-*) old age (*-ger-*).

progeria (Hutchinson-Gilford) [hŭtch′ĭn-sŭn-gĭl′fôrd] is a complex congenital anomaly which is a mixture of immaturity of some organs and tissues and degeneration of others. The result is a homunculus with the wizened appearance not merely of an old man but of a very old man.

progressiva [prō′grĕs-ī′və] and **progressive** [prō-grĕs′ĭv] are respectively the feminine singular of a New Latin adjective and an English adjective meaning going forward. The New Latin adjective appears in the title *granulomatosis disciformis chronica et progressiva.*

prosector's wart [prō-sĕk′tôrz, -tərz wôrt]. A prosector is one who (*-or*) prepares by dissection (*prosect-*, from *prosecare*, to cut up) anatomical specimens for demonstration. *Prosector* is not a word of New Latin or modern coinage; it goes back to Tertullian, a great church writer of the second century A.D., and as a Latin word it means a cutter-up, an anatomist. The wart referred to is a consequence of accidental contamination with tubercle bacilli in the process. See *necrogenic tubercle* for a fuller explanation. *Anatomic tubercle,* or *wart,* is alternate.

protein-purified derivative [prō′tē-ĭn-, -tēn-pū′rĭ-fīd də-, dē-rĭv′ə-tĭv] is a tuberculin processed from cultures of tubercle bacilli in a manner that yields a product of high protein content. See *P.P.D.*

proto-porphyria, erythropo(i)etic. See *erythropo(i)etic proto- porphyria.*

Protozoa [prōt′ə-, prō′tō-zō′ə] is a New Latin plural noun formed from Greek elements meaning first or primordial (*proto-*) living things (*-zoa,* plural of *zoon*). It is sometimes used with a small initial letter, as if it were a singular, like *protozoon* [prō′tō-zō′ŏn, -ən], for a one-celled creature. The practice is not recommended.

protuberans [prō-tū′bĕr-ănz, -tōō′bĕr-ănz, -bə-rănz] is a Latin present participle meaning swelling (*-tuberans*) forward or outward (*pro-*). It appears in the title *dermatofibrosarcoma protuberans.*

proud flesh [proud flĕsh] is a nontechnical, metaphorical or quasi-poetic term for granulation tissue so exuberant that it grows above the level of the circumscribing epithelium before it can be covered by that modestly advancing tissue. Lay persons sometimes use the term for a keloid or a hypertrophic scar.

pruriginous [proo-rĭj′ĭ-nəs] is the adjective from *prurigo* meaning full of (*-ous*) itching (*prurigin-*).

prurigo [proo-rī′gō] is a Latin word for itching. It is used in titles, as in the following entries.

prurigo (a)estivalis [ēs′-, ĕs′tĭ-vā′lĭs, -vä′lĭs, -văl′ĭs] means summer (*aestivalis*) itch (*prurigo*). A poorly defined condition of xerosis and pruritus apparently related to the heat of the summer season is so designated. *Pruritus (a)estivalis* is alternate.

prurigo hiemalis [hē′ə-, hē′ĕ-, hī′ē-mā′lĭs, -mä′lĭs, -măl′ĭs] means winter (*hiemalis*) itch (*prurigo*). A poorly defined condition of xerosis and pruritus related to the rigors of the winter season is meant. *Pruritus hiemalis* is alternate.

prurigo nodularis [nŏd′ū-lā′rĭs, -lä′rĭs, -lăr′ĭs] describes a dermatosis characterized by nodules (*nodularis*) on the extremities, usually the lower, and itching (*prurigo*).

pruritus [proo-rī′təs] is a Latin word used by Pliny and other for itching. It is one of the most misspelled words in medicine. If medical writers themselves do not misspell it, compositors who think they are being helpful set the word as *pruritis*, which inflames orthographists and causes them to itch and scratch.

pruritus (a)estivalis. See *prurigo (a)estivalis*.

pruritus ani [ā′nī] means itching (*pruritus*) of or about the anus (*ani*). This common title simply announces the symptom and the location. Causes are many and matters for determination in each case.

pruritus scroti [skrō′tī] means itching (*pruritus*) of the scrotum (*scroti*). As for pruritus ani, merely the symptom and location are told; cause remains to be determined in each case.

pruritus vulvae [vŭl′vē] means itching (*pruritus*) of the vulva (*vulvae*). As for pruritus ani and pruritus scroti, the symptom and location are stated; cause is a problem for investigation.

pseudo- [sū′-, soo′dō] is a combining form from Greek meaning false. It is very commonly used in nonce formations; several examples of more permanent uses are given below.

pseudo-acanthosis nigricans [-ăk′ăn-thō′sĭs nī′grĭ-kănz] designates a condition which looks like acanthosis nigricans (which see) but is deemed not true (*pseudo-*) because, whereas the latter is associated with covert or overt internal malignancy, the former is not. The condition seems to be a consequence of obesity.

pseudo-epitheliomatous hyperplasia [ĕp′ĭ-, ĕp′ē-thē′lē-ō′mə-təs, ōm′ə-təs hī′pêr-plā′zhē-ə, -zē-ə, -zhə] designates increased formation (*hyperplasia*) of epithelium that is not true (*pseudo-*) in the sense that it is not malignantly neoplastic, specifically not in the nature of squamous-cell carcinoma. This title would be better as *pseudo-malignant epitheliomatous hyperplasia* because the formation is truly epitheliomatous, merely not truly malignant. Such an appearance is seen in certain long-enduring dermatitides, especially granulomas and ulcerations, and in certain drug eruptions, especially bromodermas and iododermas (halodermas).

pseudofolliculitis barbae is also called sychosis barbae or barber rash, a very common dermatitis among black Africans who shave. It is caused largely by the sharp end of the curly kinky hair which acts like a hook and penetrates the skin after shaving with a razor blade. An inflammatory reaction forms around the penetrating hair to produce distinct erythematous or skin colored papules and occasionally papulo-pustules. It is an inflammatory reaction around a foreign body (ingrown hair). The term pseudo-folliculitis is used because bacteria play a secondary role. (*Regional Dermatoses in the African Race.* Olumide, Odumowo and Odiase, Int. J. Derm. Vol 29, No 9)

pseudolymphoma [sū′, sōō′dō-lĭm-fō′mə] is a term, like *pseudoepitheliomatous hyperplasia* and other false terms, that does not say what is intended. The meaning intended is *pseudomalignant lymphoma*. Clearly there are benign and malignant lymphomas. *Pseudolymphoma* in itself would deny that what is designated by it is a lymphoma at all. The fact is that what is called a *pseudolymphoma* is indeed a lymphoma but merely one that is benign, despite its fearsome histologic appearance of malignancy.

See *Lymphocytoma*. These are benign conditions but histologically look malignant e.g., arthrop bites, lymphomatoid papulosis, actinic reticuloid, Jessner's lymphocytic infiltration of the skin, some drug eruptions, borrelial lymphocytoma and angioimmunoblastic lymphadenopathy. (Lever)

Pseudomonas aeruginosa [sū′dō-mō′nəs, -năs ē-rōō′jĭ-nō′sə] is a species of bacteria which is described as falsely (*pseudo-*) of a unit (*-monas*) and bronze-colored (*aeruginosa*) in culture.

pseudopelade [sū′dō-pə-läd′] names an alopecia that resembles but is not (*pseudo-*) alopecia areata (*-pelade*). It is one of several more or less inflammatory conditions of the scalp skin and scalp hairs that result in loss of hair and scarring, unlike alopecia areata, in which hairs generally regrow and scarring does not result.

pseudoporphyria is a group of bullous photo-sensitive diseases that mimics *porphyria cutanea tarda*. It may also be called drug-induced bullous photosensitivity. (Poh-Fitzpatrick)

pseudosarcomatous fasciitis. See *nodular fasciitis.*

pseudoxanthoma elasticum [sū′dō-zăn-thō′mə ē-lăs′tĭ-kəm] names a condition in which the skin is described as infiltrated with papules or plaques that, as yellowish aggregates resemble, but are not (*pseudo-*), xanthomas. The affected skin is lax but not elastic; *elasticum* refers to defect or deficiency of elastic fibers. The condition is a generalized one. Defect of elastic fibers in the tissues of other organs occurs too; the so-called angioid streaks in the retina are one sign of the phenomenon.

Pseudoxanthoma elasticum (PXE) is a disorder of abnormal calcification of elastic fibers, with characteristic cutaneous lesions, retinopathy and vascular calcification. The primary skin lesions of PXE consist of small 2-5mm, yellow-orange papules of rhomboidal or irregular shape bounded by clinically normal skin. (Neldner, *Clin Dermatol*)

psora [sō′rə] is Greek and Latin for itch and scabies.

psoriasiform [sō′rī-ăs′ĭ-fôrm] means like or in the shape of (*-form*) psoriasis.

psoriasis [sō-, sə-rī′ə-sĭs] is New Latin from Greek word elements meaning a condition (*-iasis*) of itching (*psor-*). Of course, the modern application of the word has little to do with itch. What is designated is that common, scaly, intractable, stubborn, recalcitrant condition that comes, stays or goes unpredictably and that may be one insignificant spot, many patches or a generalized exfoliative erythroderma. Need we say its cause is unknown and it is generally difficult to treat?

psoriasis, pustular. See *pustular psoriasis.*

psoriatic [sō′rē-ăt′ĭk] is an adjective meaning pertaining to, relating to or affected with psoriasis.

psoriatic arthropathy. See under *arthopathia, arthropathic* and *arthropathy.*

pubes [pū′bēz] and **pubis** [pū′bĭs] are respectively the nominative singular and the genitive singular of the Latin word for that portion of the genital area that is covered with hair. In classical Latin, among other meanings it referred to the hair that appears on the body as a sign of puberty. The genitive form appears in a title like *pediculosis pubis*.

pubic louse [pū′bĭk lous] is a simple designation for *Phthir (i)us pubis*. *Crab louse* is an alternate.

pudoris [pōō-, pū-dō′rĭs, -dôr′ĭs] is the genitive singular of the Latin noun *pudor* and means of shame or modesty. It appears in the title *erythema pudoris*.

Pulex [pū′lĕks] is Latin for a flea. The word names a genus of fleas.

Pulex irritans [ĭr′ĭ-tănz] is the species of fleas that commonly attack human beings. It need hardly be remarked that the bite of fleas is irritating.

pulicosis [pū′lĭ-kō′sĭs] designates the condition (*-osis*) of having flea (*pulic-*) bites.

punch [pŭnch] is a word of uncertain origin. It may derive from Middle English *puncheon*, which may come from Vulgar Latin *punctio*, a pointed tool, derived in turn from classical Latin *pungere*, to prick. In any event, we use the word for a surgical instrument that cores out material in a disc by rotation of its sharp circular edge.

punch biopsy [bī′əp-, bī-ŏp′sē, -sī] is a term used for the procedure of using a punch in surgery and the specimen obtained thereby.

punctata [pŭngk-tā′tə, -tä′tə], **punctate** [pŭngk′tāt], **punctatum** [pŭngk-tā′təm, -tä′tŭm], **punctum** [pŭngk′təm, -tŭm], **puncture** [pŭngk′chĕr] are words ultimately derived from Latin *punctus*, perfect passive participle of *pungere*, to prick, to pierce into like a point. *Punctata* (feminine singular), *punctate* (an English derivative) and *punctatum* (neuter singular) derive more immediately from a Medieval Latin derivative of *punctus*—*punctare*, to work with a point or dot. Therefore, *punctata, punctate* and *punctatum* mean pointed, characterized by pointedness, pittedness, or marked with dots. *Punctum* (plural, *puncta*) is classical Latin and means a point; *puncture,* as a noun, means a wound caused by a pointed instrument, and, as a verb, it means to prick.

The classicized adjectives appear in titles like *keratoderma punctatum* (neuter) and *keratodermia punctata* (feminine).

purpura [pər′-, pûr′pū-rə] is a Latin noun meaning the color purple. We use the word exclusively for that purplish discoloration that results from hemorrhage into a tissue and with modifying words as a title for simple and complex conditions resulting from hemorrhage into tissues.

purpura annularis telangiectodes [ăn′ū-lā′rĭs, -lä′rĭs, -lăr′ĭs tĕl-ăn′jĭ-ĕk-tō′dēz] describes a condition in which purplishness (*purpura*) from hemorrhage into skin takes the form of circular (*annularis*) lesions and which is further marked by what appears to be dilatation of small end vessels or new formation of small end vessels (*telangiectodes*).

purpura, Henoch-Schoenlein [hĕn′ŏk-shûn′līn] is eponymic for a type of purpura that is also attended by episodic systemic symptoms. Araphylactoid purpura, a systemic necrotizing vasculitis of small vessels. All patients develop palpable purpura on the lower extremities and buttocks. Cause unknown, presumed to be immunologic.

purpura, nonthrombocytopenic, thrombocytopenic [nŏn-, thrŏm′bō-sī′tō-pē′nĭk] respectively describe purplishness (*purpura*) from hemorrhage in the skin that is not attended by diminution or lack of thrombocytes (*nonthrombocytopenic*) or is so attended (*thrombocytopenic*).

purpura simplex [sĭm′plĕks] describes purplishness (*purpura*) from hemorrhage in the skin that is not complicated (*simplex*) by hematologic or other subtleties.

purpuric [pər-, pûr-pū′rĭk] is an adjective meaning pertaining or relating to purpura.

pus [pŭs] is a Latin word. The gross material is well-known as more or less turbid and viscous fluid of gray-green-yellow color. Microscopically, leukocytes, necrotic tissue and micro-organisms (when the process is infectious) can be seen as solid elements within a soup of edema.

pustular [pŭs′tū-lĕr, -lər] is an adjective meaning pertaining or relating to pustules.

pustular acne. See *acne pustulosa*.

pustular bacterid. See under *bacterid*.

pustular psoriasis [sō-, sə-rī′ə-sĭs] is the title for a form or variant of psoriasis in which pustules are a prominent feature. When the appearance is seen in indubitable plaques of psoriasis there is no question of nosology but when recalcitrant and recurrent pustules of the same order appear, especially on palms and soles, with no other signs of psoriasis elsewhere, some dispute the title and relationship to psoriasis.

pustule [pŭs′tūl] is an elevated lesion on the skin that has a content which is appreciably purulent. Since the word has a suffix of diminution (-*ule*), lesions of a size up to one centimeter are reasonably designated as *pustules*; lesions of larger size are better designated as *boils, abscesses* or *furuncles*.

pustulosa [pŭs′tū-lō′sə] is the feminine singular of a Latin adjective (used by Celsus) meaning full of (-*osa*) pustules (*pustul-*). It appears in the titles *acne pustulosa, acrodermatitis pustulosa* and *miliaria pustulosa*.

pustulosis [pŭs′tū-lō′sĭs] is a generic word for any condition (-*osis*) characterized by pustules.

pustulosis palmoplantaris is a chronic skin disease of unknown etiology which occurs mainly in women and is characterized by recurrent crops of yellow pustules, erythema, and desquamation on the palms and soles. Symptoms usually appear in the fifth or sixth decade. (Rosen et al, Journal of American Academy of Dermatology Vol 19, No. 6)

Pyemotes [pī′ə-mō′tēz] is the name of a genus of mites. The derivation of the word baffles etymologists because Amerling, who coined it, left no record of what word elements he used when he concocted it.

    Pyemotes ventricosus is modern terminology for *Pediculoides ventricosus* (which see).

pyo- [pī′ō] is a combining form from Greek *pyon*, pus.

pyoderma. Group A streptococci may produce localized skin infection, e.g., impetigo or more suitable to use its full name, impetigo contagiosa.

pyoderm(i)a [pī′ō-dûr′mə, -mē-ə, -mĭ-ə] is a generic word for a condition of the skin (-*derma, -dermia*) that is marked by purulence (*pyo-*). It is also used with modifying words in titles, of which the following are representative.

    pyoderm(i)a faciale (facialis) [fā′shē-ā′lē, -ā′lĕ, -āl′ē (fā′shē-ā′lĭs, -ā′lĭs, -āl′ĭs)] specifies the location on the face (*faciale, facialis*) of a purulent (*pyo-*) process of the skin (-*derma, -dermia*) which is distinctive in that it is not quite pustular acne nor even clearly an infectious process. Even if it is related to acne and infection, it is still distinctive in its local severity and relative recalcitrance to treatment designed for those banal conditions.

    pyoderm(i)a gangrenosum (gangrenosa) [găn(g)′grə-, găn(g)′grē-nō′səm (-sə)] is a highly characteristic purulent (*pyo-*)

condition of the skin (*-derma, -dermia*) which results in ulceration (*gangrenosum, gangrenosa*). It is commonly seen in ulcerative colitis, other severe enteritides and pyogenic infections of viscera, and sometimes as a condition apparently *sui generis* although of unaccountable cause.

pyoderm(i)a vegetans [vĕj′ē-tănz] designates a condition in which purulence (*pyo-*) of the skin (*-derma, -dermia*) is further marked by exuberant (*vegetans*) growth crisscrossed by sinuses and points of issue of pus.

pyogenic [pī′ō-jĕn′ĭk] and **pyogenicum** [-ĭ-kəm] are respectively an English adjective and the neuter singular of a New Latin adjective (*-ic, -icum*) meaning giving rise (*-gen-*) to pus (*pyo-*). The English adjective describes micro-organisms that have the ability to cause purulence; the classicized adjective appears in the title *granuloma pyogenicum*.

Q

Q fever [kū fēʹvẽr, -vər] is a self-limited Rickettsial infection disease whose dermatologic sign is exanthematic erythema. The *Q* is said to stand for *query,* i.e., uncertainty of cause now known to be *Coxiella burnetii.* Should be considered in a pt with marked fever where cause can't be found. Diagnosis is by complement-fixation test. Most severe complication is endocarditis. Tetracycline and chloramphenicol are effective for treatment.

quarter-evil, or **-ill** [kwôrʹtər-ēʹvĭl, -vəl, -ĭl], is vernacular for anthrax in animals.

quartz(-)lamp [kwôrtzʹ-lămpʹ] designates an instrument that emits electromagnetic energy of a wide range of wave length. The device that is called a hot quartz-lamp generates emissions that approximately are 50% heat ($>$ 7000 Å), 25% visible light (4000 to 7000 Å) and 25% ultraviolet light (2500 to 3700 Å). The cold quartz-lamp generates a different composition, almost entirely of strong bands of ultraviolet light of the quality of 2570 Å.

Queyrat [kāräʹ], **erythroplasia of.** See under *erythroplasia.* Bowen's disease of the genitalia.

Quincke's disease [kvĭngʹkĕz, kwĭngʹkēz dĭ-, də-zēzʹ]. See *angioneurotic edema.*

Quinke's edema [kvĭngʹkē]. Angioneurotic edema; giant urticaria.

Quinquaud's disease [kăngkōzʹ dĭ-, də-zēzʹ]. See *folliculitis decalvans.*

R

R and **r.** Both the capital and the small letter are used to denote the unit of electromagnetic energy otherwise designated *roentgen.* The last we heard, the capital letter is preferred by radiotherapists.

racket nails [răk'ət, -ĕt, -ĭt nālz] is descriptive of short, broad nails in terms of a commonplace object, namely, the bat used in tennis and badminton. The nails of one or both thumbs, the great toenails and sometimes other nails may show the appearance as a hereditable phenomenon. The word *racket* derives via French (*raquette*) from an Arabic word for the palm of the hand. The equivalent title in French is *ongles en raquette* (which see).

rad [rād] was coined from the first three letters of *radiation* to designate a unit of absorbed dose of ionizing electromagnetic energy, namely, 100 ergs per gram of irradiated material.

radiodermatitis [rā'dē-ō-dûr'mə-tī'tĭs, -tē-tĭs] designates all degrees of inflammation of the skin (*-dermatitis*) resulting from excessive exposure to electromagnetic energy of wave lengths that are less than 2 Å (radium, X or gamma rays). The effects on the skin vary with the quality and quantity of that radiation, with the period of time over which delivery occurs and with the size of the area irradiated. Many exposures to small amounts of radiation over weeks, months or years to total doses of more than about 1500 roentgens tend to result in pigmentation, telangiectasia, keratoses and epitheliomatous changes of cancerous nature years later (chronic radiodermatitis).

ragweed dermatitis [răg'wēd' dûr'mə-tī'tĭs, -tē'tĭs] is a title like *poison ivy dermatitis,* but this time for allergic contact dermatitis caused by an eczematogenic allergen on the pollen of the ragweed plant. The oddity about dermatitis caused by this means is location of the process on the face, neck and arms (sometimes legs) in a pattern determined by the fall of the airborne material onto the skin. There is usually sparing of effect under the nose and chin because these areas are sheltered, and some extension of the process onto shoulders, chest and legs because a sort of chimney effect of clothes carries pollen to these places. The allergen is an oleoresin different from the protein fraction that is the cause of seasonal rhinitis, and sensitization to it does not depend upon a predisposing atopic habitus.

ranula [răn′ū-lə], deriving from Latin, literally means a little (*-ula*) frog (*ran-*). We use the word to designate a cyst on the mucous membranes of the mouth. *Mucocele, mucous cyst* and *retention cyst* are alternate terms.

rash [răsh] is a word of dubious origin. It may derive via Old French *ra* (*s*)*che*, eruption, from Latin *radere*, to scratch, and *rasus*, scraped. If so, *abrade* and *abrasion* are related to it. In any event, the word is used, more by the laity but often enough by the dermatologic cognoscenti, for an eruption on the skin. There is a sense of sudden appearance and severity of process in the word. One frequently hears it as *skin rash*, which is needlessly explicative.

rat-bite fevers. Diseases caused by *Streptobacillus moniliformis* or *Spirillum minus*. These are Gram-negative rods found in mice and rats and other animals. Lab workers are especially at risk for these diseases.

   A few days after a rat bite patient develops sudden fever (Haverhill fever) and toxic symptoms. Most will develop a maculopapular rash within the first week. About two-thirds of the patients will develop arthritis and other systemic problems occur such as pericarditis and abscesses, etc. Spirillary fever (Sodoku)

Raynaud′s disease and **phenomenon** [rānōz′ dĭ-, də-zēz′; fə-nŏm′ə-nŏn] are eponymic for an angioneurosis that appears as stark blanching of digits upon exposure of them to ordinarily tolerable cold. Pallor or cyanosis and dysesthesia of the digits paroxysmally in response to cold as a disease per se or as part of other disorders like scleroderma.

reaction [rē-ăk′shən] means response, a detectable event related to something antecedent.

reactive perforating collagenosis. Altered collagen is eliminated through the epidermis, may be secondary to trauma, i.e., often from intense pruritus seen in diabetes mellitus, renal failure and lymphoma.

reagin [rē′ă-jĭn] is a word formed from the first four letters of *reagent* plus *-in*, an agent, all of which makes it mean reagent all over again. The intent of this coinage is to specify, by the new word, reacting substances in body fluids, particularly blood, that are involved in the Wassermann and related tests for syphilis, and in seasonal rhinitis, sensitization asthma and related atopic states. The substances involved are not clearly delineated but are believed to be in the nature of antibodies and, in the case of atopic states, immunoglobulins of the IgE variety.

Recklinghausen's, (von), disease [rĕk′lĭng-hou′zĕnz, -zənz (fŭn, vŏn) dĭ-, də-zēz′]. See under *neurofibromatosis.*

recurrens [rē-kûr′-, rē-kŭr′ĕnz] and **recurrent** [rē-kûr′ənt] are respectively a Latin present participle used as an adjective and an English derivative meaning returning, happening again (*re-*). The Latin form appears in the titles *herpes simplex recurrens* and *periadenitis mucosae necrotica recurrens*; the English adjective appears in a title like *recurrent urticaria.*

"red man" syndrome refers to exfoliative dermatitis, universal erythroderma. May have any one of a number of causes from benign i.e., psoriasis, atopic dermatitis, drugs- to malignant, Hodgkin's disease and malignant lymphomas.

Serious disorder requiring prompt treatment which is usually hospitalization. (*Andrews' Diseases of the Skin*, 8th Ed., Arnold, Odom, James, W.B. Saunders Co.)

Refsum's syndrome. Autosomal recessive, generalized ichthyosis, cerebellar ataxia, progressive paresis of the extremities, and retinitis pigmentosa. Histopathology: hyperkeratosis, hypergranulosis and acanthosis; vacuoles in the basal and suprabasal cells; when stained for lipids, show their build up. (Davies et al; Lever) Histogenesis: primary metabolic defect is an accumulation of phytanic acid which results from a deficiency of alpha-phytanic acid alpha hydroxylase. (Rand & Baden)

Reiter's disease [rī′tĕrz dĭ-, də-zēz′] is eponymic for a rupial and psoriasiform dermatosis. Hyperkeratosis, conjunctivitis, urethritis, and arthritis related to gonorrheal and other microbial infection. See *keratoderma blennorrhagicum.*

Consists of urethritis, conjunctivitis and arthritis. Only onethird of patients present with the full triad. Reiter's may therefore be an episode of arthropathy within a month of urethritis or cervicitis. Additional findings may be mucocutaneous lesions such as keratodermia blennorrhagica, circinate balanitis, achilles tendonitis and plantar fasciitis. Skin findings are important and often striking.

Usually divided into two forms, endemic and epidemic. Endemic or postvenereal Reiter's is more prevalent in young males and is associated with chlamydial and mycoplasmal infections. By contrast the epidemic or postdysenteric form occurs with equal prevalence among men and women and is associated with Shigella, Salmonella, Yersinia and Campylobactera infections.

This is a seronegative arthropathy. 80% of Caucasian patients with Reiter's syndrome possess the HLA-B27 genetic marker. Usually ESR, CPR and IgA levels are elevated but may be normal. ANA and rheumatoid factor are both negative. See *keratoderm (i)a blennorrhagicum (-ca)*.

relapsing febrile nodular nonsuppurative panniculitis (Weber-Christian disease). Rare, recurrent, inflammatory nodules in adipose tissue. The microscopic features include fat necrosis, variable degrees of infiltration by lymphocytes, plasma cells and macrophages. Some perivasculitis and foreign body giant cells are not uncommon. The diagnosis is tentative unless there are documented remissions and exacerbations, showing phagocytosis of subcutaneous fat cells by macrophages.

Rendu-Osler-Weber disease [rängdōō′-ōs′lĕr-vā′bĕr, -wĕb′ ĕr dĭ-, də-zēz′]. See *Osler's disease*.

repens [rō′pĕnz, rĕp′ənz] is a Latin present participle used as an adjective and meaning creeping. It appears in the title *dermatitis repens*.

rete [rē′tē] is a Latin word for a net.

rete pegs, ridges [pĕgz, rĭj′əz, -′z, -ĭz] are descriptive of the appearance of the epidermis at the dermo-epidermal junction as seen in vertical sections of conventional histologic preparations. That appearance is likened to a network of stakes (*pegs*) or stripes (*ridges*). However, it is an illusion. Tridimensionally, the epidermis meets the papillary part of the corium as cloud and fog meet mountain peaks, i.e., the epidermis caps the papillae and fills in the "valleys" between them.

retention cyst [rē-tĕn′shən sĭst] is a simple designation for a cyst of a mucous gland. It is too simple. *Mucocele, mucous cyst* and *ranula* are alternate terms.

reticul-, reticulo- [rē-, rē-tĭk′ūl; -ū-lo] are combining forms from Latin *reticulum*, a little net.

reticular degeneration [rē-tĭk′ū-lĕr dĭ-, də-, dē-jĕn′ ĕr-ā′shən] describes a histologic appearance of epidermal cells in which intracellular edema causes cellular content to become webbed or netted (*reticular*). The phenomenon is seen in the herpes-varicella group of diseases.

reticular erythematous mucinosis (REM). Reticular erythema and dermal mucinosis. A chronic disorder characterized by a sharply marginated bluish-red eruption distributed primarily on the trunk. Appears to be related to photosensitivity. Histopathology shows a perivascular and perifollicular lymphocytic infiltrate. Dermal edema and deposition of alcian blue positive mucin is a hallmark. May be associated with disorders of immune regulation. (Braddock et al, *JAAD*, v. 19, no. 5)

reticularis [rĕ-, rē-tĭk′ū-lā′rĭs, -lä′rĭs, -lär′ĭs] and **reticulata** [rĕ-, rē-tĭk′ū-lā′tə, -lä′tə] are respectively the masculine and feminine singular of a New Latin adjective and the feminine singular of a classical Latin adjective meaning lacy, net-like, netted or webbed. They appear in titles like *pars reticularis* (feminine) and *folliculitis ulerythematosa reticulata*.

reticulin fibers [rĕ-, rē-tĭk′ū-lĭn fī′bĕrz] describes fibers that consist of lacy, netted or webbed (*reticul-*) material (*-in*). This, however, is not what is meant. Apparently *reticulin* is miswritten for *reticulum* because it is not the fiber substance that is netted; rather, the aggregate of the fibers comprises a webbed system. Perhaps French *réticuline* and Spanish *reticulina* for our *reticulum* sparked the mistake. See *reticulum fibers*.

reticulo-. See *reticul-*.

reticulo-endothelial cell, system [rĕ-, rē-tĭk′ū-lō-ĕn′dō-thē′lē-əl, sĕl, sĭs′təm]. These are terms that designate those cell units and the family of them that have so much to do with immunologic events, phagocytosis and other janitorial activities. Histiocytes in various guises and disguises (plasma cells, mast cells, etc.) derive from this source. As a system, the conception is of a fine network (*reticulo-*) cast in and about lymph and vascular structures and then laced thinly throughout the entire body.

reticulo-endothelioma [rĕ-, rē-tĭk′ū-lō-ĕn′dō-thē-lē′ō-mə] means neoplasia (*-oma*) of reticulo-endothelial cells or of the system as a whole, and of any type, benign or malignant.

reticulo-endotheliosis [rĕ-, rē-tĭk′ū-lō-ĕn′dō-thē′lē-ō′sĭs] means any abnormal condition (*-osis*) of reticulo-endothelial cells or of the system as a whole. Mycosis fungoides, Hodgkin's disease, histiocytosis X and other lymphomatoses of that nature are reticulo-endothelioses.

reticulo-granuloma [rĕ-, rē-tĭk′ū-lō-grăn′ū-lō′mə] is a word proposed to replace *nevoxantho-endothelioma*. It is a questionable improvement. The first word simply says a grain-like mass (*granuloma*) of cells of the reticulo-endothelial system, whereas the other specifies hamartomatous (*nevo-*) quality and yellow (*-xantho-*) color for the clinical lesion. Neither is completely satisfactory.

reticulohistiocytoma [rē-tĭk′ū-lō-hĭs′tĭ-ō-sī-tō′mə] as a word indicates neoplastic proliferation (*-oma*) of histiocytes that are further described as reticulated. Such lesions are known to occur solitarily (*reticulohistiocytic granuloma*) and to be of no serious consequence. There is also another condition called *multicentric reticulohistiocytosis* in which reticulohistiocytomas develop, especially on the dorsa of the hands, as part of a syndrome that may be severe in number of lesions, progression, association with mutilating arthritis, and carcinomatous degeneration. Some cases resolve spontaneously; some halt and stay stationary; a few continue to fatality.

reticulohistiocytosis is divided into two types: the singularly occurring granuloma, and multiple or multicentric reticulohistiocytosis. The granuloma type is usually a single nodule (but that is not absolute) and occurs on the head and neck. They are self-limiting. Multicentric reticulohistiocytosis nodules range from small to large and may coalesce. Is usually associated with arthritis that may be severe from cartilage and bone destruction.

reticulosis [rĕ- rē-tĭk′ū-lō′sĭs] is short for *reticulo-endotheliosis.*

reticulum [rĕ-, rē-tĭk′ū-ləm] is the Latin word for a little net.

reticulum-cell sarcoma [sär-kō′mə] is a reticulo-endothelioma that is used distinctively by some to designate the "tumor phase" of mycosis fungoides in which the cells are of a more uniform type.

reticulum fibers [fī′bērz] designates those fine, thready argyrophilic structures seen in healing wounds, granulomatous lesions and other repair processes of connective tissue. They are thought to be young collagen fibers, and in aggregate appear like a ragged network. They are part of the connective tissue of the dermis.

retiform [rĕt′ĭ-, rē′tĭ-fôrm] means in the shape of (*-form*) a net (*reti-*).

retrovirus group. Well known tumor causing RNA viruses in animals. The first of these viruses proven to cause cancers in humans was the human T-cell leukemia/lymphoma virus I [HTLV-I]. The AIDS virus now known as (HIV-I) human immunodeficiency virus earlier was designated as (HTLV-III.)

rhabdomyoma [răb′dō-mī-ō′mə] is a New Latin formation from Greek elements meaning a tumor or neoplasia (*-oma*) of striated (*rhabdo-*) muscle (*-my-*) elements.

rhagadiform [rə-găd′ĭ-fôrm] means in the shape of (*-form*) a fissure (*rhagadi-*).

rhagas, rhagades [răg′ăs, -əs; răg′ə-dēz] are the singular and plural forms of a Greek word meaning a fissure. Particularly in the plural the word is applied to fissures at the angles of the mouth, at commissures like the canthi and around pursed openings like the anus.

rheo- [rē′ō] is a combining form from a Greek verb meaning to flow. It is used in prefixed position and appears in words like *rheology* (study of flow mechanics), *rheostat* (an instrument that regulates the flow of electricity). See also *-rrhagia, -rrhea.*

rheumatic nodule [rōō-măt′ĭk nŏd′ūl, nŏj′ōōl] designates a nodular lesion, generally on an extremity associated with rheumatic fever or rheumatoid arthritis.

rhinophyma [rī′nō-fī′mə] means overgrowth (*-phyma*) of the nose (*rhino-*). The word is applied to characteristic enlargement and distortion of the nose, particularly of the bulb and wings, in the form of lobulated masses that are dotted with patulous follicular openings exuding copious sebum. Fibroplasia, hyperplasia of sebaceous glands, telangiectasia, and inflammation are prominent features. Seborrheic dermatitis and rosacea seem associated, and alcoholism is thought to be exacerbating.

rhinoscleroma [rī′nō-sklē-rō′mə, -sklə-rō′mə, -sklĕ-rō′mə] literally means a hardening (*-scleroma*) of the nose (*rhino-*). The condition results from infection with a micro-organism named *Klebsiella rhinoscleromatis.* The lesions on, in and about the nose are distinctively hard nodules that sooner or later break down, ulcerate and scar.

This is a destructive scarring granulomatous infection of the upper respiratory tract due to the Gram-negative rod *Klebsiella rhinoscleromatis.* Can lead to death from airway obstruction.

rhinosporidiosis [rī′nō-spō-rĭd′ĭ-ō′sĭs, -ĭ-ō′sĭs] denotes the condition (*-osis*) of infection with a mold termed *Rhinosporidium seeberi.* While the nose is a common site of infection (the organism must have been named from finding it there), adjacent areas like the eyelids and remote areas like the genitalia may bear the process, which appears like polypoid excrescences that develop fissures and granulations.

Rhus [rŭs] is Latin from Greek word for sumac(h). The word is now used for a botanical genus that includes the species popularly termed *poison ivy, oak* or *sumac. Toxicodendron* is an alternate designation.

Rhus dermatitis [dûr′mə-tī′tĭs, -tē′tĭs] is an alternate designation for poison ivy dermatitis for allergic contact dermatitis caused by plants of the genus *Rhus.* T cell mediated delayed type hypersensitivity dermatitis.

Riehl's melanosis [rēl]. Dyschromia of the face and neck attributed to ingestion of certain chemicals as food additives or from photosensitization to certain topically contaminating substances.

Riley-Day syndrome [rī′lē; dā]. Familial dysautonomia; tearlessness, cutaneous blotching, hyperhidrosis, postural hypotension, ticklishness, indifference to pain, emotional instability.

ringed hair [rĭngd hâr] is a literal translation of *pili annulati.*

ringworm [rĭng′wûrm′] is a word that goes back to the early fifteenth century. It is just about getting worn-out now. We don't give it more than another century because even lay people are beginning to be sophisticated enough to say, still inaccurately to be sure, "fungus" for infection with a fungus as they say "sinus" for infection of a cranial sinus. Anyway, *ringworm* has been used for the past 500 years to denote ring-shaped patches of cutaneous disease. Whether the idea in *worm* originally implied vermicular cause or referred to the creep of the process we don't know, but it is sure that many more conditions than superficial fungous infections were formerly called *ringworm.* Such words have all the disadvantages of folkways because of implications that are read into them. Physicians ought to avoid the word.

Ritter's disease [rĭt′ērz dĭ-, də-zēz′]. See *dermatitis exfoliativa neonatorum.*

Rocky Mountain spotted fever is a sometimes fatal systemic infection manifested by fever, severe headache, rash and other organ disease caused by the vasculitis induced by *Rickettsia rickettsii.* The organism is usually transmitted to humans from animal reservoirs by a tick bite. (Richard B. Hornick) The rash consisting of pink macules is a great help in diagnosis of this ultra-dangerous disease which usually starts on the extremities and spreads to the central portions of the body. Biopsy shows perivascular red cell infiltration. Special stains, fluorescent tagged antibodies to *R. rickettsii,* will show the intracellular organisms. (Hornick)

rodent ulcer [rō′dənt ŭl′sēr] is a fanciful title that describes loss of substance (*ulcer*) in terms of a gnawed (*rodent*) process. The term is applied to those basal-cell epitheliomata that have become large and eroded because they are naturally aggressive and have been too long neglected.

roentgen [rŭnt′-, rĕnt′gĕn, rənt′gən] **ray** and **unit** are named after Wilhelm Konrad Roentgen (Röntgen), a German physicist (1845–1923), who is credited with the discovery in 1895 of what he modestly called X rays. X or roentgen (röntgen) rays consist of electromagnetic energy of wave lengths in the range of 0.5 to 2.0 Å. A roentgen unit is not a quantity of electromagnetic energy but a measure of ability of energy of that type to ionize air under standardized conditions. It is even more complicated than that, but let it be further understood that roentgen unitage varies with the quality (wave length) of radiation. Roentgen units are also referred to as roentgens and R's, or r's, for short. Notice that the designation *roentgen* ordinarily begins with a lower-case letter as is the habit with eponymic designation of units in physics, e.g., *ampere, coulomb, faraday, gauss, joule, ohm, volt*, etc.

Romberg's syndrome [rŏm′bērgh]. Progressive facial hemiatrophy.

rosacea [rə-zā′-, rō-zā′shē-ə, -sē-ə, -shə] is the feminine singular of a Latin adjective meaning made of or like roses. We use the word as a noun to designate a chronic, inflammatory, acneform condition of the face marked by erythema, telangiectasia and pustules. The center of the face, especially the nose, the brows, chin and cheeks are sites of heaviest involvement. The eyes are sometimes affected by a characteristic keratitis. In *acne rosacea*, the alternate title for this condition, *rosacea* is adjectival, as originally.

rosacea-like tuberculid(e) (of Lewandowsky) [to͞o-, tū-bû-r′kū-lĭd, -lĭd ŏv lĕv′ăn-, lā′vŏn-dŭv′skē, -lou′ăn-dou′skē] is the title of a process that looks like rosacea but is thought to be caused by the tubercle bacillus within a special and specific immunologic complex. See *tuberculid (e)*.

Rosai-Dorfman syndrome is sinus histiocytosis with massive lymphadenopathy.

rosea [rō′zē-ə] is the feminine singular form of a Latin adjective meaning rosy, like the common red rose. It is found in the title *pityriasis rosea*.

roseola [rō-zē′ō-lə, -ə-lə], which is New Latin and means a little (*-ola*) rose, is applied to any exanthem that consists of rose-red macules or patches. Enteric fevers, syphilis, measles and other viral diseases may produce the appearance.

roseola infantum [ĭn-făn′təm, -făn′tŭm, -to͞om]. See *exanthema subitum*.

The most common infectious exanthem occurring during the first two years of life. Classic between the ages of 6 and 18 months.

About one-third of all children develop clinical disease. Most cases are reported in Spring or early Fall. Appears to be caused by human herpesvirus 6.

The incubation is 7 to 15 days. No prodrome. Really has a dramatic presentation. Starts with a high fever 39° C (+ −) which lasts about 3 days then breaks and out comes the rash. Amazingly none of this appears to upset the child too much, i.e., they do well but of course always with some exceptions, e.g., febrile seizures. Remember the rash appears *after* the fever has broken.

Few diseases in medicine have been more suitably named than *exanthem subitum.*

rose spots [rōz spŏts] is a term applied to exanthemata that consist of tiny red macules, particularly those of typhoid fever.

Rothmund's syndrome [rōt′mo͞ondz, rôth′mŭndz sĭn′drōm] is eponymic for a melange of genetic abnormalities that is characterized by juvenile cataracts, premature graying and loss of hair and wasting of muscles.

Rothmund-Thomson syndrome [rōt′mo͞ond; tŏm′sən]. Congenital poikiloderma and premature cataract formation.

-rrhagia [rā′jə, rā′jē-ə, -jĭ-ə] and **-rrhea** [rē-ə] are both terminal combining elements derived from Greek, the former (like -*rrhexis*; see below) from a verb meaning to break, to burst, the latter (like *rheo-*; see above) from a verb meaning to flow. As used in forming compound medical words, they refer to discharges or abnormal flow of material, e.g., *blennorrhagia*, discharge of gonorrheal pus; *osteomelorrhea*, excess of bone on a femur likened to a flow, as of wax on a lighted candle; and *seborrhea*, abnormal flow of sebum. A part of the Greek verb appears in a word like *catarrh*, literally a flowing downward; -*rrhagia* appears as -*rrhage* in words like *hemorrhage*.

-rrhexis [rĕk′sĭs] is a combining form from a Greek verb meaning to break, burst, and means rupture. It appears in words like *acanthorrhexis* and *dermatorrhexis*. Compare -*rrhagia*.

rubefacient [ro͞o′bə-fā′shənt] derives from Latin word elements and means making (-*facient*) red (*rube-*). It is used as an adjective or as a noun for a material that induces erythema.

rubella [ro͞o-bĕl′ə] is New Latin from word elements meaning something slightly (-*ella*, diminutive) red (*rub-*). We use the word to designate an acute exanthematic disease that resembles ordinary measles (see *rubeola*, below) but is milder in every respect. *German measles* is a popular alternate designation.

One of the childhood exanthems now rare due to use of live-attenuated vaccine. Incubation period from 2 to 3 weeks, an RNA togavirus. Usually a mild self-limited infection in infants and children. The rash, associated with fever and arthritis, is the most common but still rare complication.

Causes the serious congenital rubella syndrome. If exposure occurs during the first trimester, 50% of fetuses may have a major congenital anomaly.

The congenital rubella syndrome shows deafness, heart defects and cataracts.

The rash consists of discrete rose-print macules and papules 1 to 4 mm in size. Starts on the face and works down to the whole body. This fades as it spreads lasting about three days.

Definitive diagnosis is serologically determined. All infants born to mothers who had rubella during pregnancy should be observed for late-emerging manifestations of congenital rubella syndrome.

Rubella vaccine prevents the disease and should be administered as the triple vaccine at 15 months. (Bialecki et al., Journ. Am. Acad. Derm., Vol 21, No 5)

rubeola [roo-bē′ō-lə, -ə-lə, roo′bē-ō′lə] is New Latin from word elements meaning something slightly (*-ola*, diminutive) red (*rube-*). Literally, then, the word is equal to *rubella* (see above), but we use it distinctively to designate ordinary measles, that combination of exanthematic, maculo-papular erythema, conjunctivitis and coryza attended by fever and malaise.

ruber, rubor, rubra [roo′bēr, -bēr; roo′bôr; roo′brə] are Latin words in noun (*rubor*) and adjective forms (*ruber*, masculine; *rubra*, feminine) relating to redness. The adjectives appear in classicized titles, e.g., *lichen ruber planus*, a red (*ruber*) flat (*planus*) conglomerate of papules (*lichen*) and *pityriasis rubra pilaris*, a red (*rubra*) finely scaling condition (*pityriasis*) around hairs (*pilaris*). *Rubor* can be used in place of *erythema*; it is part of the well-known rhyming mnemonic combination of words describing inflammation, i.e., *calor* (fever, local warmth), *dolor* (pain, or itch of the skin), *rubor* (redness or erythema) and *tumor* (swelling or edema).

rubrifacient [roo′brĭ-fā′shənt] is a variant of *rubefacient* (which see).

ruby spots [roo′bē, -bĭ spŏts] likens to the jewel those small angiomata that appear on the trunk in some hepatoses and in old age.

Rud's syndrome. Generalized ichthyosis with hypogonadism, mental deficiency, and epilepsy.

rugose, rugous [roo′gōs, roo-gōs′; roo′gəs] derive from Latin *ruga*, a wrinkle, and mean full of (*-ose, - ous*) wrinkles (*rug-*).

"run(-)around" [rŭn′ə-round′] is colloquial for inflammatory conditions of the soft parts about nails and conveys the idea of tendency to extend circularly. *Paronychia* and *panaritium* are more learned alternates.

rupia, rupial [rōo′pē-ə, -pĭ-ə; rōo′pē-əl] are respectively a noun meaning filth and an adjective meaning filthy derived via New Latin from Greek *rhypos*, dirt, filth. The adjective particularly is used to describe lesions, especially of psoriasis and syphilis, that have an unusually dirty quality about them in the form of purulence and excessive scaling.

"rupioid" [rōo′pē-oid] is found in dermatologic textbooks but in no formal dictionaries. It is used in the former in connection with descriptions of the scales of psoriasis as though it were synonymous with *ostraceous*, which means relating to an oyster, or (in this special context) to its shell. Of course, an ostraceous scale looks dirty, and *rupial* could be reasonably applied as additionally descriptive, but *rupioid*, which would mean like (*-oid*) filth (*-rupi-*), is needless, since we have *rupial*, with which it is nearly synonymous.

S

saber shin [sā′bĕr, -bər shĭn] is descriptive, in terms of a historically commonplace object, of the shins of some patients afflicted with congenital syphilis who have suffered osteitis of the tibias caused by infection with *Treponema pallidum*. The distortion of the bones is such that between the knee and ankle the legs bow forward and produce a resemblance to the curve of a saber blade.

saddle nose [săd′l nōz] is another description, in terms of an object that is still commonplace, of the noses of some patients with congenital syphilis who have suffered failure of development of the bridge of the nose as a result of intra-uterine infection with *Treponema pallidum*. The appearance then is of a concavity between the main portion of the nose and the brow, a concavity that is broader and deeper than usual, giving a distinct impression of a miniature saddle.

sailor's skin [sā′lĕrz skĭn] is still another of those designations by occupation that are picturesque but far from exact. What is meant is weather-beaten skin, i.e., skin marked by telangiectasia, atrophy and keratoses. The effect is seen mainly in fair (blond), blue-eyed individuals and in them mainly if their occupations require them or misguided desires impel them to be exposed to strong sunshine, fierce winds and other rough weather over prolonged periods. Thus, in addition to sailors, farmers, police officers, other outdoor workers and "sun worshippers" are susceptible to the effects, given proper quality of skin and enough climatic insult. See *farmer's and sailor's skin*.

Saint Anthony's fire [sānt ăn′thə-nēz fīr] is a folk designation for erysipelas and ergotism. Lest anyone be misled, St. Anthony got into these acts not because he had anything to do with causing or describing the conditions but because severe inflammatory and gangrenous conditions were believed, during the Middle Ages, to be curable by the intercession of this saint.

Sanarelli-Shwartzman phenomenon [sā′nă-rĕl′lē; shwôrts′ mən]. A necrotic reaction in the skin upon subsequent injections of endotoxins from Gram-negative bacteria in the same site; similar necrosis may occur in the kidneys, liver, and spleen from the experiment.

sarcoid [sär′koid] literally means like (-*oid*) flesh (*sarc*-). The word is sometimes used as a noun in short form for *sarcoidosis* conceived as a disease *sui generis* and as an adjective both for things relating to sarcoidosis and for other things like, but not quite, sarcoidosis. Thus one hears terms like *sarcoid lesions* and *reactions* referring to sarcoidosis in some contexts and also to what is not deemed to be "true" sarcoidosis in other contexts. It is all confusing because the nosology of sarcoidosis is not settled.

sarcoidal [sär-koi′dəl] is nearly interchangeable with *sarcoid* in the adjectival senses.

sarcoidosis [sär′koi-dō′sĭs] literally means a condition (-*osis*) in which the lesions are like (-*oid*-) flesh (*sarc*-). We use the word to designate that disease process which is characterized cutaneously by papules, nodules, plaques or tumors of no great distinction, and histologically both in skin and other organs by infiltrations of sharply agminated epithelioid cells in arrangements that have been dubbed *naked tubercles*. Symptomatology in the disease depends in largest measure on the organ(s) affected, the amount of involvement and the functional reserve of affected organs. In the skin, the marks of the disease are visible, but otherwise there are no symptoms because the amount of process, no matter how great, can hardly cause cutaneous insufficiency, and there is no itching; in lungs, liver, heart, bones, eyes, etc. special symptoms are more likely because these organs can be heavily infiltrated and their functions can be embarrassed by even small amounts of involvement. Etiology is unknown, but alterations in the immune system are clearly involved in its pathogenens. (Fanburg)

sarcoma [sär-kō′mə] literally means a neoplasia (-*oma*) of flesh (*sarc*-). We restrict the word to malignant neoplasms that develop from tissues of mesodermal origin as distinct from malignant neoplasms that develop from tissues of ecto- and endodermal origin, which are usually termed carcinomas.

sarcoma, multiple idiopathic hemorrhagic [mŭl′tĭ-pəl ĭd′ĭ-, ĭd′ē-ō-păth′ĭk hĕm′ō-rāj′ĭk], better known under the eponymous title *Kaposi's sarcoma*, describes a highly characteristic neoplasia of blood vessels and connective tissue. The legs are a common site of the process; sometimes other areas of the skin and other organs are involved by the process. Use to be quite common in AIDS patients.

sarcoma, reticulum-cell. See *reticulum-cell sarcoma.*

sarcomatous [sär-kŏm′ə-təs] is an adjective meaning pertaining or relating to sarcoma.

Sarcopsylla [sär′kō-sĭl′ə]. See under *Tunga penetrans.*

Sarcoptes [sär-kŏp′tēz] is the name of a genus of mites. The word means flesh (*sarc-*) cutters (*-coptes*). (The two *c*'s of the word elements have been fused into one.)

Sarcoptes scabiei var. hominis [skā′bĭ-ē′ī və-r(ī′ə-tē, və-rī′ē-tăs, -täs) hō′mĭ-nĭs, hŏm′ĭ-nĭs] is a variety (*var.*, which may also represent Latin *varietas*) of that species of *Sarcoptes* that causes scabies in humans (*hominis*) obligatorily. *Itch mite* is a lay expression for this acarid. There are other species of the genus more adaptable to animals other than humans but still able to infest humans facultatively.

sarcoptic [sär-kŏp′tĭk] is an adjective meaning caused by, pertaining or related to *Sarcoptes*.

sarcoptic mange [mānj] is the title for infestation of animals with species-specific mite of the genus *Sarcoptes*. A lay designation is *barn itch*. Compare *demodectic mange* and see under *mange*.

sauriasis [sô-rī′ə-sĭs], **sauriosis** [sô′rē-, sô′rī-, sô′rī-ō′sĭs], and **sauroderm(i)a** [sō′rō-dûr′mē-ə, -mĭ-ə] are rarely used words that liken the appearance or condition (*-iasis*, *-osis*) of human skin (*-derma*, *-dermia*) to that of the lizard's (*sauri-*) skin. Some severe grades of ichthyosis are aptly described by the words, of which *sauroderm (i)a* is preferable because the other two sound in speech like *psoriasis*.

scab [skăb] is of Scandinavian and Middle English origin and is akin to Latin *scabies*, from *scabere*, to scratch. We use the word to designate that hard concretion that forms on superficial wounds of the skin and is composed of clotted blood and tissue debris, i.e., a crust for those who don't like scab.

scabetic [skə-bĕt′ĭk] and **scabeticide** [skə-bĕt′ĭ-sīd] are found in dictionaries as alternate words for *scabietic* and *scabieticide* (see both). We advise the latter as better formed etymologically from *scabies*, the parent word.

scabies [skā′bĭ-ēz, -bē-ēz, -bēz] is a Latin word for an itch, from the verb *scabere*, to scratch. We use the unmodified word restrictedly for the infestation with *Sarcoptes scabiei var. hominis*. In addition to burrows that house the female mite and her young in sites like webs of fingers, wrists, anterior axillary lines, penis, genital area generally and buttocks, nocturnal itching is a mark of the condition.

scabies, Norwegian [nôr-wē′jən] is another of those invidious and parochial titles, this time for severe scabietic infestations such as can occur in debilitated and hygienically deprived individuals and are usually immune suppressed.

scabietic [skā′bē-, skā′bĭ-ĕt′ĭk] is an adjective meaning pertaining or relating to scabies. See *scabetic.*

scabieticide [skā′bē-, skā′bĭ-ĕt′ĭ-sīd] is an agent that kills (*-cide*) organisms that cause scabies. See *scabeticide.*

scale, scaling, scaly [skāl; skāl′ĭng; skāl′ē] are words that derive from Teutonic languages through Old French (*escale,* husk) and Middle English (*skale*). A material that separates like a husk is a scale, the process of such separation is scaling and what is marked by such separation is scaly. *Scale* in the sense of a measure is not related and derives from Latin *scala,* a ladder.

scar [skär] derives via Latin and Old French from Greek *eschara,* hearth, fireplace. Hippocrates, Aristotle, Galen and others used the Greek word also for burns from a hearth or any other source of sufficient heat (compare *eschar*). *Scar,* perhaps influenced by an obsolete word of the same spelling and meaning a crack, is now used to denote a healed but still visible mark of injury of any sort. In the skin the lesion is a hard plaque consisting of dense fibrous tissue covered by atrophic epidermis. *Cicatrix* is an alternate word.

scarlatina [skär′lə-tē′nə] derives from Medieval Latin *scarlatum,* which first meant a material and then a red color. In 1676 Sydenham used *scarlatina* for the disease we now more often call scarlet fever; a century and a half before that (1527) Lancelotti had used *scarlattina,* an Italian word. The characteristic delicate red color of the exanthem no doubt is what must have suggested the name.

scarlatiniform [skär′lə-tĭn′ĭ-fôrm, -ə-fôrm] means in the character of (*-form*) scarlatina or scarlet fever.

scarlet fever [skär′lĕt, -lĭt, -lət fē′vĕr, -vər] is nowadays heard more commonly than *scarlatina* for the exanthematic disease caused by a streptococcus and characterized by fever, glossopharyngitis and a characteristic red rash. The word *scarlet* came into English via Old French *escarlate* and Medieval Latin *scarlatum* from a Persian word, *saqalat,* a kind of rich cloth.

One of the childhood exanthems. Caused by Gram-positive group A beta hemolytic streptococci resulting in high fever, rash, vomiting and sore throat. Incubation is 1 to 4 days.

The rash appears 12 to 48 hours after onset of fever. Early on abdominal pain may be severe and mimic an acute abdomen.

The rash starts as red patches below the ears and on the chest and axillae then spreads to the abdomen, extremities and face. Consists of scarlet macules and diffuse erythema.

The pharynx and tonsils are beefy red and may have an exudate. The palate may have scattered petechiae and erythematous punctiform lesions. Early the tongue has a white coat with red papillae resulting in "white strawberry tongue." After a few days the white coat is lost and a "red strawberry tongue" is formed. The white count is moderately elevated with predominantly polymorphonuclear cells. Throat cultures are positive for group A beta hemolytic streptococci.

Oral penicillin is curative. Prophylactic treatment is not recommended for individuals exposed to scarlet fever. (Bialecki et al., Journal Am. Acad Derm, Vol 25, No. 5)

schistosomal dermatitis, or swimmer's itch **(cercarial dermatitis)** may cause chronic papular dermatitis due to schistosoma manosi.

schwannoma. See *neurilemmoma.*

Schweninger-Buzzi, anetoderma of [shvān′ĭn-gēr; bōōt′zə] A type of atrophy in which the skin hangs slack and gives a sense of herniation upon pressure with a finger.

scler- [sklēr, sklĕr, sklər] and **sclero-** [sklē′rō, sklə′rō, sklĕ′rō] are combining forms from Greek *skleros,* hard.

scleredema [sklē′rē-dē′mə, sklēr′ə-dē′mə] literally means hard (*scler-*) swelling (*-edema*). The word is applied to such a condition in the skin and the implication is of hardness caused by fluid (compare *sclerodermia*). The word appears in the title immediately following.

scleredema adultorum (Buschke) [ə-dŭl′tō-, ăd′ŭl-tō′rəm, -tôr′əm (bōōsh′kĕ)] designates a brawny edema, generally of the face and upper portion of the shoulders and arms but not hands, sometimes of the lower portion of the trunk and the legs but not feet. Cause is not known for sure, but it may on occasion follow streptococcal upper respiratory infections. There is a strong tendency to ultimate resolution but recurrent attacks may lead to elephantiasic enlargement, presumably from lymphatic obstruction. The condition is not restricted to adults and the modification *adultorum* as well as the eponym could very well be omitted.

sclerema [sklə-, sklĕ-, sklē-rē′mə] is a New Latin formation from Greek word elements meaning the result of (*-ma*) hardening (*sclere-*). The final *e* of *sclere-* looks like a connecting vowel or insert (see under *zosteriform*) but its use in forming the compound *sclerema* is most probably based on analogy with, or influenced by, words like *scleredema* and *sclerenchyma*, where the *e* after the combining form *scler-* properly belongs to the following word element.

sclerema neonatorum [nē′ō-nə-tō′rəm] designates a generalized, nonpitting induration (*sclerema*) of the skin and subcutis that may occur in sickly newborn infants (*neonatorum*) and is caused by solidification of fat in the panniculus adiposus. It is a rare disorder that seems to depend on chemical oddities in the composition and ratios of human fats and upon coincidental nutritional, infectious or environmental noxae like low ambient temperature. Prognosis is bad.

sclero-. See *scler-*.

sclerodactylia [sklē′rō-dăk-tĭl′ē-ə, -ĭ-ə] is New Latin from Greek word elements meaning a condition (*-ia*) of hardened (*-sclero-*) fingers (*-dactyl-*). The phenomenon is seen in acrosclerosis and systemic sclerosis.

sclerodermatous [sklē′rō-dûr′mə-təs, -dĕr-măt′əs] is an adjective meaning relating or pertaining to scleroderm(i)a.

scleroderm(i)a [sklē′rō-dûr′mə, -dûr′mē-ə, -ĭ-ə] is New Latin from Greek elements meaning a hardened (*sclero-*) condition of the skin (*-derma, -dermia*). The word is generic and can bespeak any indurated condition of the skin caused by anything from persistent edema to scarring. Most often it is used restrictedly to denote the cutaneous involvement of systemic sclerosis.

sclerodermoid [sklē′rō-dûr′moid] is another adjective from *scleroderm(i)a* meaning like (*-oid*) the hardened condition of the skin in that disease.

scleronychia [sklē′rō-nĭk′ē-ə, -ĭ-ə] is New Latin from Greek elements meaning an excessively hardened (*scler-*) condition (*-ia*) of the nails (*-onych-*).

sclerosing hemangioma [sklə-rō′sĭng hē′măn-jē-ō′mə] describes a scarring process that obliterates a small hemangioma. Not that obliteration of largish hemangiomata of newborns and infants which occurs spontaneously over the first few years of life is meant, but that event mainly on legs and arms of grown persons which eventuates into a cutaneous nodule, a dermatofibroma or histiocytoma is denoted. Judgment of the event is histologic, not clinical.

sclerosis [sklə-, sklĕ-, sklē-rō′sĭs] is New Latin from Greek elements meaning a condition (*-osis*) of hardness (*scler-*). The word is ordinarily generic, but specific in the following title.

sclerosis, systemic [sĭs-tĕm′ĭk], is applied to that process of hardening of connective tissue and the consequences thereof which are so cutaneously characteristic in the form of scleroderm(i)a and hidebound feel and appearance of arms, face and chest, and then variably characteristic in gastro-intestinal, pulmonary and renal involvement as determined by physical signs, radiography and biochemical abnormalities.

sclerotic [sklə-, sklĕ-, sklē-rŏt′ĭk] is an adjective meaning pertaining or relating to sclerosis.

scorbutic [skôr-bū′tĭk] means pertaining or relating to scurvy. It derives from New Latin *scorbuticus*, adjective of New Latin noun *scorbutus*, scurvy, which in turn is probably derived from Old English *scurf*.

scratch [skrăch] derives from Middle English. As a verb, the word refers to that operation on the skin which consists of stroking it by design or accident, in linear fashion, gently or fiercely with fingernails or sharp instruments. As a noun the mark of the operation is denoted. Such a mark may vary from imperceptible damage to superficial, incised wound to a depth of pars papillaris.

scrofula [skrŏf′ū-lə] derives from Medieval Latin through Late Latin *scrofulae*, a word that meant swellings of neck glands and was formed by adding a suffix of diminution (*-ul-*) to *scrofa*, a breeding sow. The reason for application to tuberculosis cutis colliquativa is conjectural. In Webster's New International Dictionary, Second Edition, the surmise is "perhaps by a fanciful comparison of the glandular swelling to little pigs." The Oxford English Dictionary states that in early use *scrofulae* meant glandular swellings and that pigs were supposed to be subject to the effect. However all that may be, the word is obsolescent for that form of tuberculosis cutis that is characterized by a deep focus in a lymph node or other subcutaneous structure like a joint that becomes a cold abscess and develops a sinus through overlying structures to a point of exit on the skin.

scrofuloderma. This form of cutaneous tuberculosis is usually due to a focus of active tuberculosis in lymph nodes or in the skeletal system. The first evidence is a deep nodule which gradually enlarges, becomes attached to the skin, softens, and produces an ulcerative lesion or sinus tract that may be covered by a mass of granulation tissue. The floor of the ulcer is deeply attached to the subcutaneous tissue. (Lincoln & Sewell. *Tuberculosis in Children*. NY: McGraw-Hill, 1963.)

scrofuloderm(i)a [skrŏf′ū-lō-dûr′mə; -mē-ə, -mĭ-ə] means a condition of the skin (-*derma*, -*dermia*) characterized by what has been described under *scrofula*. *Tuberculosis cutis colliquativa* is alternate.

scrofulosorum [skrŏf′ū-lō′sō′rəm, -sôr′ŭm, -sôr′ōōm] is the masculine plural of a New Latin adjective used as a noun and means of the scrofulous or of the tuberculous. It appears in the title *lichen scrofulosorum*.

scrofulous [skrŏf′ū-ləs] is an adjective meaning pertaining or related to or afflicted with scrofula or cutaneous tuberculosis.

scrotal tongue [skrō′təl tŭng] is picturesquely descriptive of a furrowed appearance of the tongue that resembles the scrotum in contracted state. *Lingua plicata* is an alternate term.

scruff [skrŭf] is a corrupt form of *scuff*, a word of unknown origin for the nape of the neck.

scurf [skûrf] derives from Middle English and Scandinavian and is akin to Latin *carpere*, to pluck. It is an obsolete word for scales or crusts on the scalp. See *dandruff*.

scurvy [skûr′vē] derives from *scurf*. The application of the word to the condition that results from deficiency of vitamin C must be figurative rather than literal. The skin in avitaminosis C is not particularly scaly, but the general appearance of the patient is sad because of the hemorrhages in the skin and mucous membranes and because the patient is so debilitated. *Scurvy* is used as a pejorative adjective in nonmedical writing for a run-down or mean quality, as a *scurvy fellow*, *trick*, etc.

scutulum [skōō′-, skū′tū-ləm, -lŭm] is a Latin word meaning a little (-*ulum*) shield (*scut-*). The word is used to describe a tiny concave crust, especially that of a lesion of favus.

sebaceous [sē-, sĭ-, sə-bā′shəs] is an adjective from *sebum* literally meaning in the nature of (-*aceous*) tallow, grease or fat (*seb-*) and hence relating or pertaining to the sebaceous gland or its product.

sebaceous cyst [sĭst] bespeaks a circumscribed, walled structure derived from a sebaceous gland. In recent years doubt has been cast on the reality of such an origin and it is averred that what has been so long called *sebaceous cyst* is an epidermal or epidermoid cyst, i.e., derived from epidermal elements other than the sebaceous gland. We doubt the iconoclasm. Contemplating the comedo and evolution of some comedones to encystment and imagining structural and functional changes in cells of the sebaceous glands after obstruction, it is still likely that cysts develop from sebaceous glands. Moreover, sebaceous glands are epidermally derived. All maturely differentiated epidermal cells retain ability to de-differentiate to anaplasia, and then pluripotentiality to re-differentiate after resumed anaplasia. What is gained by the indefinite designations of *epidermal* or *epidermoid cyst* ?

sebaceous gland [glănd] designates the well-known structure associated with hair follicles and productive of sebum by a process of cellular alteration.

sebaceum [sē-bā′shē-əm, -sē-əm, -shəm] and **sebaceus** [-shē-əs, -sē-əs, -shəs] are respectively the neuter singular and the masculine singular of a New Latin adjective meaning pertaining or relating to sebum. They appear in titles like *adenoma sebaceum* and *nevus sebaceus.*

seborrhea [sĕb′ə-rē′ə] literally means a flow (-*rrhea*) of sebum. Flow of sebum is normal but when the word is applied an abnormal condition in terms of quality or quantity is implied.

seborrheic dermatitis [sĕb′ə-rē′ĭk dûr′mə-tī′tĭs, -tē′tĭs] names a fairly characteristic inflammatory condition of the skin that is thought, with reason, to be related to dysfunction of the sebaceous gland or poor composition of its product. The clinical marks of the condition are itching, redness and scaling. The sites of predilection in order of frequency are scalp, face, chest, back and intertriginous spaces.

"seborrhiasis" [sĕb′ə-rī′ə-sĭs] is somebody's cute coinage to suggest the clinical appearance of a dermatosis which looks like a combination of seborrheic dermatitis and psoriasis, particularly when such a process occurs on the scalp, face and chest. It is not a particularly good play on words because the element of psoriasis is really omitted entirely. As a matter of fact, the word is a good one to encompass comprehensively all variations of dysfunction of sebaceous gland structure and function because it simply means a condition (-*iasis*) relating to the flow of sebum (*seborrh-*). Perhaps a better formulation would be "*sebopsoriasis*" [sē′bō-sə-rī′ə-sĭs], which could bespeak a form of psoriasis that is greasy (*sebo-*) in appearance, or an eventuation of psoriasis by the Koebner phenomenon upon seborrheic dermatitis, or seborrheic dermatitis that is psoriasiform, or finally the simultaneous existence of seborrheic dermatitis and psoriasis.

sebum [sē′bəm] is a Latin word for tallow and grease. We apply the word to the product of the sebaceous gland or that mixture of fatty acids, waxes, alcohols, glycerides and phosphatides that issues from the pilosebaceous ostium.

secondary [sĕk′ən-dĕr′ē, sĕk′ən-dĕr-ē, -ĭ] in medical contexts has two meanings, namely, 1) obligatorily sequential to something primary and 2) merely sequential to something. The entries below illustrate the fine difference.

secondary infection [ĭn-fĕk′shən] bespeaks infection additional to or superimposed upon something pre-existing with no obligatory connection.

secondary syphilis [sĭf′ĭ-lĭs] bespeaks that stage of syphilis that obligatorily follows the primary stage.

second disease [sĕk′ənd dĭ-, də-zēz′]. In an ordinal designation of the exanthemata, scarlet fever (scarlatina) is second disease.

Senear-Usher disease [sĕ-nēr′; ŭsh′ēr]. Pemphigus erythematosus.

senile, senilis [sē′nĭl, -nĭl; sĕn-ĭ′, sĕ-nĭ′lĭs] are respectively an English adjective and the masculine or feminine singular of a Latin adjective meaning pertaining or relating to an older person or the elderly (who are now euphemistically called "senior citizens"). The Latin adjective appears in a title like *keratosis*, or *verruca, senilis* (both feminine).

senile keratosis [kĕr′ə-tō′sĭs] and **keratosis senilis** are terms for epidermal dysplasia that is clinically marked by dry scaling and histologically by squamous-cell proliferation that is suspiciously precancerous. The implication in the titles is that mere aging is promotional of such changes. Modern thinking prefers *actinic keratosis* as an alternate term that stresses the factor of damage from ultraviolet radiation. There is more to it than ultraviolet radiation alone since it is the skin of blue-eyed blonds, who do not pigment well, that is most susceptible to the damaging effects of prolonged climatic insults.

serologic [sē′rō-lŏj′ĭk] is an adjective meaning relating or pertaining to serology.

serologic test for syphilis is a straightforward enough statement of a procedure designed to test for syphilis by employing serum of blood. See *serology* for an undesirable alternate.

serology [sē-rŏl′ə-jē, -jĭ] simply means the study (-*logy*) of serum (*sero-*), the serum of blood, that is. Anything about blood serum is a proper subject of serology, be it of its chemical determination of constituents, color, viscosity, etc. However, euphemism has corrupted the word by relating it too firmly to tests for syphilis. Thus, we have such oddities as "do a serology," "positive or negative serology," etc.

serpentine [sûr′pĕn-tīn, -tēn] derives from Latin via French and refers to creeping or crawling like a snake (*serpent-*). The word is used in descriptive morphology for lesions that seem to enlarge by languidly creeping along in linear fashion, or for the borders of lesions that assume the shape of the curl of a snake at rest.

serpiginosum [sĕr-, sŭr-pĭj′ĭ-nō′səm] and **serpiginous** [sĕr-, sûr-pĭj′ĭ-nəs, -ə-nəs] are respectively the neuter singular of a New Latin adjective and an English adjective which, in about the same way as *serpentine*, describe the shape or spread of lesions in the fashion (*-ginosum*, compound noun and adjectival element) of a creep or crawl of a snake (*serpi-*; for *i* as a connecting vowel see under *zosteriform*). The classicized word appears in a title like *angioma serpiginosum*.

severe combined immunodeficiency disorders (SCID) are characterized by their apparent congenital absence of all adaptive immune function and a great diversity of genetic enzymatic, hematologic and immunologic features. There are several different subcategories. See *autosomal-recessive (SCID)*.

Sézary's syndrome [sāzărēz′ sĭn′drōm] is an erythrodermic leukemic variant of mycosis fungoides, that is characterized by a highly distinctive monocytoid cell in the peripheral blood and clinical appearance. An exfoliative erythroderma with resemblances to mycosis fungoides and characterized by a special mononuclear cell in the blood.

shagreen [shə-grēn′] derives from Turkish and names a type of processed leather. Its distinction is that it is embossed in papules by means of pellets pressed into the undersurface during tanning and then usually colored green.

shagreen skin. See *peau de chagrin.*

shampoo [shăm-pōō′] derives from a Hindi word for massaging and washing of hair with soap and water. We use the word for the operation and for a preparation to do it with. From the frivolity of cosmetology and the excesses of advertising one would think that a shampoo as a preparation is more than a weak solution of soap or other detergent, colored, perfumed and priced beyond reason, and as an operation more than an over-elaborate wash of the scalp by oneself or a "beautician."

shingles [shĭng′g′lz], a lay designation for herpes zoster, is a corruption of Latin *cingulum* meaning a belt or girdle. The Latin word is the translation of the Greek word *zone* [zō′nā], which the Greeks also used to name the disease. The word *zoster*, which too means belt, was not used by the Greeks for the disease. In classical times the Romans used the word *zona* and much later *zoster*. *Herpes zoster* first appeared in Medieval Latin.

sicca [sĭk′ə] is the feminine singular of a Latin adjective meaning dry. It appears in a title like *pityriasis*, or *seborrhea, sicca*. Let it be noted in passing that the stem *-sicc-* appears in the words *desiccate* and *desiccation*, which are often misspelled by doubling the *s* and omitting one *c*. The error comes about from failure to observe that the word element *-sicc-* has but one *s* and two *c*'s and that the prefix is *de-*, which ends in *e* and does not have an *s* at the end.

simplex [sĭm′plĕks] is a Latin adjective meaning simple or single. It appears in a title like *herpes simplex*.

sinus, dental. See *dental fistula* and *dental sinus*.

Sister Mary Joseph's nodule a skin sign of metastatic cancer, this is a deep-seated paraumbilical nodule most frequently stemming from a metastatic gastric adenocarcinoma.

sixth disease [sĭksth dĭ-, də-zēz′]. In an ordinal designation of the exanthemata, roseola (exanthema subitum) is sixth disease.

Sjögren's syndrome [shô′grĕn]. Keratoconjunctivitis sicca, xerostomia, and arthritis after menopause.

Sicca syndrome. Keratoconjunctivitis sicca, dryness of mucous membranes, telangiectases or purpuric spots on the face and bilateral parotid enlargement, seen in menopausal women, often associated with rheumatoid arthritis, Raynaud's phenomenon and dental caries. Changes in the lacrimal and salivary glands resembling those of Mikulicz's disease. There is an immunological overlap in some instances with lupus erythematosis.

Sjögren-Larssen syndrome [shô′grĕn; lärs′sŭn]. Ichthyosiforme erythroderma, spastic paralysis, mental retardation, and miscellaneous dyscrasias of structure and function.

Well established entity. Syndrome associated with ichthyosis combined neuroectodermal and mesodermal defects. Lamellar ichthyosis, mental retardation and spastic paraesis.

skin [skĭn] derives from Old Norse *skinn*. Ordinarily the word is applied to the organ that invests the bodies of mammals, birds, reptiles, amphibians and fishes; there are many metaphorical uses of it.

skin-color(ed) [skĭn kŭl′ĕr(d)] is a phrase used by most Western dermatologists in an unqualified way for "white" as though the world were populated entirely by Caucasians. Need one be reminded that there are more skins of yellow, black and red color than white or pink? Compare *flesh-color* (*ed*).

skin eruption, or **rash** [ē-rŭp′shən; răsh], are unnecessarily explicative. Volcanic events and foolhardy acts are unlikely to be suggested by the unmodified words in any conceivable dermatologic context.

slough [slŭf] derives from Middle English words meaning cast-off skin. In general medicine, separation of a membrane or of necrotic debris en masse is designated by the word. For the skin, the development of a gangrenous ulcer would have a stage of slough.

Sneddon-Wilkinson disease [snĕd′′n; wĭl′kĭn-sən]. Subcorneal pustular dermatosis.

solar [sō′lēr, -lər], **solare** [sō-lä′rē, -lä′rē, -lär′ē], and **solaris** [sō-lä′rĭs, -lä′rĭs, -lär′ĭs] are respectively an English adjective, the neuter singular and the masculine or feminine singular of a Latin adjective meaning pertaining or relating (*-ar*, *-are*, *-aris*) to the sun (*sol-*). The English adjective appears in the titles *solar dermatitis*, *solar eczema* and *solar urticaria*, simple titles which carry the implication that the shine of the sun has something to do with the development of the conditions. The Latin adjectives appear in titles like *erythema solare* (neuter) and *urticaria solaris* (feminine).

solution [sə-loo′shən], as a pharmaceutical form, designates a preparation in which active ingredients are completely dissolved in an aqueous vehicle and which is consequently clear.

sore [sôr, sōr] derives from Anglo-Saxon and Middle English words meaning, as a noun, a boil, ulcer or other localized, painful lesion of the skin and, as an adjective, painful.

sphaceloderm(i)a [sfăs′ē-lō-dûr′mə; -mē-ə, -mĭ-ə] derives from Greek word elements that mean a condition of the skin (*-derma*, *-dermia*) resulting from gangrene (*sphacelo-*). The word is rather ponderous and little used nowadays but there are still conditions of cutaneous gangrene so obscure in course and mechanism that this noncommittal word can well be used to designate and describe certain ulcers until etiologic resolution is possible and made.

Spiegler-Fendt sarcoid [shpēg′lēr; fĕnt]. See *Bäfverstedt's syndrome*.

spilus [spī′ləs] is a New Latin formation from *spilos*, a Greek word for a spot. Dictionaries define it without any qualification as *nevus*. What is meant apparently is a distinctive, flat pigmented mole. See *nevus spilus*.

spindle cell [spĭn′d'l sĕl] describes a cell that is fusiform, i.e., shaped like a spindle. Many cells are fusiform, but the reference is specific in the title immediately following.

spindle-cell carcinoma [kär′sĭ-nō′mə] describes squamous-cell carcinoma of severe grade wherein the neoplasia is marked by fusiform development of the rapidly multiplying, ordinarily squamous, cells.

spindle cell hemangioendothelioma is a recently described tumor which is composed of elements of Kaposi's sarcoma and cavernous hemangioma. Presents as multiple nodules in the dermis and subcutaneous tissue usually on the upper extremity. One case has been reported to metastasize. (Lever)

spinosum [spĭn-, spī-nō′səm] is the neuter singular of a Latin adjective meaning full of (-*osum*) thorns (*spin-*), therefore, prickly, spiny. It appears in the title *stratum spinosum*.

spinulosa [spĭn′ū-, spī′nū-lō′sə] and **spinulosus** [-səs] are respectively the feminine singular and the masculine singular of a New Latin adjective meaning spinous. They appear in the titles *trichostasis spinulosa* and *lichen spinulosus*.

spiradenoma, eccrine [spī′răd-ə-nō′mə, -ē-nō′mə, ĕk′rīn, -rēn, -rĭn] is a New Latin formation from Greek word elements that mean neoplasia, tumor or over-development (-*oma*) of the coil (*spir-*) portion of a sweat (*eccrine*) gland (-*aden-*).

spirit(s) [spĭr′ĭt(s)], as a pharmaceutical form, designates a preparation in which volatile ingredients are dissolved in alcohol.

Spirocheta [spī′rō-kē′tə] is New Latin from Greek and literally means a coiled (*spiro-*) hair (-*cheta*). The word names a genus of micro-organisms that are like fine spirals.

Spirocheta pallida [păl′ĭ-də] names the species of the genus that is the cause of syphilis. *Pallida* (from Latin) means pale. *Treponema pallidum* (which see) is newer terminology.

spirochete [spī′rō-kēt] names an individual organism of the genus *Spirocheta*.

spirochetosis [spī′rō-kē-tō′sĭs] means a condition (-*osis*) of infection with a spirochete. Usually syphilis is meant.

Spitz nevus (spindle and epithelioid cell nevus) this lesion, still widely known by the inept name of benign juvenile melanoma, occurs primarily in youth as a red tumor (papule or nodule). It consists of a nest of nevus cells at the dermal epidermal junction and in the dermis. Both Dr. Sophie Spitz and her husband Dr. Arthur Allen made splendid contributions to dermatology.

spongiosis [spŏn′-, spŭn′jē-ō′sĭs, -jĭ-ō′sĭs] means a condition (-*osis*) of sponginess. The word is used to describe intercellular edema within the epidermis to a degree that gives the area a spongy appearance.

spoon nail [spo͞on nāl] is descriptive in terms of a familiar object of a nail plate that has a concavity where it should have a convexity. See *koilonychia* for an alternate designation.

Sporotrichon, -um [spō′rō-trĭk′ŏn, -əm, spō-rŏt′rĭ-kŏn, -kəm] is the name of a genus of fungi. The ending -*on* is Greek; -*um* is Latin. The word literally means a hair (-*trich*-) sowing (*sporo*-) agent (-*on*, -*um*). In new terminology, *Sporotrichon* is replaced by *Sporothrix*, which etymologically comes to the same meaning.

Sporotrichon, -um schenckii [shĕn′kĭ-ī, -kē-ī] is a species that is pathogenic for humans. It is characterized by a blackish aerial crown in culture.

sporotrichosis [spō′rō-trĭ-kō′sĭs] is the condition (-*osis*) caused by a pathogenic *Sporotrichon, S. schenckii* in the case of a man. A chronic infection often starts in the skin and spreads by the lymphatics or blood to bones, joints and other organs. Pulmonary type may also develop from aspiration of the fungus.

Often a very characteristic skin disease with linear distribution of isolated deep-seated nodules, ulcers and abscesses, caused by the plant saprophyte *Sporothrix schenckii*. Inhalation can result in pneumonia; this is extremely rare and usually occurs as primary pulmonary sporotrichosis, although multifocal sporotrichosis with pulmonary involvement has been documented. (E. Jones)

squama, squame [skwā′mə; skwām] are respectively a Latin and an English word for a scale. The basic idea in the root of the Latin word is roughness.

squamous [skwā′məs] is an adjective meaning scaly or full of (-*ous*) scales (*squam*-).

squamous cell is descriptive of epidermal cells between the basal-cell and granular-cell layers. The flat character of the cells rather than scaliness is denoted by *squamous. Malpighian, mucous* and *spinous cell* are alternate terms.

squamous-cell carcinoma [kär′sĭ-nō′mə], or **epithelioma** [ĕp′ĭ-, ĕp′ē-thē′lĭ-ō′mə, -lē-ō′mə], is a designation for malignant development of squamous cells. Clinical marks of the condition are more or less eroded masses, and histologic characteristics are reduplication of such cells with undue numbers of mitotic figures, cellular pleomorphism and abnormal keratinization in the form of whorls within the epidermis.

stasis dermatitis [stā′sĭs dûr′mə-tī′tĭs, -tē′tĭs] is a glib designation for inflammatory processes of the legs between knees and ankles which are not incontestably psoriasis, pyoderma, trauma, etc. The implication of vascular insufficiency, particularly venous sluggishness (*stasis*, a standing still) is more assumed than provable. Inflammatory processes of any sort on the legs are worse on account of the gravitationally affected hemodynamics but it is debatable if stasis per se is a prime cause or merely promotional of them. Let it be shown that stasis of a reasonable degree and duration induced by a tourniquet or other restrictive measure can produce more than moderate edema without the intercession of other factors like trauma and secondary infection. Are varicose veins or valvular insufficiency of the veins of the lower extremities always attended by "stasis dermatitis"? Is "stasis dermatitis" always curable by re-establishment of venous sufficiency? Does not "stasis dermatitis" occur without venous insufficiency from vascular defect or gravity?

steat(o)- [stē′ə-tō] is a combining form from the stem of the Greek word *stear*, fat, tallow, genitive *steatos*.

steatocystoma multiplex [mŭl′tĭ-plĕks] bespeaks a condition in which numerous (*multiplex*) encystments develop either from sebaceous glands or look as though they did.

steatoma [stē′ə-tō′mə] literally means the result of (*-ma*) fatting (*steato-*) or a tumor (*-oma*) arising from a sebaceous (*steat-*) gland. The word is alternate for *sebaceous cyst*, but not for *lipoma*.

sterile abscess. See *abscess, sterile*.

Stevens-Johnson syndrome [stē′vənz-jŏn′sŭn sĭn′drōm]. Erythema multiforme of severe nature affecting the eyes and mouth particularly and attended by grave constitutional illness; ectodermosis erosiva pluriorificialis is a formal title. See *ectodermosis erosiva pluriorificialis*.

Stewart-Treves syndrome [stū′ert; trēvz]. Malignant degeneration of tissues following lymphedema resulting from radical mastectomy.

sting, stinging [stĭng; stĭng′ĭng] are of Anglo-Saxon derivation. A *sting* designates a sensation of sharp, momentary pain. Stinging as a noun or an adjective suggests rapid repetition of such sensations. The bites of certain insects are stings and the sensation created by weak electric currents is stinging.

stomatitis [stō′mə-tī′tĭs, -tē′tĭs] means inflammation (-*itis*) of the mouth (*stoma-*). The word is generic.

stomatitis, aphthous. See *aphthous stomatitis*.

stratum [strä′-, strā′təm, străt′əm, -ŭm, -ōōm] derives from the past participle (*stratus*) of a Latin verb (*sternere*) meaning to spread, strew, lay out or cover. It therefore means a layer. The plural is *strata* [strā′tə], which is often mistakenly used as a singular, with an erroneous plural, *stratas. Verbum sap.*

The epidermis is divided into strata as follows:

stratum corneum [kôr′nē-əm] designates the first or topmost layer of the epidermis and consists of dead cells that have been chemically altered into horn (*corneum*) i.e., largely fibrous protein.

stratum germinativum [jĕr′-, jûr′mĭ-nə-tī′vəm] designates the last or bottommost layer of the epidermis and consists of a single row of cells that regularly divide (*germinativum*, sprouting) and thus produce all cells above the basal layer.

stratum granulosum [grăn′ū-lō′səm] designates a layer that is usually seen second from the top of the epidermis (i.e., below the stratum corneum) and consists of two to three rows of cells whose contents are granular (*granulosum*, full of grains).

stratum lucidum [lōō′sĭ-dəm] describes a layer that is exceptionally light (*lucidum*) in the sense that it is hard to delineate. In fact it is not everywhere seen. It can be visualized where skin is naturally thick or thickened by hyperkeratosis as a second layer from the top of the epidermis (i.e., below stratum corneum and above stratum granulosum) consisting of a row or two of poorly outlined and poorly differentiable cells.

stratum malpighii [măl-pē′gĭ-ī, -pĭ′gē-ī] is an eponymic designation of the third or fourth layer from the top of the epidermis (third or fourth depending upon whether a stratum lucidum is present) and consists of six to ten rows of cells that are better described in aggregate by alternate designations like *stratum mucosum* and *stratum spinosum* (see immediately following).

stratum mucosum [mū-kō′səm] describes the third or fourth layer of the epidermis (*stratum malpighii* or *spinosum*) as being full of mucus (*mucosum*) in the sense that it consists of cells that are plump and juicy in their individuality and aggregate.

stratum spinosum [spĭn-ō′-, spī-, spĭ-nō′səm] describes the third or fourth layer of the epidermis (*stratum malpighii* or *mucosum*) as being full of spines (*spinosum*). The reference is to "intercellular bridges," fibrils that seem to extend from adjacent cells to each other.

strawberry angioma, or **mark, tongue** [strô′bĕr′ē, -bĕr-ē, -ĭ ăn′gē-ō′mə, mărk, tŭng]. Here are further instances of the use of a familiar object to give easy recall to the characteristics of a less familiar object. *Strawberry angioma,* or *mark,* describes a superficial hemangioma in terms of the color and size of the fruit; *strawberry tongue* describes the tongue in scarlet fever in terms of color and surface characteristics of the fruit.

stria [strī′ə] is Latin for a groove, furrow or channel. The plural is *striae* [strī′ē, -ī]. In medical application a rather shallow, linear depression takes the designation.

stria albicans [ăl′bĭ-kănz] means a furrow that is turning white (*albicans*).

stria atrophica [ə-trŏf′ĭ-kə] designates the type of furrowed depression that develops from atrophy.

stria distensa [dĭs-tĕn′sə] designates the type of furrowed depression that develops when the skin is put on stretch by events like pregnancy or obesity.

striata [strī-, strĭ-ā′tə], **striate** [strī′āt′] and **striatus** [strī-, strĭ-ā′təs, -tŭs] are (the first and third) the feminine and masculine singular of a Latin adjective meaning furnished with furrows and (the second) an English adjective meaning striped. In dermatologic context the Latin adjectives also mean striped. They appear in the titles *dermatitis pratensis striata* and *lichen striatus.*

strophulus [strŏf′ū-ləs] is New Latin from a Greek word meaning a small (-*ulus,* diminutive) twisted band or cord (*stroph-*). It is not clear etymologically how it comes to be applied to the blister that forms on the top of a wheal unless one imagines that blister to be twisted out of the underlying edema into a tense, cordlike structure.

S.T.S. is an acronym for **s**erologic **t**est *for* **s**yphilis.

Sturge-Weber syndrome [stûrj; wĕb′ĕr]. Meningo-oculo-facial angiomatosis.

sty(e) [stī] is as bothersome etymologically as is the inflammatory process in a gland of an eyelid. The modern word may be a backformation from an Anglo-Saxon word, *styang* (*e*) or *styany,* interpreted as *sty-on-eye.* But still, whence *sty* (*e*)? This word seems to stem from roots in Anglo-Saxon and other Indo-European languages that mean to rise, climb or ascend (compare modern German *steigen*). In earlier Germanic languages, apparently related nouns meant step, staircase or ladder; in a dialect of North England a *sty* means a ladder. In short, we can be sure that *sty* (*e*) has come to mean something that arises on the eye, even if we cannot be sure how the word arose.

sub- [sŭb] is a Latin prefix meaning under and has extended meanings of below in the sense of inferior or abnormal.

subacute [sŭb′ə-kūt′] is an adjective referring to what is less than (*sub-*, below) acute.

subacute lupus erythematosus [lōō′pəs ĕr′ĭ-thĕm′ə-tō′sĭs, -thē′mə-tō′sĭs] is a title used by some to designate that form of lupus erythematosus that is not as asymptomatic as discoid lupus erythematosus nor yet so severe as systemic lupus erythematosus. That is to say, there is visible spread of cutaneous lesions, reflection of systemic process in the form of leukopenia, urinary abnormalities and perhaps appearance of the LE phenomenon but no great constitutional symptoms in the form of fever, malaise or prostration.

subcorneal [sŭb-kôr′nē-əl] refers to position just under (*sub-*) the stratum corneum (-*corneal*).

subcorneal pustular dermatosis [pŭs′tū-lĕr, -lər dûr′mə-tō′sĭs] is the title of a condition of the skin (*dermatosis*) characterized by pustules that develop just under the stratum corneum (*subcorneal*) on the abdomen and in the axillary and inguinal folds. The condition is notable for chronicity and recalcitrance. Its cause and nosologic position are unclear. The pustules are sterile. May respond to sulfones and sulfapyridines.

subcutaneous [sŭb′kū-tā′nē-əs] refers to position just under (*sub-*) the skin.

subcutaneous fat necrosis of the newborn is a literal translation of *adiponecrosis subcutanea neonatorum* (which see).

subcutaneous mycoses chromomycosis, sporotrichosis, lobomycosis and various mycetomas. Some of the organisms involved in this group of diseases are not strictly fungal; the actinomyces, for example, are anaerobic Gram-positive bacilli. (E. Jones)

subcuticular [sŭb′kū-tĭk′ū-lĕr, -lər] should refer (-*ar*) to position just below (*sub-*) the epidermis (-*cuticul-*, literally the little skin) and be synonymous with *subepidermal*.

subcutis [sŭb-kū′tĭs] designates the tissue directly below (*sub-*) the skin (-*cutis*). It amounts to the upper reaches of the panniculus adiposus.

subepidermal [sŭb′ĕp-ĭ-dûr′məl] and **subepithelial** [sŭb′ĕp-ĭ-thē′lĭ-əl, -lē-əl] refer (-*al*) to position just below (*sub-*) the epidermis (-*epiderm-*, -*epitheli-*).

subitum [soo′bĭ-təm, -tŭm, -toom] is the neuter singular of a Latin adjective meaning sudden. It appears in the title *erythema, or exanthema, subitum.*

subungual [sŭb′ŭng′gwəl] refers to position under (*sub-*) a plate of a nail (-*ungal* = *ungu-* plus -*al*, pertaining to).

subungual abscess [ăb′sĕs] designates a collection of pus (*abscess*) under (*sub-*) a plate of a nail (-*ungual*).

subungual hematoma [hĕm′ə-tō′mə] designates a mass (-*oma*) of fluid blood (*hemat-*) under (*sub-*) a plate of a nail (-*ungual*).

subungual hyperkeratosis [hī′pĕr-kĕr′ə-tō′sĭs] designates a condition (-*osis*) of increased (*hyper-*) formation of horn (-*kerat-*) under (*sub-*) a plate of a nail (-*ungual*).

subungual wart [wôrt] designates a wart under (*sub-*) a plate of a nail (-*ungual*).

sudamen, sudamina [soo-, sū-dā′mən; sū-dăm′ĭ-nə] are respectively the singular and plural of a Latin word for sweating. We used the words for lesions of miliaria crystallina.

sudoriferous [soo′-, sū′dĕr-ĭf′ĕr-əs, -ə-rəs] means bearing or carrying (-*ferous*) sweat (*sudori-*).

suffodiens [sŭ-fō′dĭ-ĕnz] means digging (-*fodiens*) under (*suf-* = *sub-*). See *folliculitis abscedens et suffodiens.*

suggillation [sŭg′jĭ-lā′shən] derives from the Latin noun *suggillatio,* formed from the past participle of the verb *suggillare,* meaning to beat black and blue. The word then means a bruised condition in which swelling and particularly ecchymosis are prominent.

Sulzberger-Bloch syndrome. See Bloch-Sulzberger syndrome.

Sulzberger-Garbe disease [sŭlts′bĕrg-ĕr; gär′b]. Distinctive exudative discoid and lichenoid chronic dermatosis.

summer acne, eruption, itch [sŭm′ĕr, -ər, ăk′nē, ē-rŭp′shən, ĭch] are simple but unsatisfactory designations for conditions that are thought to be caused or influenced by the season.

sunburn [sŭn′bûrn′] designates the well-known effects of exposure to critical amounts of ultraviolet light in the range of 2600–3200 Å within the spectrum of sunshine. Erythema and blistering are the common cutaneous effects; fever and malaise may be constitutional effects.

super- [sōō'pēr] is a Latin prefix equivalent to Greek *hyper-*, meaning above, more or in excess.

superficial [sōō'pēr-físh'əl] refers to what is shallow in a physical or figurative sense.

superficial basal-cell epithelioma [bā's'l-, z'l-, -zəl-sĕl ĕp'ĭ-thē'lĭ-ō'mə, -lē-ō'mə] denotes a type of neoplasia of basal cells that does not tend downward.

superficial granulomatous pyoderma is a localized vegetative form of pyoderma gangrenosum.

superficial infection [ĭn-fĕk'shən] denotes inflammatory process caused by micro-organisms that does not tend downward.

superficial malignant melanoma [mə-lĭg'nənt mĕl'ə-nō'mə] is a title that only a pathologist could think up. What is meant is malignant melanoma still situated high in the skin around the dermo-epidermal junction and pars papillaris. In that position, the condition has a better prognosis if it has not yet metastasized, as it likely hasn't, and if it is completely extirpated locally. It is merely a matter of time, however, before "superficial" becomes "deep," a word not used to modify *malignant melanoma*. Some, but no great, comfort can be taken from the reading of "superficial."

supernumerary [sōō'pēr-nōō'mēr-ĕr'ē, -ĕr'ĭ] refers to what is more (*super-*) than the usual number (*-numerary*).

supernumerary digits, nipples, etc. denote more than the usual number of the structures cited.

suspension [sŭs-pĕn'shən], as a pharmaceutical form, designates a preparation in which ingredients are merely more or less dispersed as visible particles and which is consequently turbid.

Sutton's nevus [sŭt'n]. Leukoderma acquisitum centrifugum.

sweat [swĕt] derives from Anglo-Saxon and Middle English words. The word designates the product of the sweat gland, namely, a dilute solution of inorganic salts and even lesser concentrations of organic substances like urea and amino acids.

sweat gland [glănd] is the simple designation of the structure in the skin that produces sweat. *Eccrine* and *coil gland* are alternate terms.

Sweet's syndrome (acute febrile neutrophilic dermatosis). Inflammatory cutaneous plaques, fever and arthralgias, neutrophilia and histologic evidence of neutrophilic vessel-based dermal inflammation without infection. (Jorizzo et al., Journal of American Academy of Dermatology, Vol 19, No. 6)

swelling [swĕl′ĭng] derives from Anglo-Saxon. Enlargement by vascular dilatation and edema or of solid masses are the medical senses of the word.

swimmer's itch [swĭm′ĕrz, -ərz ĭch] is another parochial designation, this time for pruritus caused by bites of schistosomes.

sycosiform [sī-kō′sī-fôrm] and **sycosiforme** [sī-kō′sī-fôr′mē] are respectively an English adjective and the neuter singular of a New Latin adjective meaning in the form of a fig (sycosi-). The Latin adjective appears in the title ulerythema sycosiforme.

sycosis [sī-kō′sĭs] is a New Latin formation from Greek word elements that mean a figgy (syc-) condition (-osis). What is meant is a follicular pyoderma consisting of lesions that to some ancient observer suggested small figs. This is one of the less apt names utilizing a familiar object.

sycosis barbae [bär′bē, -bī] designates a follicular pyoderma (sycosis) of the beard (barbae).

sycosis vulgaris [vŭl-gā′rĭs, -gä′rĭs, -gär′ĭs] means the common (vulgaris) variety of follicular infection (sycosis).

syndactylia [sĭn′dăk-tĭl′ē-ə, -ĭ-ə] and **syndactyly** [sĭn-dăk′tĭl-ē] are respectively a New Latin noun and its English derivative formed from Greek word elements meaning a condition (-ia, -y) of joined, i.e., fused (syn-) digits (-dactyl-, finger or toe).

syndrome is from the Greek word syndrome meaning concurrence. A set of symptoms which occur together. The sum of signs of any morbid state. A symptom complex. (Stedman's Medical Dictionary, Williams & Wilkins)

synovial [sĭn-ō′-, sī-nō′vē-əl] is an adjective meaning pertaining or relating to synovium. The origin of synovium is unknown except that it was coined by Paracelsus (16th century). A sacculation or herniation of joint linings or tendon sheaths is designated by synovium.

synovial cyst [sĭst] bespeaks an enclosed structure derived from joint linings or tendon sheaths. Lesions called synovial cysts occur in interphalangeal joints of fingers. Some such lesions seem to be local degenerations of tissues around joints rather than encystments from their linings.

syphilid(e) [sĭf′ĭ-lĭd, -līd, -lēd] means any lesion within the possibilities of syphilitic process. See -id (e).

syphilis [sĭf′ə-, sĭf′ĭ-lĭs] is the main word of the title of a poem written in Latin by Girolamo Fracastoro (16th century) about a shepherd

named Syphilus, who is described as the first sufferer of the dread
disease since designated by that word. The complete title is *Syphilis
Sive Morbus Gallicus* ("About Syphilus or the French Disease").
As a word *syphilis* is patterned after similar formations like *Aeneis*,
Vergil's epic better known to us as the *Aeneid*. The Greco-Latin
ending -*is* conveys the sense of "about or concerning." Thus, *Aeneis*
is a story about Aeneas and *Syphilis* is an account of the trials and
tribulations of Syphilus, poor boy.

Caused by a motile corkscrewlike spirochete *Trepenema pallidum*, usually spread by direct contact through sexual relations. Incubation period may be less than 2 weeks to one month or more.
The first sign is the chancre followed by fever and other systemic
symptoms and a macular papular skin eruption with mucous
patches; this is secondary syphilis. Tertiary syphilis shows gummas
and cardiovascular lesions and central nervous system involvement.

syphiloderm [sĭf′ĭ-lō-dûrm′] means any cutaneous (-*derm*) process
within the possibilities of syphilis.

syphilologist, syphilology [sĭf′ə-, sĭf′ĭ-lŏl′ō-jĭst; sĭf′ĭ-lŏl′ō-jē, -ə-jī]
mean respectively a student of (-*logist*) and the study of (-*logy*)
syphilis. Like leprosy, syphilis is such a large consideration that we
designate its study and students by distinctive words.

syphilophobia [sĭf′ə-, sĭf′ĭ-lō-fō′bē-ə, -lə-fō′bĭ-ə] means unwarranted
fear (-*phobia*) of syphilis.

syring(o)- [sĭ-rĭng′gō] is a combining form from Greek *syrinx*, genitive *syringos*, a tube.

syringocystadenoma   papilliferum   [sĭ-rĭng′gō-sĭst′ăd′ə-nō′mə
păp′ə-, păp′ĭ-lĭf′ĕr-əm] describes a circumscribed, walled structure
(-*cyst*-) of the tubular portion (*syringo*-) of a sweat gland that takes
a reduplicated (-*ma*) glandular (-*adeno*-) conformation with nippled (*papilliferum*) structures within lumina.

syringoma [sĭr′ĭng-gō′mə] describes a reduplication (-*ma*) or tumor
(-*oma*) of the tubular portion (*syringo*-, *syring*-) of a sweat gland.

systematized [sĭs′tə-mə-tīzd′] is said of diseases or lesions thereof
that are widespread and seem to have some meaningful pattern
rather than haphazard distribution.

systematized nevus [nē′vəs] describes a congenital anomaloy (*nevus*) in which there is pattern and wide distribution of the lesions.

systemic [sĭs-tĕm′ĭk] refers to (-*ic*) what is placed (-*tem*-) together
(*sys*-, for *syn*-), i.e., a combination of things in obligatory relation-

ship. What pertains to the organs of the body combined in structure and function is termed *systemic*.

systemic lupus erythematosus [lōō′pəs ĕr′ĭ-thĕm′ə-tō′səs, -thē′mə-tō′səs] describes the process designated by *lupus erythematosus* as it affects many organs of the body simultaneously.

systemic sclerosis. See *sclerosis, systemic*.

T

tache [tŏsh, tăsh] is a French word for a spot. To ears accustomed
only to English, *taches blanches, bleuâtres,* or *bleues,* must sound
more expressive than do *white, bluish* or *blue spots.* One does not
hear *taches blanches* for the lesions of vitiligo, but *taches bleuâtres,*
or *bleues,* for those patches of blue color that sometimes attend pediculosis pubis is frequently used and is memorable.

tarda [tär′də], **tardus** [tär′dəs, -dŭs] are respectively the feminine singular and the masculine singular of a Latin adjective meaning late,
slow. They appear in the titles *porphyria cutanea tarda* and *nevus
tardus.*

tattoo [tă-tōō′] derives from Tahitian *tatau,* meaning puncturation.
The word is used both as a verb and noun to refer to the operation
of driving pigments into skin by puncture according to a design
and to the result of the procedure. Accidental deposition of adventitious, exogenous pigments is also designated by the word.

tegument, tegumentum. See under *integument.*

telangiectasia, -ectasis [tĕl′ăn-jē-, tĕl′ăn-jĭ-ĕk-tā′zhē-ə, -zē-ə, -zhə,
-ĕk′tə-sĭs] mean a condition (*-sia, -sis*) of dilated (*-ecta-*) end (*tel-*)
i.e., small, blood vessels (*-angi-*). In addition to designating the
general condition the words are sometimes used loosely for specific
units of dilated capillary or slightly larger end vessels.

telangiectasia macularis eruptiva perstans [măk′ū-lā′rĭs, -lä′rĭs,
-lär′ĭs ē′rŭp-tī′və pûr′stănz] is translatable as chronic or persistent
(*perstans*), eruptive (*eruptiva*), spotty (*macularis*) dilatation of end
vessels (*telangiectasia*). The title is applied to a variant of urticaria
pigmentosa in which telangiectasia is a striking clinical feature.

telangiectaticum [tĕl′ăn-jē-, tĕl′ăn-jĭ-ĕk-tā′tĭ-kəm] and **telangiectodes** [tĕl′ăn-jĭ-ĕk-tō′dēz] are New Latin adjectival formations from
Greek word elements meaning respectively consisting of (*-ticum*)
and like (*-odes*) dilated (*-ecta-*) end (*tel-*) vessels (*-angi-*). The first
appears in the title *granuloma telangiectaticum* (neuter) and the
second in *purpura annularis telangiectodes* (feminine).

telogen [tē′lō-, tĕl′ō-jĕn] literally means end (*telo-*) i.e., last, growth
(*-gen*). The word is used to refer to the "resting" stage of a hair or

final phase of a hair cycle, that more or less long period before a hair is shed or falls. See *anagen* and *catagen* for related words.

terebrans [tĕr′ə-, tĕr′ə-brănz] is the present participle of a Latin verb and means boring (through), piercing. It appears in the title *basiloma terebrans*.

tertiary [tər′-, tûr′shē-, tûr′shĭ-ĕr′ē, -ĭ, -shə-rĭ, -rē] means third in progression.

tertiary syphilis [sĭf′ĭ-lĭs] designates the stage after the secondary and is marked in the skin by nodulo-ulcerative or gummatous lesions.

tetter [tĕt′ēr, -ər] derives from Anglo-Saxon *teter*, meaning a blister or pimple. The word is obsolete now but was once widely and loosely used, as *ringworm* was, for a variety of conditions as unrelated as the eczematous, pyodermic and lupoid.

thèque [tĕk] is a French word for a box or small chest and derives from a Greek word *theke*, of the same meaning. The word is used in descriptions of cutaneous histology to designate those smallish, tight collections of melanin-producing cells belonging to nevi situated around the dermo-epidermal junction. The tendency of dermatologists who know only English is to anglicize the pronunciation to *thēk*.

The entry of *thèque* gives us an opportunity to digress in order to expatiate upon certain laws of philology and linguistics and to illustrate them by citing a number of interesting words related to *thèque*.

The Greek word *theke* (pronounced thā′kā in ancient Greek), as is, or subtly changed, is found in compound words both in original Greek and in many languages that borrowed it. Thus, from the Greek word *apotheke*, meaning a place where things are stored or laid (*-theke*) up or away (*apo-*), the Romans formed *apotheca*, also meaning a place for storing things, i.e., a repository, storehouse or warehouse, and *apothecarius*, a clerk or warehouseman. The Germans took over *apotheke* directly from Greek but gave to it a different and limiting meaning, that of a store or shop in which drugs, medicines and related items are sold—in other words a drugstore or pharmacy. The druggist or pharmacist is called an *apotheker* in German.

The English word *apothecary* (from Latin *apothecarius*) once— long, long ago—referred to a shop where drugs, preserves, spices and similar nonperishable commodities were sold. Then the use of the word was restricted to mean only a shop where drugs were compounded and prescriptions for them filled. The word then also came to be applied to the person selling these drugs and filling the prescriptions. Today, that person is more generally known as a druggist, a pharmacist or, particularly in England, a pharmaceutical chemist (chemist, for short) and, of course, the range of activities and products sold is nowadays very wide indeed. Of further interest is the fact that the French and Russians also have their words for similar meanings derived from *apotheke* or *apothecarius*.

From the very same Greek source, French and American English have *boutique*, simply a store in France but, among us in the United States, a specialty shop of off-beat women's apparel and costume jewelry, and Spanish has *bodega*, which in some Spanish-speaking countries means a storehouse, warehouse, vault, wine cellar, in others, and among Spanish-speaking persons in the U.S.A., a food store or retail grocery shop. *Boutique* and *bodega* show two common phenomena of philology, namely, aphaeresis (the removal of an initial letter, *a* for the cases in point) or that form of aphaeresis that is called aphesis (the gradual withering of an initial letter that is not pronounced) and consonantal shift from *p* to *b*. The same two modifications are seen in English *bishop* from Latin *episcopus*. Changes of this sort and others, like the appearance of *q* in the French *thèque* are exceedingly common in linguistic evolution.

Theke also appears altered in medical and botanical terminology, e.g., *theca* (a sheathed structure, especially the synovial sheath of a tendon), hence *intrathecal* (within a sheath, pertaining to the route of administration of medicine within a sheath, especially again that sheath which holds the cerebrospinal fluid) and *thecium* (a spore case, a seed pod), hence *perithecium* (the enclosing structure).

Finally, *thèque* is found as a combining form in the French word *bibliothèque*, literally a storehouse of books, a library in short, and in current English, in *discothèque* (more often without the accent mark), literally a place where playing records (*disco-*) are stored, actually a dance hall that uses recorded music to shake up the terpsichoreans. In both of these words *-thèque* is pronounced in the French manner, tĕk.

thermal, or **thermogenic, an(h)idrosis.** See *an* (*h*)*idrosis thermal,* or *thermogenic.*

thesaurismosis, thesaurosis [thĕ′sô-rĭs-, thĕ-sôr′ĭs-mō′sĭs; thĕ′sô-rō′sĭs] mean a condition (*-osis*) of storage (*thesaurism-, thesaur-,* a storing up). The word is generic for conditions in which there is excess or abnormal accumulation in the body, or in particular organs, of an endogenous or exogenous material, e.g., fats, heavy metals, phosphatides, etc.

A related word is *thesaurus*, from Greek via Latin, in which languages it meant anything stored up, a collection, especially of precious objects, hence, a treasure, and also the place where things or precious objects were stored, hence, a repository or treasury. In Latin the word also had an extended meaning—a literary storehouse. That, in effect, is the only one of its original meanings that *thesaurus* has in English today, as in Roget's *Thesaurus*, a storehouse or treasury of words. *Treasure, treasurer, treasurable*, and *treasury* come from *thesaurus* via Old French. *Treasury* has the additional meaning of a governmental department in charge of currency, funds, revenue, etc.—all a form of wealth, of course.

third disease [thûrd dĭ-, də-zēz′]. In an ordinal designation of the exanthemata, German measles (rubella) is third disease.

Thompson's syndrome [tŏm(p)′sŭnz, -s'nz, -sənz sĭn′drōm]. See under *poikiloderma congenitale*.

thrix [thrīks] is a Greek word for hair. The stem is seen in the genitive *trichos*, whence comes the combining form *trich* (*o*)-.

thrush [thrŭsh] has cognates in Danish, Dutch and Swedish words meaning rotten wood. We use the word to designate superficial fungous infection with *Candida albicans* of the mucous membranes of the mouth and the rest of the gastro-intestinal tract. The off-white, spongy appearance of the mucous surfaces in that condition must have suggested the allusion to rotten wood.

thymic hypoplasia (DiGeorge Syndrome) results from dysmorphogenesis of the third and fourth pharyngeal pouches, leading to hypoplasia or aplasia of the thymus and parathyroid glands, resulting in T-cell immunodeficiency disorder. (Buckley)

tick [tĭk] derives from a Middle English word for an arachnid, i.e., a spider or other eight-legged creature. We use the word for certain members of the order of *Acarina* in the class of *Arachnida*.

tincture [tĭngk′tūr, -chēr] derives from a Latin word element relating to dyeing. We use the word to designate a pharmaceutical preparation that is an alcoholic solution or extract of a nonvolatile, vegetable substance (compare *spirit*). There are three exceptions to this definition, namely, tincture of iodine, ferric chloride and cantharides, which are not of vegetable origin.

tinea [tĭn′ē-ə] is a Latin word for a moth and a worm. We use the word for superficial fungous infections generically and somewhat more specifically with modifying adjectives (except in the first of the entries following). The allusion to a moth is said to stem from the appearance of affected skin to moth-eaten cloth. The *worm* idea appears in *ringworm*. A selection of still current titles employing *tinea* appears below.

tinea amiantacea [ăm′ē-, ăm′ĭ-ăn-tā′shē-ə, -sē-ə, -shə] would seem to mean a superficial fungous infection (*tinea*) that has the clinical appearance of asbestos (*amiantacea*). It does not, however, have anything to do with fungous infection. The title is applied to any scaly condition of the scalp, other than fungous, in which the scales are seemingly lamellar and strongly adherent like asbestos. Severe cases of psoriasis of the scalp and pityriasis sicca are described by the title most aptly.

tinea capitis [kăp′ĭ-tĭs] means superficial fungous infection (*tinea*) of the scalp (*capitis*).

tinea circinata [sûr′sĭ-nā′tə, -nä′tə] describes superficial fungous infection (*tinea*) in the form of circular or round (*circinata*) lesions.

tinea corporis [kôr′pō-rĭs, -pô-rĭs] means superficial fungous infection (*tinea*) of the body (*corporis*) generally.

tinea cruris [kroo′rĭs] means superficial fungous infection (*tinea*) of the region of the upper portion of the thigh (*cruris*).

tinea favosa [fə-vō′sə] means superficial fungous infection (*tinea*) in which the aggregate of scutular lesions is in the form of a honeycomb (*favosa*). It's fanciful. Specifically, infection with *Trichophyton schoenleinii* is meant. See *favus*.

tinea glabrosa [glă-, glə-brō′sə] means superficial fungous infection (*tinea*) of the generally smooth (*glabrosa*), i.e., hairless, skin.

tinea imbricata [ĭm′brĭ-kā′tə, -kä′tə] means superficial fungous infection (*tinea*) in which the lesions appear like laid-out tiles (*imbricata*). Infection with *Trichophyton concentricum* produces such an appearance.

tinea inguinalis [ĭng′gwĭ-nā′lĭs, -nä′lĭs, -năl′ĭs] means superficial fungous infection (*tinea*) of the groin (*inguinalis*). It is about the same as *tinea cruris*.

tinea pedis [pĕ′-, pē′dĭs] means superficial fungous infection (*tinea*) of the foot (*pedis*). The commonest event is infection between the toes but infection of the rest of the foot is encompassed by the term.

tinea tonsurans [tŏn′soo-, tŏn-sū′-, tŏn′sū-rănz, -sə-rănz] designates a superficial fungous infection in which a shearing (*tonsurans*) of hair is specified. Infection of the scalp by any uncommon *Trichophyton (crateriforme, sulfureum* and *violaceum*).

tinea trichophytica [trĭk′ō-fĭt′ĭ-kə, trĭk′ō-fĭ′tĭ-kə] means superficial fungous infection (*tinea*) by a *Trichophyton (trichophytica*).

tinea unguium [ŭng′gwĭ-əm] means superficial fungous infection (*tinea*) of the nails (*unguium*). *Onychomycosis* is a commoner alternate.

tinea versicolor [vûr′sĭ-kō′lôr] means superficial fungous infection (*tinea*) that is characterized by a change of color (*versicolor*). That common infection with Pityrosporum orbrinlare whose lesions are characteristically tan to brown in the spring and then whitish in the fall after sun-tanning is described. *Pityriasis versicolor* is an alternate title.

tomato tumor [tə-mā′tō, -mä′tō tōō′-, tū′mẽr] is a homely designation, in terms of a familiar vegetable, of a large lesion of the condition more subtly termed *cylindroma*. *Turban tumor* is an alternate title when the conglomerate of lesions simulates that form of headdress.

tonsurans [tŏn′sōō-, tŏn-sū′-, tŏn′sū-rănz, -sə-rănz] is the present participle of a Late Latin verb meaning shearing, clipping, trimming. It appears in the title *tinea tonsurans*.

tophus [tō′fəs] is a Latin word (also written *tofus* in Latin) for a calcareous deposit, such as is found in certain springs. We use the word to designate those hard papules that contain urates and are to be found in sufferers from gout, particularly on the pinnae of the ears.

torti [tôr′tī] is the masculine plural of a Latin adjective (past participle of verb *torquere*, to twist) meaning twisted. It is found in the title *pili torti*.

Torula [tôr′ū-lə] derives from Latin *torus* and means a little (*-ula*) knot or bulge (*tor-*). We use the word to designate a species of yeast-like fungi. One of the morphologic characteristics of the organism in culture is knottiness to a small degree. The modern designation for the genus is *Cryptococcus*; *Torula capsulatum* and *histolytica* are now termed *Cryptococcus neoformans*.

torulosis [tôr′ū-lō′sĭs] means a condition (*-osis*) caused by a pathogenic species of *Torula*. *Cryptococcosis* is more modern.

torus [tō′rəs, tôr′ŭs] is Latin for a knot or bulge. The basic idea in the word is a swelling or protuberance.

torus palantinus [păl′ə-tī′nəs] designates a characteristic, bony protuberance on the vault of the palate.

totalis [tō-tā′lĭs, -tä′lĭs, -tăl′ĭs] is the masculine or feminine singular of a Latin adjective meaning total or entire. It appears in the title *alopecia totalis* (feminine).

toxic-. See **toxic(o)-.**

toxic [tŏk′sĭk] means relating to a poison or toxin (which see). The word was not, however, fashioned from *toxin*. It first appeared in print in 1664 whereas *toxin*, strange as it seems, was not coined until more than 200 years later (1886).

toxic epidermal necrolysis [ĕp′ĭ-dûr′məl nə-krŏl′-, nĕk-rŏl′ĭ-sĭs] a condition in which the epidermis dies (*necro-*) and separates (*-lysis*). It would seem often to be caused by drugs. The clinical appearance has been aptly likened to scalded skin because the epidermis peels after blistering in the manner of a second-degree burn. The outcome is sometimes fatal.

Toxic epidermal necrolysis (TEN) (Lyell's syndrome), a very severe type of erythema multiforme that starts suddenly with high fever, extensive erythematous, blotchy skin and marked debility. Huge bullae develop which soon denude, giving the appearance of scalded skin. This is the subepidermal type or true TEN. It may be like Stevens-Johnson syndrome and is identical histopathologically with epidermal type erythema multiforme.

toxic shock syndrome. This important acute febrile disease is due to toxins elaborated by *Staphylococcus aureus* organisms usually but also by Streptococci toxins. Mainly reported in women using tampons during menses. Also occurs with post surgical infections. There is an erythematous macular dermatitis which blanches with pressure but even bullae have been reported.

Systemic symptoms include but are not limited to vomiting, hypotension, renal insufficiency and renal failure.

toxic(o)- [tŏk′sĭk; tŏk′sĭ-kō] is a combining form from Greek meaning pertaining or relating to a poison.

Toxicodendron (-um) [tŏk′sĭ-kō-dĕn′drŏn (-drəm)] is the name of the genus of plants that includes poison ivy, posion oak and sumac(h). The ending *-on* is Greek; *-um* is the corresponding Latin ending (both endings are neuter singular).

toxicosis [tŏk′sĭ-kō′sĭs] means a condition (*-osis*) of poisoning (*toxic-*). The word is generally applied to the state that supervenes in diphtheria, tetanus, botulism and insect or snake venenation rather than poisoning by ordinary chemicals.

toxin [tŏk′sĭn] derives via Latin from a Greek word for a bow and also an arrow. Like archers before and since, Greek warriors sometimes dipped their arrows in poisonous drugs and the business was referred to as *toxikon pharmakon*. As has often happened in such phrases, the word for drug (*pharmakon*) evolved in a logical direction but the word denoting the carrier of the drug (*toxikon*) gave rise to words relating to poison. Thus, first *toxic* appeared, then *toxin* and most recently *toxoid* and *toxic* (*o*)- as a combining form (see specific entries).

toxoid [tŏk'soid] means like (*-oid*) poison (*tox-*). When used as a noun, the best sense of this word is that of a poison rendered weaker by artificial processing.

transient acantholytic dermatosis [trăn'shənt ăk'ăn-thō-lĭt'ĭk dûr'mə-tō'sĭs] describes a condition in which lesions develop that show in the microscope acantholysis of epidermal cells, reminiscent of the same appearance in pemphigus vulgaris. The condition resolves spontaneously in a reasonable time, a transiency that clinically belies pemphigus vulgaris.

Treponema [trĕp'ō-nē'mə] is New Latin from Greek elements meaning a turning (*trepo-*) thread (*-nema*). The word aptly designates the genus of micro-organisms that have the appearance of tiny pieces of fine, spiral threads in motion. With a small initial letter, *treponema* designates an individual organism.

Treponema carateum [kăr'ə-, kā'rə-tē'əm] designates the species of *Treponema* that causes carate or pinta. *Carateum* is a New Latin formation from a Spanish word of South American origin, *carate,* meaning brown ("liver") spots on the skin.

Treponema pallidum [păl'ĭ-dəm] designates the species of *Treponema* that causes syphilis. *Pallidum* is the neuter singular of a Latin adjective meaning pale.

Treponema pertenue [pĕr-, pûr-tĕn'ū-ē, -ŏŏ-ē] designates the species of *Treponema* that causes yaws. *Pertenue*, a Latin neuter singular adjective, means very (*per-*, intensive) thin (*-tenue*).

treponeme [trĕp'ō-, trĕp'ə-nēm] is an anglicized form for an individual organism of the genus *Treponema,* like *spirochete* from *Spirocheta*. One saw the word in print and heard it in speech long before it appeared in a dictionary (Webster's Third New International Dictionary).

trich-, or **tricho-** [trĭk; trĭk'ō], is a combining form from the Greek word *thrix,* hair, genitive *trichos,* of hair. The element is used in many words relating to hair or what looks like hair; there are, in fact, too many *trich*(*o*)'s and too much synonymy. The following selection is of dermatologic interest.

trichatrophy [trĭk-ăt'rə-fē, -fĭ] means malnutrition (*-atrophy*), therefore deterioration, of the apparatus of hairs (*trich-*).

trichauxis [trĭk-ôk′sĭs] means increase (-*auxis*) in size and number of hairs (*trich-*). It is rarely heard; *hypertrichosis* is a more common alternate. Perhaps inordinate thickness and coarseness of hair rather than mere increase in number are better designated by the word.

trichiasis [trĭ-kī′ə-sĭs] literally means a condition (-*iasis*)—any abnormal condition—of hair (*trich-*), but is not used that way. The word is restricted to the ophthalmologic complication in which eyelashes become inverted and irritate the eyeballs. Such an event occurs in entropion, such as is nearly inevitable in ocular pemphigus (essential shrinkage of the eye).

Trichina [trĭ-kī′nə] names a genus (-*ina*) of hairlike (*trich-*) nematodes, one species of which (*T. spiralis*) is pathogenic for humans. *Trichinella* is alternate, but less used.

Trichinella [trĭk′ĭ-nĕl′ə] is taxonomically preferred to *Trichina* and describes the members of a genus (-*in-*) of nematodes as little (-*ella*) hairs (*trich-*).

trichinelliasis [trĭk′ĭ-nĕl-ī′ə-sĭs], **trichinellosis** [trĭk′ĭ-nĕl- ō′sĭs], **trichiniasis** [trĭk′ĭ-nī′ə-sĭs] and **trichinosis** [trĭk′ĭ-nō′sĭs] all mean infestation with pathogenic species of *Trichinella* or *Trichina*. The dermatologic interest in the condition lies in edema of the eyelids that sometimes attends the infestation when it is localized in the ocular muscles, as, in addition to elsewhere (e.g., the diaphragm), it is likely to be.

trichitis [trĭ-kī′tĭs, -kē′tĭs] means an inflammatory (-*itis*) condition of the hair (*trich-*) apparatus. The word is rarely used.

tricho-. See *trich-*.

trichoclasia, trichoclasis [trĭk′ō-klā′zhē-ə,-zē-ə, -zhə; -klā′sĭs] are words meaning a condition (-*ia*, -*is*) of broken (-*clas-*), hairs (*tricho-*). The words are general and may be used to designate breakage of hair that may be artificial as in trichotillomania or for brittleness and inevitable breakage as in monilethrix and trichorrhexis nodosa. *Trichorrhexis* is an alternate word.

trichocryptomania [trĭk′ō-krĭp′tō-mā′nē-ə, -nĭ-ə, -nyə] means a compulsion (-*mania*) to hide (-*crypto-*), i.e., store or swallow, hair (*tricho-*). *Trichophagy* is an alternate word for the neurosis when swallowing is the means of hiding. Also see *trichocryptotillomania* and *trichokleptomania*. The dermatologic interest in the psychopathy is the artificial alopecia caused by the habit; of general interest is the possibility of formation of trichobezoars.

trichocryptosis [trĭk′ō-krĭp-tō′sĭs] literally means a condition (*-osis*) of hidden (*-crypt-*) hairs (*tricho-*). It is a learned alternate, like *pili incarnati*, for ingrown hairs.

trichocryptotillomania [trĭk′ō-krĭp′tō-tĭl′ō-mā′nē-ə, -nĭ-ə, -nyə] is extended from *trichocryptomania* and designates a compulsion (*-mania*) to pluck out (*-tillo-*) and hide (*-crypto-*), i.e., store or swallow, hair (*tricho-*). See *trichocryptomania, trichokleptomania* and *trichophagy*.

tricho-epithelioma [trĭk′ō-ĕp′ĭ-thē′lĭ-ō′mə, -lē-ō′mə] names a condition in which there is reduplication (*-ma*) or neoplasia (*-oma*) of epidermal elements (*-epithelio-, -epitheli-*) of the hair (*tricho-*) structures. The clinical mark is an indifferent papule; the histologic marks are more characteristic in the form of numerous rudimentary formations of hair follicles. The condition is benign. *Epithelioma adenoides cysticum* is an alternate title.

trichofolliculoma [trĭk′ō-fə-lĭk-ū-lo′mə] is still another of those formations with *-oma* in the sense of tumor, this time to designate benign hamartomatous dysplasia of that part of the epidermis that makes up the infundibulum (*-follicul-*) of a hair (*tricho-*) apparatus. The clinical appearance is indifferent enough, but the histopathology is characteristic in multiplicity of malformed, abortive hair follicles spreading from the main anomaly like a caput medusae.

trichoglossia [trĭk′ō-glŏs′ē-ə, -ĭ-ə] is a learned alternate for hairy (*tricho-*) tongue (*-glossia*). See *black hairy tongue*.

trichokinesis [trĭk′ō-kĭ-nē′sĭs, -kī-nē′sĭs] is as learned as *pili torti* for a condition of twisted (*-kinesis*) hairs (*tricho-*).

trichokleptomania [trĭk′ō-klĕp′tō-mā′nē-ə, -nĭ-ə, -nyə] means a compulsion (*-mania*) to steal (*-klepto-*) i.e., pluck out and hide by storing or swallowing, hair (*tricho-*). The word is related in its psychopathic connotations to *trichocryptomania, trichocryptotillomania* and *trichophagy*.

trichoma [trĭ-kō′mə] is given in dictionaries as alternate for *trichiasis* and *plica polonica*. If anything, it should be synonymous with *hypertrichosis* or *trichauxis* in line with the commonest meanings of *-ma* and *-oma*. It's enough to make one's hair stand on end.

trichomatosis [trĭk′ō-mə-tō′sĭs] is a word that should be treated like *trichoma* (which see).

trichomycosis [trĭk′ō-mī-kō′sĭs] means a fungous infection (*-mycosis*) of hairs (*tricho-*). While the word is general, it is hardly heard except in the following title:

trichomycosis axillaris nodosa [ăk′sĭ-lä′rĭs, -lä′rĭs, -lär′ĭs nō-dō′sə], or **nodularis** [nŏd′ū-lä′rĭs, -lä′rĭs, -lär′ĭs], which describes a characteristic fungous infection of the hairs (*trichomycosis*) of the armpits (*axillaris*) that has the clinical appearance of very many knots (*nodosa*) or of little knots (*nodularis*). Other characteristics, like yellow, red, brown or black color of the concretions, are not encompassed in the title. Species of *Nocardia* are the cause.

trichonocardiosis [trĭk′ō-nō-kär′dĭ-ō′sĭs, -ē-ō′sĭs] designates trichomycosis axillaris nodosa, or nodularis, by cause, i.e., by a species of *Nocardia*, specifically *N. tenuis*.

trichonodosis [trĭk′ō-nō-dō′sĭs] bespeaks a condition (*-osis*) of hair (*tricho-*) affected by knots or bulges (*-nod-*). *Beaded hair* is alternate.

trichonosus [trĭk′ō-nō′səs] is given in dictionaries as meaning a disease (*-nosus*) of hair (*tricho-*). It is a useless word subject to misunderstanding; *trichopathy* and *trichosis* are better alternates.

trichopathophobia [trĭk′ō-păth′ō-fō′bē-ə, -ĭ-ə] means a morbid fear (*-phobia*) of disease (*-patho-*) of the hair (*tricho-*). Inordinate fear of baldness is the usual form the madness takes.

trichopathy [trĭ-kŏp′ə-thē, -thĭ] means an abnormality (*-pathy*) of hair (*tricho-*).

trichophagy [trĭ-kŏf′ə-jē, -jĭ] means chewing or swallowing (*-phagy*, eating) of hair (*tricho-*).

trichophobia [trĭk′ō-fō′bē-ə, -bĭ-ə] means a morbid fear (*-phobia*) of hair (*tricho-*). It is applied to abnormal revulsion to the sight of loose hair on clothes and thereabouts. It might also be applied to a fear of too much hair, especially on the face and especially among women.

trichophytica [trĭk′ō-fĭt′ĭ-kə] and **trichophyticus** [-fĭt′ĭ-kəs] are respectively the feminine singular and the masculine singular of a New Latin adjective meaning relating to *Trichophyton* (*-um*). They appear in the titles *acne trichophytica* and *lichen trichophyticus*.

trichophytid(e) [trĭk′ō-fĭ′tĭd, -tīd, -tēd, trĭ-kŏf′ĭ-tĭd] means any clinical process within the family (*-id, -ide*) of lesions caused by infection with a *Trichophyton*. See *-id* (*e*).

trichophytin [trĭ-kŏf′ĭ-tĭn, trĭk′ō-fĭ′tĭn] is an "antigen" crudely processed from any of the common *Trichophyta*. In manner of production, use and reading it is similar to tuberculin and other agents of the class.

Trichophyton, -um [trĭk′ō-fī-, trĭ-kŏf′ĭ-tŏn; -təm, -tŭm, -tōōm] names a genus of fungi. The hairy (*tricho-*) characteristic of this class of primitive plant (*-phyt-*) life is recorded in the word. The ending *-on* is Greek neuter singular; *-um* is the corresponding Latin ending. Many species are pathogenic for humans and are named eponymically or for another cultural characteristic, e.g., *gypseum* (calcareous), *purpureum* or *rubrum* (purple or red), *schoenleinii* (of Schoenlein), *sulfureum* (yellow, like sulfur), *violaceum* (violet), etc.

trichophytosis [trĭk′ō-fī-, trĭ-kŏf′ĭ-tō′sĭs] means a condition (*-osis*) caused by a *Trichophyton*.

trichoptilosis [trĭk′ō-tĭ-lō′sĭs, trĭ′kŏp′tə-lō′sĭs] describes a condition (*-osis*) of hairs (*tricho-*) in which they are feathered (*-ptil-*), i.e., longitudinally split into two or more strands.

trichorrhea [trĭk′ə-, trĭk′ō-rē′ə] literally means a flow (*-rrhea*) of hair (*tricho-*). Abnormal fall or shedding of hair is meant.

trichorrhexis [trĭk′ə-, trĭk′ō-rĕk′sĭs] means breakage (*-rrhexis*) of hairs (*tricho-*). Transverse fracture is meant.

trichorrhexis invaginata, see **bamboo hair.**

   trichorrhexis nodosa [nō-dō′sə] names a condition in which hairs (*tricho-*) bear knots or bulges (*nodosa*) and have breaks (*-rrhexis*) at those points. The fracture is characteristic in the form of impaction as of brushes.

trichorrhexomania [trĭk′ō-rĕk′sō-mā′nē-ə, -nĭ-ə, -nyə] means a compulsion (*-mania*) to break (*-rrhexo-*) hairs (*tricho-*). The word is less used than *trichotillomania*, which is nearly equivalent.

trichoschisia, -schisis [trĭk′ō-skĭ′zhē-ə, -zē-ə, -zhə, -sē-ə, -sĭs] mean a condition (*-ia, -is*) of cloven or split (*-schis-*) hair (*tricho-*). The word is nearly equivalent to *trichoptilosis*, but not to *trichorrhexis*.

trichoschisis means clean fracture of the hair shaft.

trichosis [trĭ-kō′sĭs] means an abnormal condition (*-osis*) of hair (*trich-*). It is a generic word.

Trichosporon, -um [trĭk′ō-spō′rŏn, trĭ-kŏs′pə-rŏn; -rəm, -rŭm, -rōōm] names a genus of fungi whose characteristic of sporulating (*-spor-*) on hairlike (*tricho-*) structures is told by the word. Pathogenic species of the genus are the cause of white piedra. The ending *-on* is Greek; *-um* is Latin; both are neuter singular.

trichosporosis [trĭk′ō-spō-rō′sĭs, -spə-rō′sĭs] means a condition (*-osis*) caused by a pathogenic *Trichosporon*.

trichostasis spinulosa [trĭk′ō-stā′sĭs spĭn′ū-, spī′nū-lō′sə] means a persistent condition (*-stasis*) of hairs (*tricho-*) that is finely spinous (*spinulosa*). This trivial condition consists of bundles of lanugo hair issuing from a common ostium. Clinically, the bundles are not seen as such and are not palpably spinous. Under the microscope the appearance is that of a tiny brush of a dozen to a score of fine hairs surrounded by a sheath of keratinized material.

trichothiodystrophy syndrome consists of brittle hair with a markedly reduced sulfur content. Short stature, mental deficiency, ichthyosis, nail dystrophy, ocular dysplasia and infertility. Autosomal recessive.

trichotillomania [trĭk′ō-tĭl′ō-mā′nē-ə, -nĭ-ə, -nyə] means a compulsion (*-mania*) to pluck (*-tillo-*) out hair (*tricho-*).

Trombicula [trŏm-bĭk′ū-lə] means a genus of mites whose larvae have ability to infest humans. The word seems to have been formed to mean a little (*-cula*) brown cloth (*trombi-*, from *thrombus*).

    Trombicula irritans [ĭr′ĭ-tănz] names a particular species of the genus. *Irritans* specifies the particularly disagreeable quality of this mite for humans.

trombidiasis, trombidiosis [trŏm′bĭ-dī′ə-sĭs; -bĭd′ĭ-ō′sĭs, -ē-ō-sĭs] designate the condition (*-iasis, -osis*) of infestation with mites of the family of *Trombidiidae.*

trop-. See *troph* (*o*)-, *trōp* (*o*)-.

troph(o)- and **trop(o)-** [trō′fō; trō′pō] are combining forms from Greek whose consistent uses and subtle meanings in compound words are difficult to specify. Appearing as they do at the beginning, within, or at the end of words and having essential meanings of turning, attracting or stimulating for *trop* (*o*)-, and nourishing for *troph* (*o*)-, they cause confusion, for they also have active and passive senses and because the figurative interchangeability of the meanings of stimulating and nourishing has resulted in the substitution of one for the other in many English and even in some Greek words. Therefore, utterly consistent logic and unambiguous meanings for the elements and their compounds are difficult to establish and maintain. Following are two illustrative words that are not troublesome: *dermatrophy*, a condition (*-y*) of under- (*a-*, alpha privative) -nourishment (*-troph-*) of the skin (*derm-*); *dermotropic*, attracted to or by (*-tropic*) the skin (*dermo-*).

tropical acne. See *acne, tropical.*

tropical anhidrotic asthenia [trŏp′ĭ-kəl, -k′l ăn′hĭ-drŏt′ĭk ăs-thē′nē-ə, -nĭ-ə, -nyə] describes the enfeeblement that is a consequence of failure of the sweating function in severe cases of miliaria rubra as may occur in regions of high temperature and humidity.

tropical ulcer or **tropical phagedenic ulcer** tissue necrosis may be due to fusobacterium releasing an exotoxin or a cytoxic factor. Complications which may result are tibial osteomyelitis and squamous cell cancer. (Adriaans)

tubercle [tōō′-, tū′bĕr-k′l] derives from Latin *tuberculum*, a little knob, lump or swelling. We have tubercles in both macro- and microscopic frames of reference. Dermatologically, we are interested particularly in the microscopic, i.e., a compact collection of epithelioid cells admixed and surrounded by small round cells that is so characteristic of some lesions of tuberculosis and other granulomatous diseases.

tubercle, naked. See *naked tubercle*.

tubercular [tōō-, tū-bûr′kū-lĕr, -lər] means pertaining to (*-ar*) a tubercle and to tuberculosis.

tuberculid(e) [tōō-, tū-bûr′kū-lĭd, -lĭd, -lĕd] literally means any lesion within the family (*-id, -ide*) of lesions of tuberculosis. See *-id* (*e*).

tuberculin [tōō-, tū-bûr′kū-lĭn] designates a material (*-in*) derived from the tubercle bacillus. Specified as *P.P.D.* (protein-purified derivative), this is widely used as a skin test to verify exposure to TB. If positive would result in a T cell mediated delayed type hypersensitivity reaction.

tuberculoderm [tōō-, tū-bûr′kū-lō-dûrm′] means a tuberculous process in or of the skin.

tuberculoid [tōō-, tū-bûr′kū-loid] means like (*-oid*) a tubercle or like tubercular processes.

tuberculoid leprosy. See under *leprosy*.

tuberculosis cutis [tōō-, tū-bûr′kū-lō′sĭs kū′tĭs] means tuberculosis of the skin (*cutis*). Following are varieties with titles in classical form:

tuberculosis cutis colliquativa [kŏl′ĭk-, kŏ-lĭk′wə-tī′və, -tē′və] designates cutaneous tuberculosis that takes the form of a "cold" abscess in a lymph node, bone joint or other underlying structure that usually discharges a thick pus through a sinus to the skin surface. *Colliquativa* carries an idea of liquefaction or dissolution. *Scrofuloderm* (*i*)*a* is an alternate title. See under *actinomycosis*.

tuberculosis cutis indurata [ĭn′dū-rā′tə, -rä′tə], or **indurativa** [-rə-tī′və], designates cutaneous tuberculosis that takes the form of hardened (*indurata, indurativa*) nodules. The condition is fairly characteristic in the common location of the lesions on the posterior aspect of the legs, deep-seated position, redness, tendency to ulcerate and healing by scarring. *Erythema induratum* and *Bazin's disease* are alternate titles.

tuberculosis cutis lichenoides [lī′kə-noi′dēz] designates cutaneous tuberculosis that resembles (*-oid*) a lichen, i.e., an agmination of papules. *Lichen scrofulosorum* is an alternate title.

tuberculosis cutis luposa [lōō-pō′sə] designates cutaneous tuberculosis that takes the form of a superficially eroded and scarred process (*luposa*; see *lupus*). This process is highly characteristic in its common location on the face in the form of intermingled "apply-jelly" nodules and scarring. *Lupus vulgaris* is an alternate title.

tuberculosis cutis miliaris [mĭl′ĭ-ā′rĭs, -ä′rĭs, -är′ĭs] designates cutaneous tuberculosis that takes the form of scattered papules and nodules in a person gravely ill with tuberculosis and one in which there has been a sudden hematogenous spread of organisms. *Acute miliary tuberculosis* is an alternate title.

tuberculosis cutis orificialis [ôr′ĭ-fĭsh′ĭ-ā′ĭs, -ē-ā′lĭs, -ä′lĭs, -ăl′ĭs, -fĭsh-ăl′ĭs] designates cutaneous tuberculosis that is seated in or around the mouth, anus or urinary meatus (*orificialis*, of an opening) in a person, usually gravely ill, with pulmonary, gastro-intestinal or genito-urinary tuberculosis.

Due to the excretion of tubercle bacilli about the mouth. Also seen about the anus.

tuberculosis cutis papulonecrotica [păp′ū-lō-nē-krō′tĭ-kə, -nĕ-krŏt′ĭ-kə] designates cutaneous tuberculosis that takes the form of papules that crust and ulcerate (*papulonecrotica*) and then heal by varioliform scarring. The extensor surfaces of the arms, legs and buttocks are common sites of the process. *Papulonecrotic tuberculide* is an alternate title.

tuberculosis cutis verrucosa [vĕr′ōō-kō′sə] designates cutaneous tuberculosis that takes the form of warty excrescences (*verrucosa*) usually on acral locations like fingers. Necrogenic tubercle, anatomic tubercle, or wart, butcher's tubercle and prosector's wart are of that nature.

tuberosum [tōō′bĕr-, tū′bĕr-ō′səm] is the neuter singular of a Latin adjective meaning full of (*-osum*) lumps (*tuber-*), knobby. It appears in the title *xanthoma tuberosum*.

tumefaction [too̅′-, tū′mə-făk′shən], derived from Latin, means the process of (-*tion*) making (-*fac*-) a swelling (*tume*-).

tumor [too̅′-, tū′mĕr, -mər] is a Latin word for a swelling. There is no inherent meaning of malignancy or cancer in the word.

tumor, glomus. See *glomus tumor*.

tumor, tomato. See *tomato tumor*.

tumor, turban. See *turban tumor*.

tumoricidal [too̅′mər-, tū′mĕr-ĭ-sī′d′l,-dəl] is a poorer word than *cancericidal* or *cancricidal* for the reason that it equates tumor with malignancy.

Tunga penetrans [tŭng′gə pĕn′ə-trănz] names a species of the genus *Tunga* of the class Hexapoda which causes a characteristic infestation by burrowing (*penetrans*). *Jigger, sand fly* or *chigo* (*e*) are vernacular names. *Tunga* is the Portuguese equivalent of the Greek *Sarcopsylla* and the latter name means a fleshy (*sarco*-) flea (-*psylla*).

tungiasis [tŭn-jī′ə-sĭs] is the condition (-*iasis*) of infestation with *Tunga penetrans*. The infestation is characteristic in the form of a shallow burrow, roofed in part by the body of the insect, usually located on the feet and particularly in the webs of the toes.

A parasitic skin infestation caused by the *Tunga penetrans* sand flea, which is prevalent in tropical Africa, Central and South America, the Caribbean Islands, Pakistan, and the West Coast of India. (Sanusi et al. *J. Am. Acad. Dermatol.* May 1989. 20: 941-944.)

tunnel. See *burrow*.

turban tumor [tûr′bən too̅′-, tū′mĕr] is picturesquely descriptive of extensive development of cylindromas on the scalp in the form of a turban, that is, a headdress of wrappings. See *tomato tumor*.

twisted hair [twĭs′tĕd, twĭst′ĭd, -əd hâr] is a straightforward descriptive term for the anomaly of hairs that have unusual bends. *Pili torti* is the title in classical form.

tyloma [tī-lō′mə], from Greek, means a development or formation (-*oma*) of callus (*tyl*-), therefore, a corn or callosity.

tylosis [tī-lō′sĭs] means a condition (-*osis*) of heavy callus (*tyl*-) formation.

Tyroglyphus [tĭ-rŏg′lĭ-fəs] names a genus of mites that are characterized as cheese (*tyro*-) carvers (-*glyphus*). Species named *T. longior* (comparative of *longus*, long), and *T. siro* (probably describing the organism as cordlike), can cause a minor infestation in food handlers who deal in cheese.

Tzanck test. [tzônk] Search for acantholytic epidermal cells in smears from the bullae and vesicles of some diseases and for enlarged or baloon cells in viral diseases.

U

ulcer [ŭl′sĕr, -sər] derives from Latin, *ulcus*, a sore. We use the derived word to designate loss of substance, from a surface downward, that is slow to heal or tends not to heal at all.

ulcer, amebic, decubital, decubitus, diabetic, phagedenic, rodent. See *amebic, decubital, decubitus, diabetic, phagedenic, rodent ulcer*.

ulcerate, ulceration [ŭl′sĕr-āt; -ā′shən] refer to the process and result of loss of substance in the formation of an ulcer.

ulcerative [ŭl′sĕr-ā′tĭv, -ə-tĭv] means tending to ulceration.

ulcerous [ŭl′sər-, ŭl′sĕr-əs] means characterized by ulceration.

ulcus [ŭl′kəs] is the Latin word used by Pliny and Celsus, among others, in much the same sense as we use *ulcer* (which see) today.

ulcus vulvae acutum [vŭl′vē ə-kū′təm] is a title that describes an ulcer (*ulcus*) that develops on the vulva (*vulvae*) in sudden and severe (*acutum*) fashion. It is an unsatisfactory story-title that could fit lesions of aphthosis, herpes simplex and many another condition in the designated site, but was coined specifically for lesions that are thought to be none of the latter, rather a condition *sui generis* and idiopathic in virgins.

ulerythema [ū′lĕr-ē-, -ə-, ū′lĕr-ĭ-thē′mə] derives from Greek word elements that mean scarring (*ul-*) redness (*-erythema*). The word is applied with modifying adjectives to vague inflammatory processes that eventuate in atrophy or scarring. Following are some examples of titles in which the word is used.

ulerythema acne(i)forme [ăk′nē-fôr′mē; ăk-nē′ĭ-fôr′mē] is descriptive of inflammatory process that is marked by scarring and redness (*ulerythema*) in the manner (*-forme*) of acne (*acne-, acnei-*). Scarring such as occurs in ordinary acne is not so designated but consequences of rosacea, tuberculids on the face and even exanthemata like smallpox and chicken pox might take the title descriptively.

ulerythema ophryogenes [ŏf′rĭ, ŏf′rē-ŏj′ə-nēz] is a title describing inflammatory process arising (*-genes*) on the eyebrows (*ophryo-*)

and resulting in scarring and redness (*ulerythema*). Certain folliculitides of the site eventuate that way.

ulerythema sycosiforme [sĭ-kō′sĭ-fôr′mē] describes an inflammatory process in which the scarring and redness (*ulerythema*) are in the shape or manner (*-forme*) of a fig (*sycosi-*). It's very fanciful. Severe pyodermas, particularly on the face and in the nature of sycosis barbae, eventuate that way.

ulerythematosa [ū′lĕr-ĭ-thĕm′ə-tō′sə, -thē′mə-tō′sə] is the feminine singular of a New Latin adjectival formation meaning full of scarring and redness. It appears in the title *atrophodermia ulerythematosa*.

-um [əm, ŭm, o͞om] is the ending of Latin neuter singular nouns and adjectives (of the second declension) and is equivalent to the Greek *-on*, e.g., *phylum, phylon*.

Uncinaria [ŭn′sĭ-nǎr′ē-ə, -ĭ-ə, -nā′rē-ə, -rĭ-ə] is the name of an order of helminths that are characterized (*-aria*) by the structure of a hook (*uncin-*).

uncinariasis [ŭn′sĭ-nə-rī′ə-sĭs] means a condition (*-iasis*) of infestation with a capable genus of the order *Uncinaria*. The dermatologic marks of the condition are vesicles or pustules at the point of entry of the larvae of *Ancylostoma* or *Necator*.

ungual, unguinal [ŭng′gwəl; ŭng′gwĭ-nəl] are adjectives from Latin *unguis*, nail, and mean relating to (*-al*) the nail.

unguent [ŭng′gwənt] as a pharmaceutical form means a preparation (*-ent*) designed to be rubbed in (*ungu-*). It is used equivalently with *ointment*, which is etymologically related. *Salve* is an old-fashioned alternate word.

unguis [ŭng′gwĭs] is the nominative and genitive singular of a Latin word for nail (of a digit). The genitive plural is *unguium* [ŭng′gwĭ-əm], of (the) nails, which appears in the titles *atrophia unguium, defluvium unguium, dystrophia unguium, fragilitas unguium* and *tinea unguium*.

unguis incarnatus. See under *ingrowing, ingrown hair, nail*.

uni- [ū′nĭ, -nē] is the combining form from Latin *unus*, one.

unilateral [ū′nĭ-lăt′ēr-əl] means pertaining to (*-al*) one (*uni-*) side (*-later-*).

unilateral nevoid telangiectasia. Myriads of scattered telangiectasias occur very strikingly over one-half of the body and usually not on the opposite side. May be congenital but is most often associated with high estrogen levels of pregnancy or underlying liver disease. These are punctate and stellate telangiectases and may also involve the gastric and oral mucosa. (Anderson and Smith)

unius [o͞o-, u̅-nī′əs, -nē′əs, u̅′nĭ-əs, -nē-əs] is the genitive of Latin *unus,* one. It appears in the title *nevus unius lateris.*

universalis [u̅′nĭ-ver-sä′lĭs, -sä′lĭs, -ver-säl′ĭs] is the masculine or feminine singular of a Latin adjective meaning belonging to all or everywhere. In medicine it has the sense of widespread in or on the body. It appears in the title *alopecia universalis.*

Unna('s) boot [o͞on′ä(z) bo͞ot] is eponymic for a type of dressing applicable to foot and leg. It is an occlusive dressing, somewhat like a plaster cast but composed of gauze bandage impregnated with a mixture of gelatin and zinc oxide paste. It is therefore more flexible and porous and more easily removable than a plaster cast. It has uses in dermatitides and ulcerated conditions of feet and legs.

Unna-Thost disease [o͞on′ä; tōst]. Keratoderma palmare et plantare.

Urbach-Wiethe syndrome [o͞or′bäk; vē′te]. Hyalinosis cutis et mucosae.

ur(h)idrosis [u̅′rĭ-drō′sĭs; u̅r′hĭ-drō′sĭs] derives from Greek word elements that mean a condition (*-osis*) in which sweat (*-idr, -hidr-*) contains large amounts of constituents ordinarily excreted in the urine (*ur-*).

uroporphyrin [u̅′rō-pôr′fə-rĭn, -pôr′fĭr-ĭn]. Porphyrin in the urine seen in some of the porphyrias. Large amounts are associated with porphyria cutanea tarda.

urtica [u̅r′tĭ-kə, u̅r-tī′kə] is Latin for a nettle, i.e., any of the weeds that have stinging hairs. In Medieval Latin the word designated a wheal or hive, as it does today too.

urticaria [u̅r′tə-, u̅r′tĭ-kär′ē-ə, -kär′ē-ə, -kä′rē-ə, -rĭ-ə] means a condition that is characterized by (*-aria*) wheals (*urtic-*).

urticaria, acute [ə-ku̅t′] is simply descriptive of whealing that is sudden, explosive and of short duration as a complete episode. Of course each wheal is of that general nature but what is meant by the title is relative severity and relative brevity of the entire condition (days to a week or two).

urticaria, cholinergic [kō′lĭn-, kŏl′ĭn-ĕr′jĭk] is the title of a form of whealing that is predicated upon abnormal reaction to acetylcholine. The clinical feature is sudden eruption of edematous papules that are clearly urticarial in their rapid evolution and equally rapid devolution. As wheals go they are not very pruritic. For individuals who are susceptible, heat, as from emotion or exercise, seems to be a provocative factor.

urticaria, chronic, or **recurrent** [krŏn′ĭk; rē-kûr′ənt], is just as simple as *acute urticaria* in its description of attacks of whealing that appear and reappear over a long period of time in terms of weeks, months or years.

urticaria, cold. See *cold urticaria*.

urticaria factitia [făk-tĭsh′ə] is another title for urticarial derm(at)ographism. The element of artifice (*factitia*) as by stroke, friction or pressure is emphasized by this title.

urticaria, papular. See *papular urticaria*.

urticaria perstans [pĕr′-, pûr′stănz] simply says persistent (*perstans*) whealing (*urticaria*). Angioneurotic edema and annular, figurate and gyrate erythemas are of the class.

urticaria, physical [fĭz′ĭ-kəl] is descriptive of whealing that is provoked by caloric heat, cold, light or mechanical trauma. The mechanism may or may not be immunologic. See *urticaria factitia*.

urticaria pigmentosa [pĭg′mĕn-tō′sə] is the title of a highly characteristic clinical condition that is marked in its commonest forms in children by patches of brownish coloration (*pigmentosa*) and whealing (*urticaria*) when the affected areas are rubbed. There are forms that are bullous, papular and even nodular. The histologic mark of the condition is conglomeration of mast cells whose content of histamine and serotonin and release of these substances upon degranulation of the cells are thought to be related to local whealing and sometimes generalized blushing.

urticaria, recurrent. See *urticaria, chronic,* or *recurrent.*

urticaria, solar, and **solaris.** See under *solar, solaris.*

urticarial [ûr′tĭ-kâr′ĭ-əl, -kā′rē-əl, -ĭ-əl] is an adjective meaning pertaining or relating to urticaria.

urticarial derm(at)ographia (-ism). See *derm (at)ographia (-ism), urticarial.*

urticata [ûr′tĭ-kā′tə, -kä′tə] and **urticatus** [ûr′tĭ-kā′təs, -kä′tŭs] are respectively the feminine singular and the masculine singular of a New Latin adjective meaning related to whealing. They appear in the titles *acne urticata* and *lichen urticatus.*

V

vaccination [văk′sə-nā′shən] is the process of exhibiting a vaccine and inducing immunologic changes thereby. The exhibition may be by enteral or parental routes and the materials may be the natural agents of diseases, attenuated, killed or related agents of diseases, or antigenic materials processed from agents of diseases.

vaccine [văk′sēn, -sĭn] derives from Latin *vaccinus*, pertaining to *vacca*, a cow. From its original application to material taken from a cow or calf afflicted with pox and used, as such or processed, for immunization, we now apply the word to any material, from any source, used for immunization.

vaccinia [văk-sĭn′ē-ə, -ĭ-ə] literally means a condition (*-ia*) relating to (*-in-*, from *-inus*) a cow (*vacc-*). The particular condition designated is cowpox in the animal or that minor disease induced in humans by accidental contagion or by the artifice of deliberate inoculation with virus of the disease. The disease no longer exists.

vacuole [văk′ū-ōl] derives via French from Latin *vacuus*, empty. The word means a small (*-ole*, diminutive) circumscribed unit or area of seeming emptiness (*vacu-*).

vacuolization [văk′ū-ŏl′ĭ-zā′shən, -ĭ-zā′shən] designates the process of development (*-ization*) of small, empty spaces (*vacuol-*).

vacuolization, basket-weave [bās′kət, -kĭt wēv] designates a type of development of small, empty spaces in cells or tissue resembling reticulation reminiscent of woven baskets. The phenomenon is seen in epidermal cells affected by the viruses of certain warts.

vagabond's (vagrant's) disease [văg′ə-bŏndz (vā′grənts) dĭ-, də-zēz′] is another of those invidious designations, this time for pediculosis corporis. *Vagabond* derives from a Latin word meaning to wander, and *vagrant* from Teutonic influenced by Latin via Old French. The reminder that the rootless, homeless and displaced are likely to be dirty and infested is thoughtlessly haughty. Lice do not discriminate and the ordinarily well-domiciled may receive their attention, given the chance in times and places of social disorder.

vanillism [və-nĭl′ĭz'm] does not mean a condition caused by vanilla; rather it refers to infestation with *Pyemotes* (*Pediculoides*) *ventrico-*

sus, which may be found among vanilla pods as well as cereals like grain. *Grain itch* is the same sort of designation by source or occupation. *Vanilla* is etymologically interesting in its derivation via Spanish *vainilla*, diminutive of *vaine*, a sheath, ultimately from Latin *vagina*. The exquisite reference is to the contents of the little pods.

variabilis [văr′ē-, văr′ĭ-ā′bĭ-lĭs, -ä′bĭ-lĭs, -ē-ə-bĭl′ĭs] is the masculine or feminine singular of a Latin adjective meaning variable, changeable. It appears in the title *erythrokeratodermia figurata variabilis* (feminine).

varicella [văr′ĭ-sĕl′ə] is New Latin and derives from Medieval Latin *variola*, which in turn derives from classical Latin *varius*, which means various, variegated or spotted in color. The diminutive *-ola* in *variola*, then, describes smallpox as a small spottedness. *Varicella* is said to have been coined as a diminutive (*-cella*) of *variola* and thus to designate a still smaller spottedness, namely, chicken pox. It is strange coinage but the word is easy to say and well sanctioned by time.

varicelliform [văr′ĭ-sĕl′ĭ-fôrm] describes what is in the shape or form of varicella or chicken pox.

varicose [văr′ĭ-kōs] derives from Latin *varicosus*, which in turn derives from *varix*, a dilated vein. It is an adjective and pertains or relates to dilated veins with the force of much or many (*-ose*, full of).

varicose eczema [ĕk′sə-mə] is applied to a superficial dermatitis of the legs that is thought to be related to faulty hemodynamics resulting from dilated and therefore incompetent veins. Such a relationship is an unproved hypothesis. See under *stasis dermatitis*.

varicosity [văr′ĭ-kōs′ĭ-tē, -ə-tē, -tĭ] designates a single dilated vein or the general state (*-ity*) of dilated veins (*varicos-*).

variegata [vā′rĭ-, văr′ĭ-ē-gā′tə, -ĕ-gä′tə] and **variegated** [văr′ĭ-ə-gāt′ĕd, -ĭd, -əd, -văr′ĭ-, văr′ē-gāt′ĕd] are respectively the feminine singular of a Latin perfect participle and the corresponding English past participle, both used as adjectives and meaning mottled. The Latin word appears in a title like *parapsoriasis variegata*.

variola [və-rī′ō-lə, -rē′ō-lə] is Medieval Latin from classical Latin *varius*, various, variegated or spotted in color. By addition of the diminutive *-ola*, the word means a small spot and by extension describes smallpox as a small spottedness.

varioliform, -formis [vâr′e-, vâr′ĭ-ŏl-ĭ-fôrm, -ō′lĭ-fôrm; văr′e-, văr′ĭ-ō′lĭ-fôr′mĭs] are respectively an English adjective and the masculine and feminine form of a New Latin adjective meaning what is in the shape or form of variola, i.e., smallpox. The classicized forms appear in the titles *acne varioliformis* and *parapsoriasis acuta et varioliformis.*

varix [văr′ĭks, vä′rĭks] is a Latin and English word for a dilated vein. Ultimate derivation is from *varus*, bent, stretched or awry. *Varix* appears in the writings of Celsus, Cicero and Pliny.

varnish [vär′nĭsh], as a pharmaceutical form, designates a preparation of an active ingredient in a vehicle, which upon evaporation, leaves a fine film.

vascular [văs′kū-lẽr, -lər], **vasculare** [văs′kū-lä′re, -lä′re, -lär′e] and **vascularis** [văs′kū-lä′rĭs, -lä′rĭs, -lär′ĭs] are respectively an English adjective, the neuter singular and masculine or feminine singular of a New Latin adjective, all meaning pertaining to blood vessels. The New Latin adjectives appear in the title *poikiloderma vasculare atrophicans* (neuter), or *poikilodermia vascularis atrophicans* (feminine).

vasculitis [văs′kū-lī′tĭs, -le′tĭs] means inflammation (*-itis*) of small (*-ul*) blood vessels (*vasc-*).

vasculitis, allergic [ə-lûr′jĭk] and **vasculitis, nodular** [nŏj′oo-, nŏd′ū-lẽr, -lər] are titles of which the first designates an inflammation of small blood vessels that is ascribed to an allergic mechanism and the second, the same thing as morphologically nodular. Neither is significantly meaningful.

vasculitis, necrotizing. See *necrotizing angiitis, vasculitis.*

vegetans [věj′ə-, věj′e-tănz] is the present participle of the Latin verb *vegetare*, to arouse or invigorate. It carries the idea of growing lushly.

vegetans, dermatitis [dûr′mə-tī′tĭs, -te′tĭs] describes an inflammatory process that is probably infectious and results in tumid plaques that seem to grow lushly (*vegetans*). See *dermatitis vegetans.*

vegetans, pemphigus [pĕm′fĭ-gəs, pĕm-fī′gəs] describes a type of pemphigus in which the bullous lesions are obscured by lush (*vegetans*) and tumid inflammation. It occurs chiefly in intertriginous places and in the folds of fatness. See *pemphigus vegetans.*

vegetans, pyoderma [pī′ō-dûr′mə] describes a type of purulent inflammation of the skin in which lush (*vegetans*) tumefaction is characteristic. See *pyoderma vegetans.*

veld, or **velt, sore** [vĕlt, fĕlt sôr] is parochial for ulceration seen in South African fields, pastures or grasslands that are designated by the Afrikaans word taken from Dutch, *veld,* or *velt,* which is akin to *field.* See *Barcoo rot.*

vellus [vĕl′əs] is a Latin word for wool or fleece. The word is applied to fine hairs or the system of very fine, less visible hairs among a coarser, more obvious variety of an animal. Lanugo hairs on human beings constitute a vestigial vellus.

venenata [vĕn′ē-nā′tə, -nä′tə] is the feminine singular of a Latin perfect passive participle used as an adjective and means filled with poison, hence, venomous, poisonous. It appears in the title *dermatitis venenata.*

venerea [və-, vĕ-nēr′, vē-nĕr′ē-ə] and **venereum** [-əm, -ūm, -ōŏm] are respectively the feminine and neuter singular of a Latin adjective (written with a capital initial letter in Latin texts) meaning related to Venus as the goddess of love, hence, to venery. The first form appears in the title *lymphopathia venerea* and the second in *lymphogranuloma inguinale,* or *venereum.*

venereal [və-nēr′ē-əl, -ĭ-əl] derives from the Latin adjective *venereus* (masculine; see *venerea* above), which is formed from the stem *vener-* as seen in *Veneris,* genitive of *Venus,* the name of the goddess of love. The word *venery* in the sense of unrestrained or promiscuous sexual indulgence, has the same derivation. *Venereal* itself means pertaining to sexual love, and, by secondary ascription, implies lasciviousness.

venereal disease [dĭ-, də-zēz′] designates any disease whose mode of transmission is usually by sexual intercourse. Chancroid, gonorrhea, lymphogranuloma inguinale, or venereum, AIDS and syphilis are of the group.

venereal wart [wôrt] is an alternate designation for verruca acuminata or condyloma acuminatum that specifies venereal transmission, a disputed concept.

ventricosus [vĕn′trĭ-kō′səs] is the masculine singular of a New Latin adjectival formation meaning full of (*-osus*) belly (*ventri-,* from *venter*). It appears in the designation *Pyemotes ventricosus.*

vermilion [vēr-mĭl′yun] is a color variously stated to be carmine, bright or brilliant red, and red-brown. Material derived from cochineal insects and cinnabar (red sulfide of mercury) are vermilion.

verruca [vē-, vĕ-rōō′kə] is a Latin word for a warty excrescence. While we may use the word for a warty excrescence of any nature, e.g., verruca senilis, we generally use the word unmodified or with modifying adjectives in classical form to designate conditions caused by papilloma viruses. The plural of the word is *verrucae* [vĕ-rōō′kē] in the Latin manner and *verrucas* in the English convention. Modifying Latin adjectives require corresponding changes in the plural when lesions of the diseases are referred to in classicized form, e.g., *verrucae acuminatae, vulgares*. Following are common examples of titles containing the word.

verruca acuminata [ə-kū′mĭ-nā′tə, -nă′tə] describes a wart that is pointed (*acuminata*). *Condyloma acuminatum* and *venereal wart* are alternate. The pointedness of warts in the genito-anal region, to which this title is exclusively applied, is more imaginary than real. Inevitable maceration from moisture in the region tends to modify what would otherwise be filiform or digitate characteristics. Friction alone does the same for common warts in exposed positions on hands and feet.

verruca digitata [dĭj′ĭ-tā′tə] describes a wart that looks as though it consists of extended fingers (*digitata*). There is more point to this description than to the one above. Particularly about the face and in other places where viral warts grow out undisturbed by friction or maceration, some warts tend to develop one or more finger-like projections upward. See *digitate warts*.

verruca filiformis [fĭ′lĭ-fôr′mĭs] describes a wart that is in the form of a thread (*filiformis*). As in digitate warts, when development is not disturbed by trauma or maceration, the surface may consist of thread-like formations.

verruca peruviana. See *verruga peruana*.

verruca plana (juvenilis) [plā′nə (jōō′vĕ-, jōō′və-nĭ′lĭs)] describes a wart whose surface is plane or flat (*plana*) and usually occurs in the young (*juvenilis*). This type of wart is distinctive in tendency to multiplicity, small size of units and common location on face, arms and hands.

verruca plantae, plantaris [plăn′tē; plăn-tā′rĭs, -tă′rĭs, -tăr′ĭs] describes a wart as being of or on the sole of the foot (*plantae, plantaris*). *Verruca plantaris* is the commoner expression used.

verruca senilis [sĕ-nĭ′lĭs, -nĭl′ĭs] is not a viral infection. The title bespeaks a verrucous excrescence of the elderly (*senilis*) and is interchangeable as a title with *keratosis senilis* and *actinic keratosis*. It denotes that flat, scaly hyperkeratosis which is marked histologically by epithelial cell proliferation and disorder of cellular morphology that forebode squamous-cell carcinoma.

verruca vulgaris [vŭl-gā′rĭs, -gă′rĭs, -găr′ĭs] is the common (*vulgaris*) wart. Warts in general are common, but what is meant here is that ordinary one—or more—on hands or elsewhere whose characteristic is to be about pea-sized, domed and rough-surfaced but not acuminate, digitate, filiform or plane.

verruciform [vĕ-rōō′sĭ-fôrm] and **verruciforms** [vĕ-rōō′sĭ- fôr′mĭs] are respectively an English adjective and the feminine singular of a New Latin adjective meaning in the shape of (*-form, -formis*) warts. The New Latin adjective appears in the titles *acrodermatitis verruciformis* and *epidermodysplasia verruciformis*.

verrucosa [vĕr′ōō-kō′sə], **verrucose** [vĕr′ōō-kōs], **verrucosus** [vĕr′ōō-kō′səs] and **verrucous** [vĕr′ōō-kəs] are Latin (first and third) and English (second and fourth) adjectives meaning full of, or in the nature of (*-osa, -ose, -osus, -ous*), warts or roughness. The Latin forms appear in titles like *tuberculosis cutis verrucosa* (feminine) and *nevus verrucosus* (masculine).

verrucosa cutis is a localized form of tuberculosis of the skin. Due to superinfection with tubercle bacilli in a previously infected individual. It usually appears on the fingers or dorsum of the hands. May be confused with common warts.

verruga peruana [vĕr-rōō′gä pä-rwä′nä], or **verruca peruviana** [pē-rōō′vĭ-ä′nə], are titles in Spanish and New Latin forms respectively of an infectious disease endemic to Peru. The causative organism is a species of *Bartonella* which is inoculated by the bite of sand-fly vectors. In addition to cutaneous involvement in the form of verrucous excrescences, there are constitutional signs and symptoms.

versicolor [vûr′sĭ-kō′lôr] is a Latin adjective meaning turning, or changing (*versi-*) color, or of many colors. It has been taken over directly into English (with pronunciation vûr′sĭ-kŭl′ẽr, -ər, vər′sə-kəl′ər). As a Latin adjective it appears in the designation *tinea versicolor*.

vesica [və-, vē-sī′kə, vĕs′ĭ-kə] is a Latin word for a bladder and a blister. In dermatologic context, if the word is to be used at all, it should be in connection with large blisters.

vesicant [vĕs′ĭ-kănt, -kənt] as an adjective means pertaining or relating to blisters and as a noun, an agent that causes blisters.

vesication [vĕs′ĭ-kā′shən] means the act of blister formation.

vesicatory [vĕs′ĭ-kə-tō′rē, -tôr′ē, -ĭ, vē-sīk′ə-tō′rē, -tẽr′ĭ] has the same senses as *vesicant*.

vesicle [vĕs′ĭ-k′l] derives from Latin *vesicula* or French *vésicule* and means a small (*-le*, diminutive) blister (*vesic-*). In an everyday frame of reference, a lesion up to one centimeter in diameter is reasonable. Beyond that size, *bleb, bulla* and *vesica* seem more appropriate.

vesicular [və-, vĕ-sĭk′ū-lēr] is an adjective meaning pertaining or relating to a vesicle.

vesiculation [və-, vĕ-sĭk′ū-lā′shən] designates the process of formation of vesicles.

vesiculo-bullous [və-, vĕ-sĭk′ū-lō-bŭl′əs] is a formation like *maculopapular, papulo-pustular, papulo-vesicular* and *vesiculo-pustular* which may mean composed of both vesicles and bullae or being of a size between a vesicle and a bulla.

vesiculo-pustular [və-, vĕ-sĭk′ū-lō-pŭs′tū-lēr, -lər] is a formation like the one above which may mean composed of vesicles and pustules or having characteristics of vesicles and pustules, a matter of clinical indecision about morphology.

vestimentorum [vĕs′tĭ-mĕn-tō′rəm, -tôr′əm, -ōͼom] is the genitive plural of the Latin noun *vestimentum*, clothing. It appears in the title *pediculosis . . . vestimentorum*.

vibex [vī′bĕks] is a Latin word for the mark of a blow. We apply the word only to a linear hemorrhage such as might appear from a whiplash. The plural is *vibices* [vī′bĭ-sēz].

Vidal's disease [vēdäl′]. Lichen chronicus simplex.

Vincent's angina [vĭn′sĕnts, -sənts ăn-jī′nə]. Stomatitis and pharyngitis caused by a combination of a spirillum and fusiform bacillus. See *angina, Vincent's.*

vitiligo [vĭt′ĭ-lī′gō] is found in the writings of Celsus and others as a word for a cutaneous eruption, "a type of tetter." The word is presumably derived from Latin *vitium*, a fault (the *l* in this word is unaccountable). We use the word to designate the characteristic leukoderma caused by destruction of melanocytes most likely of autoimmune origin.

vitiligoidea [vĭt′ĭ-lĭ-goi′dē-ə] is found in medical dictionaries for *xanthoma*, meaning something like (-*oidea*) vitiligo. It is obsolete.

Vogt-Koyanagi syndrome [fōgt; kō′yä-nä-gē]. Uveitis, iritis, glaucoma, premature graying and alopecia, vitiligo, and dysacusia.

von Recklinghausen's disease See Recklinghausen's disease.

von Zumbusch's disease See Zumbusch's disease.

vulgaris [vŭl-gä′rĭs, -gä′rĭs, -gär′ĭs] is the masculine and feminine singular of a Latin adjective meaning belonging to the multitude, hence, common, ordinary, usual, everyday. It appears in many titles, e.g., *acne vulgaris, verruca vulgaris*, etc.

vulvae [vŭl′vē, -vī] is the genitive singular of the Latin noun *vulva*, covering, as of a seed, integument, also womb, matrix. We, however, do not relate vulva to the womb, but to the genital lips collectively, which are a sort of covering. *Vulvae*, then, in the sense of belonging to the labia majora and minora, appears in many titles, e.g., *kraurosis vulvae, pruritus vulvae*, etc.

W

Waldenström's syndrome [väl'dĕn-strŏm]. Hypergammaglobulinemic purpura.

wart [wôrt] derives from Anglo-Saxon *wearte*, a callosity. We use the word mostly for certain excrescences of papilloma viral cause and also for lesions that resemble those of viral cause but are not so caused. *Verruca* is an alternate word derived from classical Latin.

wart, common. See *verruca vulgaris.*

wart, flat. See *verruca plana (juvenilis).*

wart, mosaic. See *mosaic wart.*

wart, periungual. See *periungual.*

wart, plantar. See *verruca plantae, plantaris.*

Wassermann test [väs'ĕr-män]. Predicated upon competition for complement by a serum that is or is not from a syphilitic and by a sheep red cell system.

weal [wēl], meaning a hive or urtica, is a modern variant of Old English *wale*, which has several meanings, namely, in geotopography, a ridge or raised part; in nautical language, a piece of timber extending horizontally around the top of the sides of a boat (compare *gunwale*) and finally the mark of a whiplash, i.e., a swelling. *Wheal* (see below) used in any of the senses of *weal* is a misspelling. *Weal* in the sense of welfare (e.g., the common weal) is of still another origin.

Weber-Christian disease [wĕb'ĕr; krĭs'chən]. Relapsing febrile nodular nonsuppurative panniculitis.

Weber-Cockayne disease [wĕb'ĕr; kŏk-än']. Epidermolysis bullosa hereditaria.

weeping [wēp'ĭng] is said of superficial inflammatory processes in which there is considerable exudation of clear serum from rupture of vesicles or discontinuity of the epidermis. *Oozing* is an alternate word with less emotional connotation.

Wegener's granulomatosis [vā'gə-nēr]. See *granulomatosis, Wegener's.*

Vasculitis with granulomatosis. A systemic disease in which necrotizing vasculitis is seen in association with necrotizing granulomas primarily in the upper and lower respiratory tract and in other organs, and focal necrotizing glomerulitis, etc. Formerly fatal now very treatable with immunosuppressive agents.

welt [wĕlt] is a word derived from Middle English and means a linear wheal or a vibex (which see).

wen [wĕn] derives from Anglo-Saxon *wenn*, a lump or tumor. The word is old-fashioned and was once commonly used to designate benign lumps, particularly on the scalp, that are epidermoid cysts, i.e., either sebaceous cysts or atheromata.

Werlhof's purpura [vĕrl′hōf]. Essential thrombocytopenic purpura.

Werner's syndrome [vĕr′nĕrz, wûr′nĕrz sĭn′drōm] is eponymic for a dysplasia that is marked by dwarfism, progeria, a characteristic facies (beaked and peaked nose) and ulcers over points of friction and pressure.

Werther's nevus [vĕr′tĕr]. Syringocystadenoma papilliferum.

wheal [hwēl], derived from Old English *hwele* and Middle English *whele*, would mean a pimple or pustule. However, the modern word meaning a hive or urtica developed from a misspelling of *weal* (see above), which has that meaning originally.

white frontal forelock. See *forelock, white frontal.*

whitehead [hwīt′hĕd′] is alternate for *milium* (which see). Lay people also apply the word to a kind of superficial pustule on a face marked by acne that is small, tense and quite white in its purulent content.

white piedra. See under *piedra.*

whitlow [hwĭt′lō] is of dubious origin, possibly not from English at all but from early modern Dutch or Low German. Guesses like origin from *white* and *flaw* or *quick* and *flaw* are interesting, but still only guesses. However, the word is old-fashioned, as is its alternate, *felon*, for an abscess on the ball of a finger or under a nail. It is also found in:

whitlow, melanotic [mĕl′ə-nŏt′ĭk], which is sometimes applied to a malignant melanoma arising in a finger tip, especially under a nail.

Wickham's striae [wĭk′əmz, -′mz strī′ē, -ī] is eponymic for whitish cross-hatching seen on lesions of lichen planus.

"widow's peak" [wĭd'ōz pēk] describes a sharp remainder of scalp hair in the middle frontally when considerable recession at the temples has occurred.

Willan's disease [wĭl'ən]. Psoriasis.

winter itch [wĭn'tēr, -tər ĭch] is a direct translation of *pruritus hiemalis* (which see).

Wiskott-Aldrich syndrome [wĭs'kŏt; ôl'drĭch] is a rare, immunologic, sex-linked, recessive condition featuring eczema, repeated infections, and thrombocytopenia. Platelet count is decreased, with a bleeding tendency. There is a marked susceptibility to infections (e.g., bacteria, viruses, fungi, *Pneumocystis carinii*). Serum IgM is decreased. Serum IgA is normal or may be markedly increased. Serum IgG is normal or increased. Blood lymphocytes are usually decreased in number, especially the small lymphocytes. Incidence of malignancy of the lymphoid system is increased, i.e., eczema, susceptibility to infection, thrombocytopenia, and dysgammaglobulinemia in a fatal combination. (Wallach)

Wood's light [woŏdz līt] designates electromagnetic energy with a wave length of about 3650 Å and an apparatus that produces ultraviolet light of that quality. It is named after Robert W. Wood, an American physicist. The dermatologic interest in this photo-emission lies in the fluorescence it induces in certain conditions, especially certain fungous infections.

woolly hair nevus [woŏl'ē hâr nē'vəs] is a designation for a congenital anomaly of scalp hair in which the hairs in mass look or feel like wool.

Woringer-Kolopp disease is one of the cutaneous T-cell lymphomas. (Lever)

wrinkle [rĭng'k'l, -kəl] derives from both Old and Middle English and as a noun means a crease, fold or furrow. The skin is finely wrinkled naturally; as age advances, wrinkles in the skin become coarser, deeper and more visible.

X

xanth-, xantho- [zănth; zăn'thō] are combining forms from Greek *xanthos*, yellow.

xanthelasma [zăn'thĕl-āz'-, zăn'thə-lăz'mə] is New Latin from Greek word elements meaning a yellow (*xanth-*) plate (*-elasma*). We use the word to designate those yellow plaques in eyelids that contain cholesterol and signify a lipoidosis of minor import.
Soft, yellow-orange, irregular plaques found about the eyes (xanthoma palpebrarum). Xanthelasmas are probably the most common of all xanthomas. They do not always signify hyperlipoproteinemia but, more often than not, some elevation in low-density lipoprotein is present. (Fredrickson)

xanthelasmoidea [zăn'thĕl-ăz-, zăn'thə-lăz-moi'dē-ə] means something (*-oidea*, a class of things) of the order of xanthelasma. The word is used as an alternate for *urticaria pigmentosa* when the lesions are distinctly yellow (*xanth-*) plaques (*-elasm-*).

xantho-. See *xanth-*.

xanthochromia [zăn'thō-krō'mē-ə, -mĭ-ə] is New Latin from Greek word elements meaning a condition (*-ia*) of yellow (*xantho-*) coloration (*-chrom-*). *Aurantiasis* and *chrysoderma* are near alternate terms.

xanthoderm(i)a [zăn'thō-dûr'mə; -mē-ə, -mĭ-ə] is New Latin from Greek word elements meaning a condition (*-ia*) of yellow coloration (*xantho-*) of the skin (*-derma, -dermia*).

xanthogranuloma [zăn'thō-grăn'u-lō'mə] is a term preferred by some for *nevoxanthoendothelioma* (which see). Sometimes *juvenile* is added adjectivally because the condition commonly occurs in the young, in the very young in fact, for whom *infantile* in the term would be more to the point.

xanthoma [zăn-thō'mə] is New Latin from Greek elements meaning a yellow (*xanth-, xantho-*) tumefaction (*-oma*) or process (*-ma*). The word is used in titles as follows:

xanthoma dissemination [dĭ-sĕm'ĭ-nā'təm, -nä'tō͞om] is a title for a condition in which yellow tumors develop in a dispersed (*disseminatum*) arrangement.

xanthoma, eruptive [ē-rŭp′tĭv] is a title for a condition in which yellow tumors appear as a sudden development. Xanthoma diabeticorum is of that nature.

xanthoma, hypercholesteremic [hī′pēr-kō-lĕs′tēr-ē-mĭk, -kə-lĕs′tēr -ĕm-ĭk] is a title for a condition in which yellow tumors are associated with increased levels of cholesterol in the blood.

xanthoma, hyperlipemic [hī′pēr-lĭ-pĕm′ĭk] is a title for a condition in which yellow tumors are associated with high levels of blood lipids.

xanthoma, normocholesteremic [nôr′mō-kō-lĕs′tēr-ē-mĭk, -kə-lĕs′-tēr-ĕm-ĭk] is a title for a condition in which yellow tumors are associated with normal levels of cholesterol in blood.

xanthoma palpebrarum [păl′pē-brā′rəm] is a title for a condition in which yellow tumefactions are seated on the eyelids (*palpebrarum*). *Xanthelasma* is alternate.

xanthoma striata palmaris (or **xanthochromia striata palmaris** when they are not elevated) usually indicate the presence of the forms of hyperlipoproteinemia associated with florid obstructive liver disease, dysglobulinemia or type 3 hyperlipoproteinemia. (Fredrickson)

xanthoma tendinosum [tĕn′dĭ-nō′səm] is a title for a condition in which yellow tumors are seated over tendons (*tendinosum*).

xanthoma tuberosum [tōō′bēr-, tū′bēr-ō′səm] is a title by which yellow tumors are described as knobby (*tuberosum*).

xanthomatosis [zăn-thō′mə-tō′sĭs] is New Latin from Greek word elements meaning a condition (*-osis*)—any condition—characterized by yellow tumor.

xanthomatous [zăn-thŏm′ə-təs, -thō′mə-təs] is an adjective meaning pertaining or relating to xanthoma.

xer(o)- [zē′rō] is a combining form from Greek *xeros*, dry.

xeroderm(i)a [zē′rō-dûr′mə, -dûr′mē-ə, -mĭ-ə] means an unusually dry (*xero-*) condition of the skin (*-derma, -dermia*).

xeroderma pigmentosum [pĭg′mĕn-tō′səm] designates a characteristic dermatosis in which the skin is more troubled than the literal title describes. In addition to being unusually dry (*xero-*) and hyperpigmented in spots, it is marked by telangiectasis and an inevitable tendency to develop keratoses and ultimately malignant epitheliomata. The defect is in DNA repair after ultraviolet irradiation.

Rare heterogeneous group of diseases with hereditary deficiencies of enzyme systems in the skin that repair ultraviolet-induced damage to keratinocyte and melanocyte DNA. This inability to maintain the integrity of DNA leads to extreme sun sensitivity and multiple freckles over the face, lip, conjunctivae and extremities which evolve into variably sized pigmented papules interspersed with hypopigmented areas. Keratoses, basal and squamous cell carcinomas and malignant melanomas evolve and frequently lead to early death. (Frank Parker, *Cecil Textbook of Medicine*, 18th Ed., Wyngaarden and Smith, Editors, Saunders Co.)

xerosis [zē-rō′sĭs] is New Latin from Greek elements meaning a dry (*xer-*) condition (*-osis*). It is a generic word which in dermatology is applicable to any condition of the skin where dryness is more than its normal dry state.

xerostom(i)a [zē′rō-stō′mə, -stō′mē-ə, -mĭ-ə] is New Latin from Greek word elements meaning a dry (*xero-*) condition of the mouth (*-stoma, -stomia*).

xerotica [zē-rŏt′ĭ-kə] is the feminine singular of a New Latin adjective derived from a Greek word meaning dry, and means dried out. It appears in the title *balanitis xerotica obliterans*.

X(-)ray(s) [ĕks′ rā(z)′]. When this term is used as a noun, no hyphen should appear in it, but when it is used as an adjective, the hyphen is required. In both instances it is preferable to write *X* as a capital letter. Electromagnetic energy of wave lengths between 0.5 and 2 Å are designated as X rays; X-ray therapy is less used in dermatology now than formerly.

Y

yaws [yôz] is a word of Cariban origin. The Caribans are an Amerindian people of the northern part of South America, the Lesser Antilles, Guatemala, Honduras and British Honduras. The word *yaws* is akin to *yaya*, a name for the disease in the language of the Calinagos, a Caribbean people who live in the Lesser Antilles. In any event, yaws is a spirochetosis caused by a treponema (*T. pertenue*) which resembles the micro-organism that causes syphilis. The commonest cutaneous lesions of yaws are comparable to nodular lesions of syphilis.

Z

zirconium granuloma. See *granuloma, zirconium.*

zit [zĭt] is a parochial word of unknown origin for a pimple, which is a parochial word of uncertain origin for a papule. It is used by feisty young folk for the inflammatory papules and pustules that develop from the comedones of acne.

zona [zō'nə] is Latin from Greek *zone* (pronounced zō'nā), a girdle or belt. This word was more commonly used than *zoster* or *herpes zoster* in the remote past and is still common enough in some modern languages (e.g., French, *le zona*). See *herpes zoster, shingles* and *zoster.*

zoonosis [zō-ŏn'ō-sĭs]. The meaning of this word can be derived from its Greek word elements as a disease (*-nos-* from *nosos*, disease, plus *-is*, noun ending) of animals (*zoo-* from *zoon*, an animal) or a diseased condition (*-osis*) of an animal (*zoon-*). In dermatology another meaning is applied, namely, a disease of human beings caused by a metazoal ("animal") parasite and in general medicine, still another meaning, to wit, a disease communicated to humans by an animal.

Zoon's disease [zōōn]. Plasmocytoma penis.

zoster [zōs'-, zŏs'tĕr, -tər] is a direct borrowing from Greek *zoster*, a girdle. See *herpes zoster, shingles* and *zona.* Some modern dermatologists prefer this word to all other designations for the disease.

zosteriform [zōs-, zŏs-tĕr'ĭ-fôrm] is an adjective meaning in the shape of (*-form*) a girdle (*zosteri-*).

Zumbusch's disease [tzōōm'bōōsh]. Severe, generalized pustular psoriasis.

APPENDIX ON EPONYMY

Eponymic Methodology and Practice

The word *eponym* literally means an additional (*ep-*, from Greek *epi-*, upon) name (*-onym*, from Greek *onyma*, name). It thus encompasses ordinary family names or surnames (*sur-*, French, = *super-*, Latin, = *epi-*, Greek); nicknames (derived from *ekename*, in which *eke-* means additional, by misdivision of *an ekename* to *a nekename*, eventually pronounced and spelled *nickname*); and any other similarly additional nominal ascription to a person, place, phenomenon, etc.

Relevant to medicine, science in general, and the humanities, an eponym is a designation of a thing (a datum, disease, doctrine, etc.) by the name of a person or place (real or mythical) with whom or with which that thing is strongly or long associated.

Every now and then one hears someone say that eponymic designations for diseases, syndromes, signs, symptoms, and miscellaneous related matters are inadequate, uninformative or unnecessary. Yet, medical eponyms persist because in so many instances they are as adequate, informative or necessary as formal terms and phrases. If persons who say we should dispense with all eponyms were to persuade us all to do so, they and we would many times have to stand mute.

Eponymic methodology and practice are bound up with the development of language: everyday language, learned language, and the language of nomenclature and taxonomy in all sciences from astronomy to zoology. The creation of eponyms will go on despite carping or peevish objections because eponyms serve instantly defining and mnemonic purposes.

Eponymous words are abundant in everyday language. Readers may be amused by recalling or looking up the eponymic sources of frequently used words like aphrodisiac, boycott, leotard, masochism, sadism, serendipity, and many, many more. Mathematics, physics, and chemistry abound in eponyms and could not get along without them. Instance, ampere, Avogadro's number, Brownian movement, Fermat's last theorem, Newton's laws, Planck's constant, and roentgen. In the nomenclature and taxonomy of botany, microbiology, and zoology, eponymic practice has long been standard in Latinized form, particularly in designations of genera and species. For example, *Begonia semperflorens* and *Macadamia ternifolia; Escherichia coli* and *Rickettsia rickettsii; Ancylostoma brasiliense* and *Dermacentor andersonii.*

The Linnean schema of designating species eponymously by the names of persons requires and deserves more explanation. The convention is to Latinize names of any provenance in the nominative and then to use the genitive singular cases of the classicized names with small initial letters after the genus names capitalized.

Simple rules for forming genitive singular cases in Latin from names as they are may be formulated as follows:

1. For names ending in *a* as a sole vowel, add *e.*

2. For names ending in any other single vowel (*e, i, o,* or *u*), add *i.*

3. For names ending in any other letter, except *r* preceded by *e,* and *j, w* or *y,* add *ii.*

4. For names ending in *r* preceded by *e,* add *i.*

5. For names ending in *j,* drop the *j* and add *ii.*

6. For names ending in *w,* substitute *v* for *w* and add *ii.*

7. For names ending in *y,* drop the *y* and add *ii.*

8. For names ending in more than one vowel, insert a *v* after the last vowel and add *ii.*

The following table may further clarify.

Rule	Conventional Names	Latinized Forms	
		Nominatives	Genitives
1.	Avicenna	Avicenna	avicennae
2.	Kyrle	Kyrleus	kyrtei
2.	Kaposi	Kaposius	kaposii
2.	Pedroso	Pedrosous	pedrosoi
2.	Rendu	Renduus	rendui
3.	Galen	Galenius	galenii
4.	Osler	Oslerus	osleri
5.	Kogoj	Kogoius	kogoii
6.	Shaw	Shavius	shavii
7.	Ducrey	Ducreius	ducreii
8.	Thoreau	Thoreauvius	thoreauvii

When place names are used to designate species in the Linnean schema, the names are Latinized as adjectives and then used in correspondence with the gender of the genus name. Examples are *Leo africanus* (masculine), *Pieris japonica* (feminine), and *Amblyomma americanum* (neuter).

In ordinary medical discourse, eponymic methodology and practice are relatively simple. In English, the commonest convention is to use the possessive case, e.g., Addison's disease and islands of Langerhans. When the possessive case is not used for a single name, the definite article precedes the name, e.g., the Kveim test. When more than one person's name is used, the names are joined by hyphens, not apostrophized in any way, and preceded by the definite article if a syndrome is specified, e.g., the Peutz-Jeghers syndrome, but not preceded by the definite article if a disease is specified, e.g., Mucha-Habermann disease. A hyphenated and apostrophized name would signify a single person, e.g., Baden-Powell's movement.

In some instances in which a last name is banal or exceptional, eponyms have been made out of full names, e.g., Campbell de Morgan spots and the Cornelia de Lange syndrome, or out of middle and last names, e.g., (J.) Ferguson Smith's epithelioma and the (E.) Treacher Collins syndrome; and finally, there is that most unusual instance of

the Argyll Robertson pupil, fashioned from the penultimate and last names of the sesquipedalian complete name
of Douglas Moray Cooper Lamb Argyll Robertson. Occasionally one sees an eponym placed in a parenthesis after
the title of a disease, e.g., porokeratosis (Mibelli). The
words *disease* and *syndrome* are frequently used interchangeably, syndrome more often than disease when the
condition is complex.

In French and German literature, the word *morbus* (disease) is sometimes used with an eponym following, e.g.,
morbus Darier. The French also use their possessive preposition *de* in terms like *mal,* or *maladie, de Méléda* and *maladie de Raynaud;* the Germans use *von* in the same way.
The Germans also frequently make an adjective out of a
suitable name and say, e.g., *das Boecksche Sarcoid* and *die
Brightsche Krankheit.* English also makes adjectives out of
proper names, and thus we have Cushingoid facies and
Hunterian chancre; or uses a name as an adjective unex-
tended by adjectival suffixes, as in Unna boot. English is
also peculiar in making nouns like bartholinitis for inflammation of Bartholin's glands and leishmaniasis for infection
with any of the *Leishmania.*

In recent times, a new and commendable modesty has
fostered a habit of naming diseases and related phenomena
after the names of patients in whom the pathology was discovered (Christmas's factor, Hartnup's disease); or after the
names of places where discovery was made (Australia antigen, Philadelphia chromosome).

For some conditions, formal titles tend to multiply in
synonymy until there are several, none completely comprehensive or satisfactory because no one of them can encompass all that is important in those conditions. This is especially true of hereditary and dysplastic syndromes. By
way of example, a dermatologist will speak of adenoma sebaceum; a neurologist, of tuberous sclerosis; and perhaps a
"compleat" physician, of epiloia. It depends on what aspect of the disease looms largest in a particular context.

Nor are the names of Balzar, Bourneville, or Pringle satisfactory for the disease in point. Some eponyms suffer from much the same trouble of multiplicity either from priority disputed or discovered *post factum,* or by later accretions of names because different individuals added something of importance about a condition. An example is the Osler-Weber-Rendu-Goldstein syndrome for familial hemorrhagic telangiectasia which, by the way, has a dozen other formal titles. Sometimes a title that is too long to remember easily or difficult to keep straight in mind promotes eponymy. The Sulzberger-Garbe syndrome for distinctive exudative discoid and lichenoid chronic dermatosis is an example. If an original or later observer names a condition too well, eponymic designation tends not to be made or, if once made, tends to be forgotten. In some instances, neither formal titles nor eponyms are felicitous, and in such cases there is little to choose between them. Moreover, the order of words in some formal titles or of names in cp onyms is frequently different in different sources. Finally, eponyms are still sometimes used as euphemisms or disguises, e.g., Hansen's disease for leprosy; and once were often used to mock and insult, e.g., the French disease for syphilis.

In short, while it is true that some eponyms are ill-chosen, trivial, parochial, invidious, pejorative, or out of date, the principles and practices of eponymy are nevertheless universal, more or less useful, and often absolutely necessary whenever quick codification and nomenclature are required and no more-appropriate words or terms are available for the purposes. Then, even when more-precise designations become possible because more information has been garnered, many eponyms tend to persist for sentimental reasons or because they are more memorable or as memorable.